The Working Woman's Pregnancy Book

A Yale University Press Health & Wellness book is an authoritative, accessible source of information on a health-related topic. It may provide guidance to help you lead a healthy life, examine your treatment options for a specific condition or disease, situate a healthcare issue in the context of your life as a whole, or address questions or concerns that linger after visits to your healthcare provider.

Joseph A. Abboud, M.D., and Soo Kim Abboud, M.D., *No More Joint Pain*

Thomas E. Brown, Ph.D., *Attention Deficit Disorder: The Unfocused Mind in Children and Adults*

Marjorie Greenfield, M.D., *The Working Woman's Pregnancy Book*

Ruth H. Grobstein, M.D., Ph.D., *The Breast Cancer Book: What You Need to Know to Make Informed Decisions*

James W. Hicks, M.D., *Fifty Signs of Mental Illness: A Guide to Understanding Mental Health*

Steven L. Maskin, M.D., *Reversing Dry Eye Syndrome: Practical Ways to Improve Your Comfort, Vision, and Appearance*

Mary Jane Minkin, M.D., and Carol V. Wright, Ph.D., *A Woman's Guide to Menopause and Perimenopause*

Mary Jane Minkin, M.D., and Carol V. Wright, Ph.D., *A Woman's Guide to Sexual Health*

Arthur W. Perry, M.D., F.A.C.S., *Straight Talk about Cosmetic Surgery*

Catherine M. Poole, with DuPont Guerry IV, M.D., *Melanoma: Prevention, Detection, and Treatment*, 2nd ed.

E. Fuller Torrey, M.D., *Surviving Prostate Cancer: What You Need to Know to Make Informed Decisions*

Barry L. Zaret, M.D., and Genell J. Subak-Sharpe, M.S., *Heart Care for Life: Developing the Program That Works Best for You*

The Working Woman's Pregnancy Book

MARJORIE GREENFIELD, M.D.

Illustrations by BETH HALASZ *and* LINDA Y. C. CHAO

Yale University Press 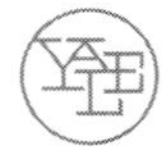 NEW HAVEN & LONDON

The information and suggestions contained in this book are not intended to replace the services of your physician or caregiver. Because each person and each medical situation is unique, you should consult your own physician to get answers to your personal questions, to evaluate any symptoms you may have, or to receive suggestions for appropriate medications.

The author has attempted to make this book as accurate and up to date as possible, but it may nevertheless contain errors, omissions, or material that is out of date at the time you read it. Neither the author nor the publisher has any legal responsibility or liability for errors, omissions, out-of-date material, or the reader's application of the medical information or advice contained in this book.

Published with assistance from the Williams Memorial Publication Fund and from the Louis Stern Memorial Fund.

Set in Quadraat and Scala by Tseng Information Systems, Inc., Durham, North Carolina.
Printed in the United States of America.

Library of Congress Cataloging-in-Publication Data
Greenfield, Marjorie.
The working woman's pregnancy book / Marjorie Greenfield ; illustrations by Beth Halasz and Linda Y. C. Chao.
p. cm. — (Yale University Press health & wellness)
Includes bibliographical references and index.
ISBN 978-0-300-11310-5 (cloth : alk. paper) —
ISBN 978-0-300-11324-2 (pbk. : alk. paper)
1. Pregnancy—Popular works. 2. Pregnant women—Employment—Popular works. I. Title.
RG525.G7293 2008
618.2—dc22 2007044543

A catalogue record for this book is available from the British Library.

10 9 8 7 6 5 4 3 2

To my best friend and husband, Dr. Tony Post

Contents

Preface

In planning *The Working Woman's Pregnancy Book*, I wanted to create a resource that would be comprehensive, reassuring, and relevant. I looked at the popular pregnancy books and found very little about working; their recommendations often didn't seem to fit with the complexities of modern life. In my own experience of having a child, a practical book called *The Working Woman's Guide to Breastfeeding* was more applicable to my life than the regular breastfeeding books seemed to be. I knew I'd have to go back to work shortly, and this one book didn't assume my son and I would be glued together every moment during the first few years. I thought: Wouldn't it be great to write an all-inclusive pregnancy book that would speak to the 60 to 80 percent of women who hold jobs while they are pregnant?

Once I had decided to create a book for women in the workforce, I needed to choose a title. Recognizing that all mothers are working mothers, I tried to find a name that didn't use the term "working woman" but still reflected the book's purpose. I just couldn't hit upon anything that said it all. In the end, I decided to trust that "The Working Woman's Pregnancy Book" will capture my goal for this book: meeting the needs of any mother-to-be with a busy life on the job—or at home.

The range of pregnancy experiences is vast, with many opportunities for learning "mom to mom." The anecdotes and advice included in this book come from mothers with a wide range of backgrounds and experiences. Although their insights can't possibly represent the full diversity of the American maternal workforce, they are as varied in age, race, religion, economic status, sexual orientation, marital status, and types of work as was practical to obtain. I would love to hear more pregnancy stories from readers as a way of learning further about the breadth of experiences of working parents-to-be.

I also want to explain what may seem like assumptions about gender and sexual orientation. In this book, I used the male gender for the partner, since that is the most common arrangement, and alternated male and female for the baby (by chapter). In places, I assumed that the mom was heterosexual and in a long-term relationship, but I tried to address other arrangements when it made a difference. In other words, I have tried to speak to a variety of readers, while recognizing that no book can meet everyone's needs on every page. Although this book is written to mothers-to-be, fathers will find lots of useful information in it as well. In the recommended reading section, I have listed a few resources created just for dads.

The Working Woman's Pregnancy Book starts with your decision about when (and whether) to have a baby, and takes you through getting off of birth control, fertility treatment, each trimester of pregnancy, labor and birth, the first few months after the baby arrives, and the return to work. While it can be read cover to cover, I imagine most readers will check out the sections that seem relevant, perhaps relying on the index to find specific information and advice. I hope that this book informs, reassures, and empowers you. You are starting a most amazing adventure.

Part 1

Strategic Planning (Before Conception)

When is the best time in life to have children? I get asked this question all the time, and usually there is no perfect answer. If you are wondering when you should get started, taking stock of your relationship, job demands, age, finances, general health, and personal desires can help you decide if you are ready to have a baby. In this section, you'll find a quiz to help you figure out if the time is right, along with information about pre-pregnancy emotional and physical wellness, pre-conceptual medical care, and how to provide the healthiest environment for your early embryo. Pregnancy may temporarily compromise your performance at work and it will certainly complicate your life, but for most of us who have ventured down the path to parenthood, the experience has made life immeasurably richer and more meaningful.

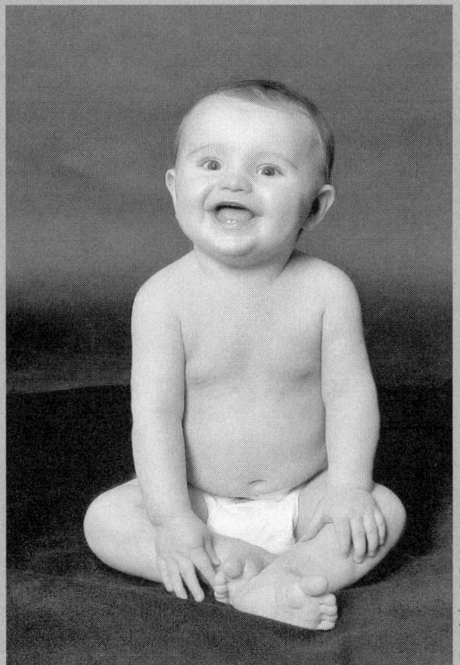

LeRoy Dierker, M.D.

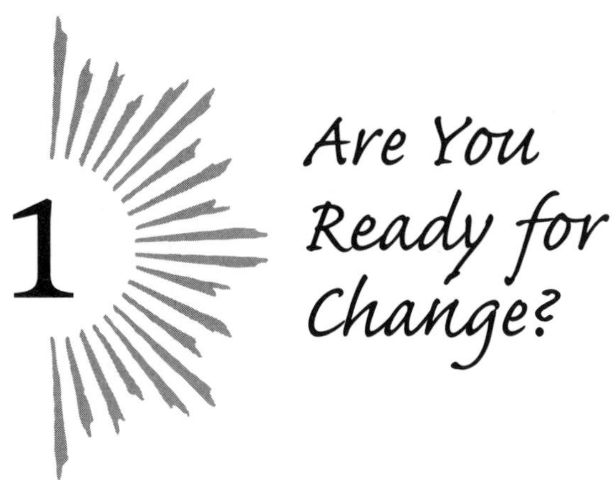

1 Are You Ready for Change?

How do people know they are ready to take on the challenges of pregnancy and parenting? The question—and its answers—come up in different ways. Maybe you're wondering about that special glow you felt after holding your sister's newborn, or you can't wait to see your husband as a dad. Whatever your reason for considering motherhood, the decision usually starts with a feeling—which may run up against practical considerations.

This quiz is designed to help you weigh the importance of those different "heart and head" factors that might influence your decision. You may want to try running through the quiz, reading the rest of the chapter, talking to your partner and others close to you, and then taking it again to see if your answers change after thinking through all the issues.

Deciding Whether to Have a Baby

In today's society, women have children at a great range of ages and within all sorts of different family structures, but having children isn't for everyone. How do pregnancy and motherhood fit into your dreams, self-image, relationships, financial plan, and twenty-four-hour day? Career constraints, lifestyle choices, relationship issues, personal health problems, the demands of fertility treatment, and many other dynamics can put baby plans on hold, for a while or forever. The first step toward figuring out *when* you want to get pregnant, then, is to decide *if* you want to have children at all.

I always knew that I wanted to be a mother. I would have gone to the ends of the earth to have a child—in vitro, adoption, whatever it took. (Maggie P., administrator)

QUIZ: Do You Want to Have a Baby?

		A	B	C
Do you want to have children at some time?				
1	Do you want to be a mom?	yes	maybe	no
2	Is it important to you to continue the family name or bloodline?	yes	a little	no
3	Do you want to make a family with your partner?	yes	maybe	no or n/a
4	Do you want to experience pregnancy and childbirth?	yes	maybe	no
5	Do you have any medical conditions that will make pregnancy risky for you or the baby?	no	unsure	yes
Is now the time?				
	EMOTIONAL READINESS			
6	When you think about having a baby, do you feel mostly positive or mostly negative?	positive	unsure	negative
7	Are you willing to take the best care of yourself while you are pregnant?	yes	maybe	no
8	Are you ready to make the compromises necessary to raise a child?	yes	maybe	no
	RELATIONSHIP READINESS			
	(single mothers skip this section and give yourself four extra points)			
9	Is your relationship stable and loving?	yes	unsure	no
10	Do you and your partner both feel ready for children?	yes	unsure	no
11	Do you and your partner generally agree on who will care for the baby, and how tasks, including earning a salary, will be distributed between you?	yes	unsure	no
	YOUR JOB			
12	How will your working conditions affect your ability to safely carry a pregnancy?	no problem	unsure	may be a problem

		A	B	C
13	How will pregnancy and motherhood affect your career?	no problem	unsure	negatively
14	Do you have successful pregnant or parenting role models at work?	yes	sort of	no
15	Is your workplace family-friendly?	yes	sort of	no
	CHILDCARE OPTIONS			
16	Do you have a good support system for after the baby comes?	yes	sort of	no
17	Have you thought about how you (or your partner) will arrange for childcare, and what childcare options are available to you given your financial situation and personal beliefs?	yes	sort of	no
	FINANCES			
18	Are you financially ready to have a child?	yes	unsure	no
19	Do you have paid maternity leave?	yes	unsure	no
20	Does your health insurance cover prenatal care?	yes	unsure	no
	YOUR HEALTH			
21	Are you healthy enough to have a baby now, or do you need to make some changes?	healthy enough	unsure	not healthy enough
22	Do medical problems or a history of a difficult pregnancy make it likely that you will have pregnancy complications?	no	unsure	yes
23	Have you had a preconception appointment with your doctor or midwife?	yes		no
	PARENTAL AGE			
24	How old are you?	over 38	32–38	under 32
25	How old is your partner? (skip and score as one point if not applicable)	over 45	35–45	under 35

Scoring: Give yourself two points for every A answer, one for each B, and none for each C.

35–52: Time to get moving!

21–35: In the "negotiation phase."

Less than 20: Not ready.

My husband and I knew we wanted to have children, but we got off to a late start. So we decided to let nature take its course. Our first two children were sixteen months apart, followed by a miscarriage and a third child twenty-nine months later. This was very difficult in the short term, but worth it. A sibling is the best thing to give your child beyond parental love. I look at my children and see that they've learned how to negotiate in the world by learning how to negotiate with each other. (Deb L., writer)

Timing

Once you have decided that you want to have children, the question becomes when. Of course, in the heat of the moment or through contraceptive method failure the decision is sometimes made without a plan, but many people do have the opportunity to choose when they will start a family.

I got pregnant while I was getting ready to take the bar exam; my husband and I were debating whether to have children right away or let me establish my career first. I think we got a little lazy (with birth control) hoping the decision would make itself. (Brenda W., lawyer)

I was on the birth control pill, but I hated it, so I got off it. And I thought, "If I get pregnant, then I get pregnant." I laugh at people who try to do all that planning. With the first one, we were at a party, and had a good time, and that's how that happened. (Helene L., teacher)

I had a miscarriage. I was so devastated, and I hadn't even thought that I wanted to have a baby. It's amazing how you can feel the loss of something you didn't even know you wanted. The loss of that baby made us realize we really wanted one, so we got pregnant with my daughter. (Shani M., student)

Emotional Readiness

Being a good parent involves sacrifices—putting someone else's needs above your own. Children are a lot of work. Even though men may share duties in the home more than they did in previous generations, women still carry the pregnancy, and often take on most of the day-to-day family responsibilities. Are you ready to take good care of yourself during pregnancy, including not smoking or drinking? Do you have love to give when you get home from work? Nearly all women find that pregnancy and children affect their sleep, their capacity to work, the time and energy available for recreation or travel, and their personal relationships. Most parents, particularly mothers, must alter their lifestyles to accommodate children.

I think men tend to be more ready than women, because they don't really envision the amount of work involved. (Zoe B., inventory manager)

Many women worry that their work demands will prevent them from being good mothers, and conversely that having children will hamper their work. While no one can be completely prepared for the changes that parenting will bring, it may help to talk to friends about how having a baby has transformed their lives and how they have managed the demands. If you start to get discouraged, don't forget to also ask them what they like about having children and whether they would do it all over again!

My mom put the children first and put off her career until we were in school. When I was growing up, she told me to get my career established and not to do it the way that she did. She was a great mom though, always there for us, so I have that in my mind as the model of being a good mother. I am torn between different images of how to be a mom. (Naomi B., attorney)

Relationship Readiness

The quality of your relationship with your partner will influence your experience as a parent as well as your child's life in your new family. Love and respect between parents help children feel secure; unresolved conflicts complicate the important task of parenting as a team. Consider how you communicate and resolve disagreements within your relationship. If your partnership is unstable or unhealthy, having children together is not likely to make it better or easier.

As you negotiate baby-making, talk about your own families, their values, and how you were raised, with the goal of discovering if your ideals conflict. For example, do you want the satisfaction and financial security of working, expecting to use daycare or a sitter, while he (and his parents) think that only the mother should be home with the children? Does your partner want you to earn a salary, while you anticipate staying home for an extended time? Do you expect that since your partner works from home, he will take care of the baby? While every little decision doesn't need to be made now, starting a dialogue will serve you well through the many decisions you will make together as parents.

My best advice for success combining working and being a mother: choose who you marry and choose who you work for. (Cheryl P., radiologist)

One more note: raising children is a team effort, and I believe it should be a team decision. Some women get "accidentally" pregnant on purpose. Although this strategy may net them a baby, in the long run the adjustment will be easier if both parents are enthusiastic participants. Women who choose to be single mothers will need to enlist the support of their friends and family—the responsibilities of parenting are too intense to manage alone.

Your Job

Large corporations and companies with predominantly female employees often have maternity policies in place, but planning for pregnancy and birth isn't always easy. In many jobs, there is no good time to have children. You will need to decide what is right for you personally and professionally. Ask around to find out what benefits are available for pregnant and parenting employees, who has used them, and how becoming a parent has affected their career paths. Seek out role models who have successfully combined motherhood and career and learn how they managed.

Many working women recommend banking "brownie points" at work ahead of any change to your family plans. A stockpile of goodwill among your coworkers and supervisors can pay off later if you are feeling poorly during pregnancy or when you need to run out for a childcare emergency. Now is the time to offer to help others, cover for coworkers, and go the extra mile for the organization. Pregnant women who are seen as hard-working team players often can coast a bit on their reputations when necessary, without loss of respect. If you pull more than your weight now, your coworkers will know that when they need help, you will be there.

I felt a bit guilty during the four months I took off because my three colleagues in my unit had to cover my work, but since then we have all covered for each other in so many different ways that there are no hard feelings. (Janet G., attorney)

In the past, women hesitated to get pregnant in my job—but after I had my son there was a baby boom. I don't think I was a trailblazer, but everyone was waiting to see how the firm handled a pregnancy. I was treated so well that it gave others the confidence to go ahead. (Kendra F., civil litigator)

I felt guilty about trying to get pregnant right after starting a new job, so I waited a year before trying. I was fortunate in that I didn't have any difficulty getting pregnant, but it was frustrating and stressful worrying about what was an acceptable time in a new job before getting pregnant. (Cheryl T., pharmaceutical sales rep)

I job-shared in my second pregnancy, with someone who had a child a year younger than mine. We occasionally met for lunch, so I chose that time to tell her that I was pregnant again. We shut the door, and before I had a chance to tell her, she said to me that she was pregnant. I wanted to say "no fair," that since my daughter was older, I was entitled to the next pregnancy. We knew that we had a problem. (Jan R., state attorney)

Pregnancy may well affect your work, but how will your working conditions affect the pregnancy? Are you exposed to radiation, toxic chemicals, or contagious infections at your workplace? Are your current hours compatible with pregnancy and parenting? Do you have heavy travel requirements? Look at your partner's work hours, too—although babies can do well within a variety of child-care arrangements, many parents feel deprived if they can't spend enough time with their children. Leaving the house before the children wake up and coming home after they are asleep might make it hard to be the kind of parent you want to be.

If having time with your family is important to you, plan ahead by choosing a workplace where having a family life is valued, or at least possible. Some jobs just aren't made for combining work and family. If your workplace has a reputation for being family-unfriendly, you might consider changing jobs now, before having children.

Childcare

Taking care of young children is a 24/7 job, and you'll need to plan ahead to make sure a responsible, loving adult is there for your child around the clock. Explore your caregiving options as early as possible: depending on your situation, you might choose to have one parent stay home, stagger both parents' work schedules so one can always be with the children, have a grandparent help out regularly, hire a nanny for in-home care, find a family daycare (in someone's home) or daycare center, take your newborn to work (in the right sort of job), or some combination of arrangements. Each plan has worked successfully for some families—you just need to identify the alternatives that are possible given your resources, and decide what feels right to you.

The agency that I worked for had implemented some very progressive family-friendly policies, including allowing new mothers to bring their newborns to work with them. I was the first one to actually test it out. I went back to work part-time (twenty hours) after only eight weeks, but it was easier (than with my first child) because I could bring Aron with me—I set up a little nursery for him in an unused storeroom with a portable crib and a baby monitor and he would nap in there. When he was awake he was with me, in a baby sling or backpack. In general, it worked pretty well as he used to take these marathon four-hour naps every day, so I could actually get a lot done. He came to work with me until he was about eight months old and then graduated to a small family daycare. We had a "retirement party" for him with a big cake. (Lisa H., community planner)

My first baby was colicky, and I had a hard time feeling good about leaving him alone because he cried inconsolably for hours. When he was four months old and I needed to return to teaching, the director at my school hired a babysitter to watch just him and one other teacher's child. Having my baby right next door and looked after so closely was a relief—to focus on my job, I really needed to know that he would be with someone who could hold and try to comfort him as much as I would. (Julie J., preschool teacher)

Finances

Childcare is just one of the baby-related decisions influenced by your financial situation. Although the Family and Medical Leave Act (FMLA) requires large employers to hold a pregnant woman's job for up to three months, this leave is often unpaid, so many parents need to save ahead to cover the lost earnings. You might also find that complications of pregnancy limit your ability to work or that your priorities shift once you're home with your little one, so that you make career decisions based more on quality-of-life issues than income. Having a baby costs money—an estimated $7,000–13,000 during the first year of life and $127,000–254,000 over eighteen years, not including college. So tidy up your finances before you start a family: try to cut down your credit card debt and stockpile some savings so that your maternity leave will be as stress-free as possible. And be sure your health insurance covers pregnancy and birth!

Health

Pregnancies go best, on average, for mothers at normal body weight who are free of major medical conditions. Doctors assess weight using the body mass index or BMI, which takes height into account. (Appendix A includes a body mass index calculator.) At the start of pregnancy, a BMI of 18.5 to 26 is considered optimal. If you have any medical problems, seeing your doctor or midwife ahead of time is particularly important, so you can be prepared for how the pregnancy may affect your health and how any health conditions might affect your pregnancy. High blood pressure, for example, can complicate pregnancy, increasing the chance that you will need bed rest or hospitalization. My advice: *before* you get pregnant, achieve your best possible health and become informed about how your medical conditions may influence the course of your pregnancy.

Age

While many of the topics in this chapter support delaying pregnancy, getting older creates some pressure to hurry the process along. Hitting a certain age can make couples eager to start a family, as they think about their fertility, how much energy they'll need to play with their little ones, and how old they'll be when their kids go on to college.

Both pregnancies were planned. I was thirty, and I wanted to have kids, and I didn't want to get old. (Kathy C., family therapist)

My pregnancy was planned. I was thirty-nine, and I said I would have a baby by the time I was forty. (Myra K., courtroom assistant)

Medically, there are four effects of advancing age: preexisting health problems, the likelihood of pregnancy complications, genetic risks, and infertility. Conditions like high blood pressure and uterine fibroids occur more frequently as we get older, and gestational diabetes is diagnosed more often in older mothers-to-be. Down syndrome and other genetic conditions become more common with age (see the table in Chapter 17). And most important, fertility diminishes and the risk of miscarriage increases as the years pass. Overall, fertility starts to drop in the early thirties, and rapidly diminishes around age forty.

Does this make you wonder how so many famous women in their late forties and fifties are able to have babies? Spontaneous pregnancies after age forty-four are rare; most of these famous pregnancies are achieved through in vitro fertilization with donor eggs. To protect their privacy, families often don't publicize how they got pregnant. Unfortunately, without that information, the rest of the world is falsely reassured that age doesn't matter—until people find themselves struggling to conceive. That's why if having a baby is important to you, you should try get started by your early thirties, or as soon as it is feasible in your life.

What next? Some of you will be ready at this point to dive into Chapter 2, which will help you prepare your body for a healthy pregnancy. Or you may want to take the quiz again, talk with your partner, gather information from friends and colleagues, evaluate the facts, and do a little more soul-searching. Trust your instincts. The decision about whether and when to start a family is just the first step in an awe-inspiring journey.

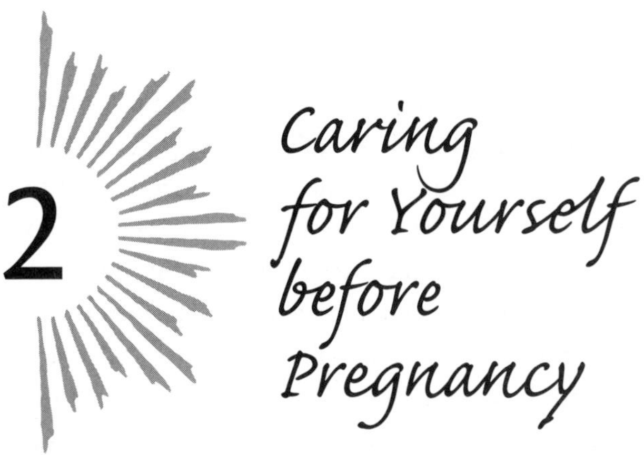

2 Caring for Yourself before Pregnancy

Do you really need to "go into training" before you get pregnant? It depends. If you are already in good health, you'll probably only need to make two simple changes: add a daily folic acid supplement (at least 400 micrograms) to your diet, and see your doctor or midwife for a preconception visit. But if you aren't in perfect health or may be exposed to chemicals or radiation that could endanger your pregnancy, you should make some changes now for the health of your future baby.

Practice Good Health Habits

Normal body weight, strength, and stamina make pregnancy easier and healthier. Now is a great time to start toning up. Strong abdominal muscles will help to prevent low back pain, and regular aerobic exercise can make labor easier. Being fit from the outset helps you stay comfortable as you carry your growing baby, and will jumpstart your recovery after childbirth.

Although overweight women usually have healthy pregnancies too, complications like gestational diabetes, overly large babies, and cesarean births are more common among women who start off heavy. Underweight women must also be careful, in this case to gain extra pounds to help the baby get enough nutrition. Approaching your recommended body weight before you conceive, if possible, will get you off to the best start.

Diet

One of the easiest and most important ways you can help prevent birth defects is to take a folic acid supplement every day starting at least three months before conception. Four hundred micrograms (0.4 milligrams) of folic acid is now recommended for all women in their childbearing years, regardless of whether they are trying to get pregnant. Why? Because the amount of folic acid most women get in their diets just isn't enough, and the birth defects it prevents occur before many women even realize they've conceived. Four hundred micrograms a day can be found in folic acid supplements, women's multivitamins, and over-the-counter prenatal vitamins—and will cut the chances of some birth defects in half. But a word to the wise: more folic acid is not better. Mega-doses of any vitamin or mineral are not good for a developing embryo and should be avoided unless prescribed by your physician.

Another word of caution about your pre-pregnancy and early pregnancy diet: some fish high in mercury content should be avoided for three months before conception and throughout pregnancy. Other foods that are best to pass up in pregnancy, as well as a list of specific fish that often contain high amounts of mercury, are listed in Chapter 10.

Caffeine, Cigarettes, Drugs, and Alcohol

Everyone who has had a few cups of coffee knows this: caffeine is a drug. Although one or two caffeinated beverages a day is probably fine, studies have shown that excessive caffeine is associated with miscarriage. While a cause-and-effect relationship isn't totally clear, it makes sense to diminish your daily caffeine intake, including coffee and soft drinks, before conception. This is especially true if you have a heavy caffeine habit—so you aren't stuck dealing with "cold turkey" withdrawal headaches during early pregnancy. Moderate caffeine use (one or two cups of coffee a day) is probably safe, especially after the first trimester.

I gave up caffeine and it wasn't as difficult as I anticipated it would be, though I did experience headaches in the beginning. (Jen R., fashion merchandiser)

Although the effects of caffeine on pregnancy are debatable, cigarettes clearly increase the odds of having a bad pregnancy outcome. During smoking, oxygen molecules are replaced by carbon monoxide in the mother's blood, so less oxygen gets to the baby. Nicotine also causes the mother's blood vessels to spasm, which diminishes blood flow, reducing the amount of oxygen and nutrients that are delivered to the uterus and fetus. Toxins in cigarette smoke cross the placenta into the baby's bloodstream, and babies of smokers are more likely than babies of nonsmokers to be born preterm and smaller than they should be. Infertility and miscarriage are more common in smokers. And we now know that the chance of sudden infant death syndrome (SIDS) is greater if the mother smoked during the pregnancy. Even second-hand smoke poses a risk to your newborn.

My best advice, then, is to do whatever you can to start your pregnancy as a nonsmoker. If you need help quitting, talk to your doctor or midwife, get the number of your local telephone quitline service by calling 1–800-ACS-2345, or check out the helpful information from the U.S. Centers for Disease Control online at www.cdc.gov/tobacco/how2quit.htm. Although it may be hard to quit, it is better to deal with the problem head-on now, rather than risk having to deal with serious pregnancy complications later.

Alcohol, like nicotine, is a commonly used drug that can be dangerous for the developing embryo. Many women come to their first prenatal appointment upset that they had some drinks before they knew that they were pregnant. Although it may be reassuring to know that a rare glass of wine probably won't cause harm, experts advise that no amount of alcohol can be considered safe. Daily moderate drinking or episodic heavy binge drinking can cause fetal alcohol syndrome (FAS), with mental retardation, unusual facial features, and poor growth. And milder forms of FAS, which can be caused by far less alcohol, can result in learning disabilities and behavioral problems.

Other drugs can also be dangerous to the developing baby. Cocaine causes spasms of the blood vessels, and can lead to miscarriage, preterm delivery, poor fetal growth, and even fetal death. Marijuana probably has some of the same risks as cigarettes, because toxins get into the bloodstream and reach the baby, and in men who smoke it daily, marijuana can decrease fertility. Narcotics like codeine, oxycodone, morphine, and heroin may be addicting to mother and baby if used for more than a few weeks. Miscarriage or fetal death can occur if narcotics are stopped abruptly during pregnancy, and a baby exposed to weeks of narcotics may suffer from withdrawal after birth.

If you wouldn't put a cigarette or joint in your baby's mouth or a needle in her arm, you shouldn't take street drugs during pregnancy. If you need help quitting, seek assistance. And be sure to discuss even your prescription medications and herbal supplements with your doctor or midwife before becoming pregnant. By controlling the substances that your little embryo is exposed to, you can get off to a good start on being a great mom.

Medical Care

Medical conditions like high blood pressure, anemia, and diabetes can complicate pregnancy. The diseases themselves can cause problems, and some medications that treat them can be toxic to the developing fetus. All women with medical conditions should see their doctors before getting pregnant. Seeing the dentist is a good idea, too. Dental problems, especially gum disease, seem to increase the chances of having pregnancy complications, possibly due to the effects of inflammation, or maybe just because tooth and gum problems often go hand in hand with poor overall health.

Workplace Safety

Many workplaces are perfectly safe for pregnant women; as a matter of fact, women who work generally have healthier pregnancies than women who don't. Some working conditions, though, require special consideration: exposures to toxic (or potentially toxic) chemicals, radiation, and germs can affect you and your baby-to-be.

Chemicals can get into your system by breathing them in, ingesting them, or having them pass through your skin. By law, your employer is responsible for providing information about chemicals in your workplace and for informing you about how to protect yourself. Your task is to request a material safety data sheet, or MSDS, for every chemical with which you may have contact. The data sheet will identify the chemical, describe what is known about its risks, and explain what to do if you are exposed. Unfortunately, most chemicals haven't been tested for safety in pregnancy, so information about risk usually isn't clear-cut. Take the time to ask your practitioner for more individualized information, and if you know that you work in a potentially hazardous environment, follow these general guidelines to help keep you and your baby safe:

- Ask about all potential hazards at your workplace.
- Use protective equipment and follow proper safety practices, including working under a hood when recommended.
- Wash your hands with soap and water before eating, drinking, and going home.
- Store chemicals in sealed containers when not in use.
- Avoid skin contact with chemicals.
- If you are exposed to any hazardous substance, follow the directions on your workplace's material safety data sheet, which will probably include changing out of contaminated clothing and washing with soap and water.
- Store your clothes from home in a protected place at work.
- Wash your work clothes separately from other laundry.
- If possible, avoid bringing contaminated items home.

Most employees exposed to radiation at work are monitored closely with radiation-sensitive tags. The Occupational Safety and Health Administration, OSHA, sets workplace standards for safe radiation exposures, and in general, exposures above safe levels for pregnancy aren't allowed for any worker.

You may know that airplane flights expose workers and passengers to low levels of radiation from being higher in the atmosphere. Infrequent air travel is safe, but pregnant pilots and flight attendants should be sure to follow their industry's safety guidelines.

Overall, the risk of radiation exposure in early pregnancy is believed to be all or nothing, meaning that high doses may cause pregnancy loss, while smaller amounts probably won't create significant problems.

Infections at Work and at Home

Women who work in healthcare or with children are often exposed to infections. The best protection against developing an infection yourself is good hand washing—cleansing your hands thoroughly with soap and water, or using a topical hand sanitizer between contacts with patients or children, before you eat, and before and after you go to the bathroom. These precautions will help protect you from infections that can harm a developing embryo. They may also help cut down on how many sick days you have to use—so you can instead stay home on a queasy morning during your first trimester, or extend your maternity leave by a day or two.

Immunizations can also protect you from infections. All adults who have not had rubella (German measles) or varicella (chicken pox) should be immunized. If you aren't sure, blood tests can determine if you are immune. The hepatitis B vaccine is recommended for healthcare workers and people with multiple sexual partners. And if you would normally be a candidate for a flu shot, planning to get pregnant shouldn't deter you; flu shots are now recommended for all pregnant women. Be aware, though, that vaccines made from live viruses, such as immunizations against rubella and measles, are not safe during pregnancy or in the month before conception. Before taking any vaccine, tell your practitioner if you think you might be pregnant.

Some infections—like cytomegalovirus (CMV) and parvovirus (fifth disease)—can be dangerous to a developing fetus, yet no vaccines are available. Blood tests can determine if you are susceptible to these germs, which are most likely to be caught from children—but routine hand washing is your best protection, since most individuals are infectious before they have symptoms. Toxoplasmosis, found in wildlife and cats, can also endanger fetuses. Most experts recommend that pregnant women don't change cat litter, to avoid exposure to this infection.

In general, if you discover that you have been exposed to a potentially serious infection and you might be pregnant, call your practitioner promptly for advice and treatment.

Preparing to Conceive

It can be hard to imagine being pregnant if you've never experienced it before. The joys of knowing—and eventually feeling—that a new life is growing inside you may be overshadowed on some days by fatigue, morning sickness, and feeling heavy on your feet. Planning ahead for a little less lifting or travel, or less standing on the job (to name just a few examples) can make the transition into pregnancy at work smoother and safer for both you and your baby. Start now to think about what changes you may need to make at work and at home when you are expecting, and talk to your practitioner to get specific recommendations.

Menstrual Cycle Chart

Year ________________

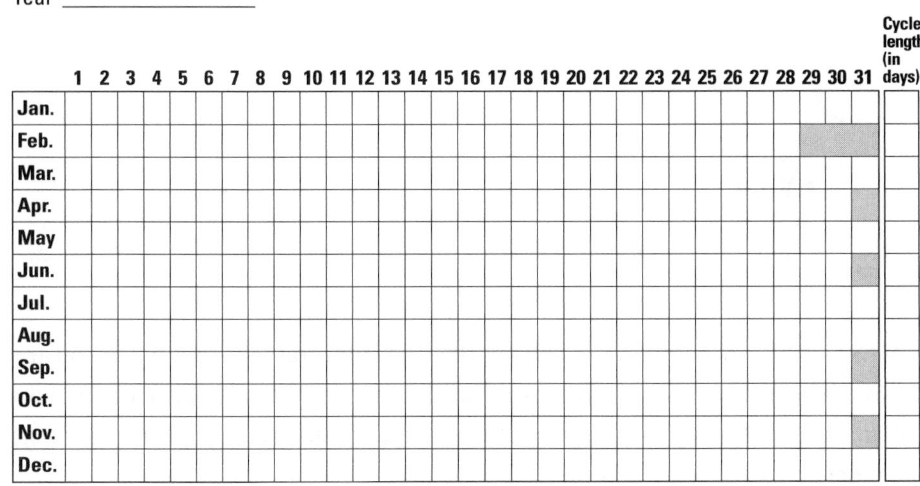

	1	2	3	4	5	6	7	8	9	10	11	12	13	14	15	16	17	18	19	20	21	22	23	24	25	26	27	28	29	30	31	Cycle length (in days)
Jan.																																
Feb.																																
Mar.																																
Apr.																																
May																																
Jun.																																
Jul.																																
Aug.																																
Sep.																																
Oct.																																
Nov.																																
Dec.																																

FLOW: **Normal** ☒ **Light** ⊡ **Heavy** ■

Menstrual cycle calendar. You can use a copy of this chart to track your cycles over the year.

Another way to start the process of planning for your baby is to begin writing down the dates of your periods, so that an accurate due date can be calculated once you conceive. Charting your cycles also allows you to see the normal pattern of your periods, which may help you to know right away when you are pregnant—so you can start taking even better care of yourself.

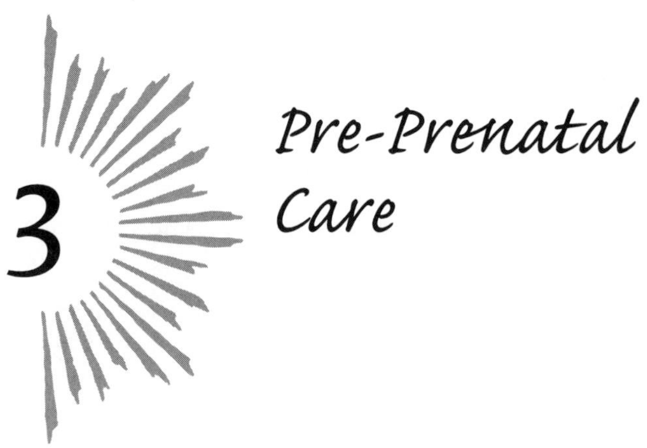

3 Pre-Prenatal Care

Most prenatal care begins some time in the first trimester—usually when you are six to ten weeks along. But if you wait until then to get good health advice, you will miss a valuable opportunity to take the best possible care of yourself during the most crucial stage, when the early embryo is developing.

The little embryo's organs start to form just a few weeks after the egg meets the sperm—around the time of the first missed period. But many mothers-to-be don't realize they are pregnant until weeks or sometimes months later, and take chances without knowing it. Rarely, a medical problem in the mother is so dangerous that pregnancy should never be attempted. More commonly, medical conditions can be managed with professional care; women with diabetes, for instance, can avoid many problems if they are at their healthiest with entirely normal blood sugars before a baby is conceived. Several serious genetic conditions can be prevented altogether if the parents are known to carry the gene before they get pregnant. For all these reasons, every woman would be wise to see her doctor or midwife for a "pre-prenatal" or preconception appointment.

Who provides preconception care? If your current gynecologist, family doctor, or nurse-midwife practices obstetrics, he or she can provide this service. If you're unsure where to turn, consult Chapter 11 for a worksheet to help you choose a practitioner.

The Preconception Appointment

Although all practitioners have their own ways of organizing the preconception consultation, the basic history and physical will often include a review of:

- Your personal health history. Bring a list of any conditions for which you see a doctor or take medicines. Try to remember all previous major illnesses, surgeries, and hospitalizations as well. If you have medical problems, you may be referred back to your primary doctor to ensure that you are in your best possible health before pregnancy, and to plan for extra care after you conceive.

  Problems with a previous pregnancy, too, like preterm birth or recurrent miscarriage, can indicate the need for special care during your next pregnancy. Some causes of complications, like a septum (dividing wall) inside the uterus, can be identified and treated only when the woman isn't pregnant.
- Your family medical history. Your doctor or midwife will use your family medical history to help assess your risk of developing complications during pregnancy, such as gestational diabetes or high blood pressure. A fun tool that you can use to document, save, and review your family medical history can be found at www.hhs.gov/familyhistory.
- The personal health history of your future baby's father. It is a good idea to have the father-to-be with you for this appointment. If that isn't possible, try to know as much as you can about his health and his family's medical history. Knowing the father's health history as well as your own will help you avoid genetically based diseases such as cystic fibrosis, sickle cell anemia, muscular dystrophy, and hemophilia. Blood tests during the visit, which are given based on family medical history and ancestry (because some diseases predominantly affect members of certain racial and ethnic groups), can prevent your baby from being afflicted by some causes of mental retardation, like fragile X syndrome, and other genetic problems. Many other genetic conditions, though, like most cases of Down syndrome, don't run in families and can only be tested in the fetus; parental age can help to estimate the risk, but testing must wait until pregnancy.
- Any medications and supplements that you normally take. Bring a list with you—or better yet, bring the actual containers, especially if you take any herbals, homeopathic treatments, or vitamins.
- Risks for infection. If you have a copy of your immunization record, bring it. (Rubella vaccination is the most important.) If you don't

remember having chicken pox, see if you can find out from your parents. If you have any risk factors for HIV, now is a good time to get tested. Your practitioner may order blood testing to check for immunity from significant infections if you are not sure you have been vaccinated.

As well as asking for your medical and family histories, the doctor or midwife will perform a physical examination if you haven't had a check-up and Pap smear in the past year. And they may provide information about

- The importance of maintaining a healthy diet and engaging in regular exercise.
- How to avoid cigarettes, alcohol, and drugs during pregnancy. If you think that you may have trouble quitting, now is the perfect time to get help.
- The best strategy for discontinuing birth control.
- Why you should keep a written record of your menstrual cycles. Tracking the first day of your period will help you to know when you are pregnant and allow your due date to be more accurately calculated.
- The importance of starting to take a daily folic acid or women's multivitamin supplement *before* you conceive. Folic acid supplementation can decrease the risk of spina bifida and some other birth defects by 50 percent, but it must be in your body by the time the baby's spine is forming—which is before most women even know they are expecting. Since many pregnancies are unplanned, all women in their childbearing years, even those using a birth control method, should take a daily folic acid supplement. Spread the word!
- The significance of possible occupational risks. Occupational health isn't always addressed in the preconception appointment, so don't be shy: bring up any concerns you have about exposures to infections, chemicals, or radiation, or other physical challenges in your workplace. Armed with this information, your doctor or midwife should be able to tell you if you are likely to have to make changes at work or take time off to accommodate your pregnancy. (Most mothers-to-be can work through pregnancy with only minor job modifications.)

Meeting with your doctor or midwife ahead of time can help you start pregnancy in the best possible shape, prepare you for what's to come, and allow you

GENETICS 101

We have two genes for each characteristic, one from our mother, and one from our father. Many genetic conditions are recessive, meaning that it takes two "bad" genes to cause the problem; each parent can carry one bad gene without having the disease. If both parents carry a recessive gene for a disease, on average:

- One in four of their children will inherit two bad copies of the gene and will get the disease
- One child of the four will be altogether free of the bad gene
- Two of the four children will be gene carriers like the parents

Recessive conditions often strike in families where no one has had the disease and the parents have no symptoms. Screening is recommended if there is a family history of a serious genetic disease, or if the ethnicity or race of one or both parents puts them in an at-risk group.

to prevent some potential problems. But if you get pregnant before having a pre-pregnancy appointment, don't worry: many of these issues can be addressed during your first prenatal visit. Whether you are pregnant or "just wishing," seek advice and support from your doctor or midwife early, to get your baby and you off to a strong and healthy start.

Part 2

Mergers and Acquisitions (Getting Pregnant)

It can be exciting, if a little strange, to switch from avoiding pregnancy to trying to conceive. In this section, I recommend strategies for stopping birth control and explain the sexual practices and timing that are most likely to make a baby. If you have trouble conceiving, as sometimes happens, you'll also find timely advice: you'll learn when to seek the help of a fertility specialist, the basics of fertility care, and some tips for juggling the demands of fertility treatments with a busy career.

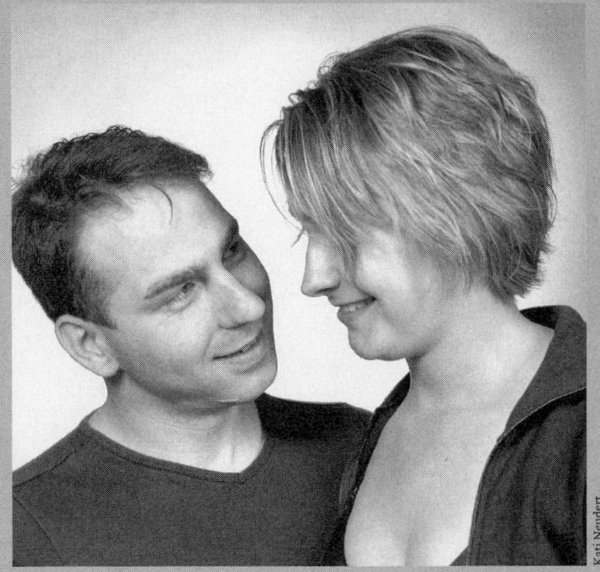

Kati Neudert

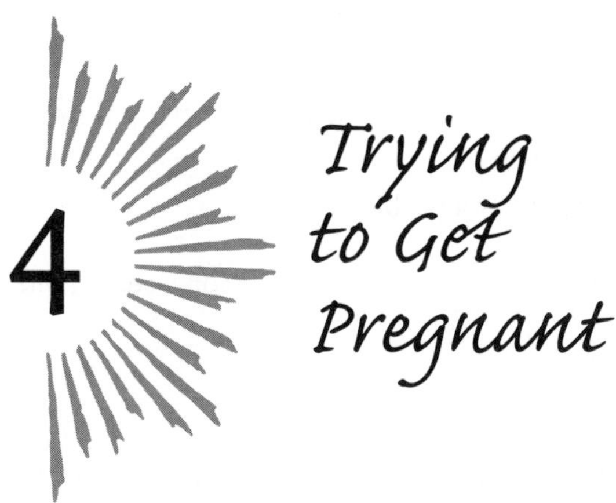

4 Trying to Get Pregnant

So you've made the decision to try to become pregnant—now what? If your natural pattern is to have sex twice a week or more, one good option is not to "try" but rather to let nature take its course. Of couples who have sex this frequently, 85 percent will be pregnant within a year. If your natural pattern of intimacy is less frequent, intercourse every other day for a week starting four or five days before ovulation (the release of the egg) will improve your odds.

How will you know when you are most fertile? Some women have a characteristic pain at ovulation, or notice a change in their vaginal secretions, but most women must use a calendar to figure out their optimal time for making a baby. Writing down the dates of your periods will allow you to track the pattern of your cycles.

Why Keep Track of Your Periods?

There are several reasons why you should begin writing down the starting dates of your periods:

- You will know when you might be pregnant, so you can get an early start taking extra good care of yourself and your baby-to-be.
- If months have gone by and you haven't conceived, you can use the pattern of your periods to help determine your most fertile days.
- Once you are expecting, your doctor or midwife will use the first day of your last period to figure out how far along you are in pregnancy, and to calculate your due date. An accurate due date will help with the timing

of certain prenatal tests, and lead to better decision-making if problems come up during your pregnancy.

- Irregular periods can be a sign of a problem.

For a simple menstrual tracking calendar that you can copy, see Chapter 2.

When Are You Most Fertile?

Ovulation, the ovary's release of the egg, occurs about 14 days before a period begins. Women with regular cycles will find this easy to calculate: if your cycle is 28 days, the first day of your period is day one, and ovulation will occur around day 14; if your cycle is 32 days, the egg is released about day 18; if your cycle is 25 days, you ovulate day 11. Just subtract 14 from the length of your cycle—in other words, the number of days between the first day of one period and the first day of the next period—to figure out the approximate day when you will ovulate.

Since the sperm live as long as five days in the woman's body but the egg lives for only a day or so, having sex a few days before ovulation provides the best chance of pregnancy. By two days after the egg's release, the window of opportunity for that month is closed.

Ovulation Testing

Some couples benefit from ovulation testing, but this scientific, unspontaneous approach to getting pregnant isn't usually necessary and can turn the joy of sex into, as a friend's husband put it, "the job of sex." Before you invest financially and emotionally in ovulation testing and the obsessiveness that it often creates, consider allowing a few months of natural, spontaneous, unprotected lovemaking, to see if you can get pregnant the old-fashioned way.

If you do end up needing to know exactly when you are most fertile, ovulation testing can be very helpful. The test is based on the fact that ovulation is caused by an interplay of hormones made by the pituitary gland (in the brain) and the ovary. After the ovary signals that an egg is ready, the pituitary gland sends out a surge of luteinizing hormone, or LH, which tells the ovary to release the egg. Ovulation predictor kits measure LH in the urine to determine when the brain

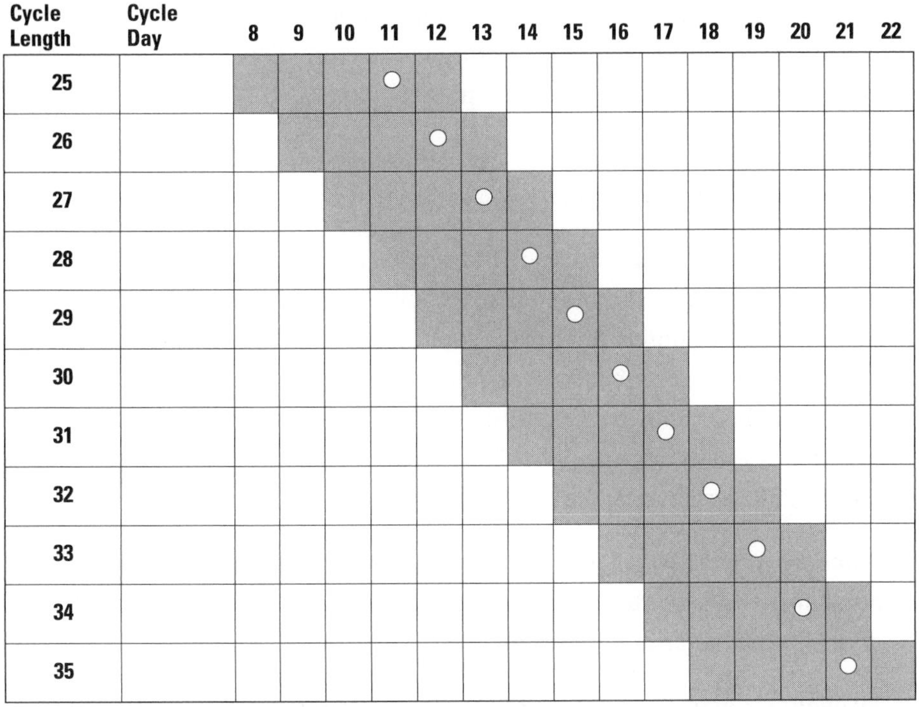

Cycle Length	Cycle Day	8	9	10	11	12	13	14	15	16	17	18	19	20	21	22
25					o											
26						o										
27							o									
28								o								
29									o							
30										o						
31											o					
32												o				
33													o			
34														o		
35															o	

Most likely fertile days based on cycle length. *The most fertile days are highlighted; ovulation is marked with an "o." The cycle length is measured from the first day of one period to the first day of the next period, with cycle day 1 being the first day of menstrual flow. Women with irregular cycles will not be able to predict ovulation by counting days.*

is giving the "go ahead" signal to the egg. Each day, starting three or four days before ovulation is expected, you will test a morning urine sample. Once the color change (or other signal) occurs, you will know that the egg will be released within twelve to twenty-four hours. Further testing of the urine after that point doesn't help—the test may stay positive for a few days, or turn negative right away. In other words, it is the *first* time the test turns positive that identifies the LH surge, indicating that ovulation is about to occur. For timing intercourse, ideally you should have sex a day or two before the test turns positive. You can stop "trying" by two days after the color change.

Ovulation test kits can be purchased at your local drugstore. The array of choices on the store shelves can be overwhelming. Your practitioner may recommend one system, or you can try a few and see which one you like best. But stay with one brand of test each cycle, since you may need to compare results day to day in order to identify when the LH surge is starting. Expensive, reusable "fertility monitors" are not better than disposable kits.

Measuring Basal Body Temperature

Taking your temperature each morning is another way of assessing ovulation. A woman's temperature tends to be low during the first half of the cycle, and about a degree higher after ovulation. Unfortunately, the temperature rises only *after* the egg is released, so by the time you see the change, your fertile days have passed. Basal body temperature, or BBT, is most useful for looking backward at a previous cycle to see what happened. BBT charting can help you anticipate the fertile days during the next month.

> ***When we were "trying," Jonathan would sometimes ask me (hopefully) if my temperature was up yet. Maybe he just felt like watching TV—without all the pressure. (Elisa R., ob-gyn)***

> ***By about six months of not conceiving I was getting a little worried, so we did the thermometer thing. I found out we were not timing it right—we had been practicing the rhythm method, successfully! Since I have always had short menstrual cycles (twenty-one to twenty-three days), I suspect I'm the most fertile shortly after my last period has ended. So no wonder I didn't conceive right away. (Jan R., state attorney)***

Because of the "after the fact" nature of temperature readings, most women find ovulation kits more immediately helpful for determining the best time to try for a baby.

Conception

Knowing a bit about how conception and implantation occur can clarify why it may take a few months—and a bit of luck—to successfully launch a pregnancy. The process starts, as you might have guessed, with a romantic encounter between the sperm and the egg. After they meet, one sperm penetrates the egg in a process called fertilization. Once fertilization occurs, all of the other sperm are prevented from entering the egg, and the cells of the fertilized egg start to multiply, forming a ball. This little "conceptus" is slowly swept down the fallopian tube and into the uterus. By five to seven days after ovulation, the conceptus will have begun to burrow into the wall of the uterus, a process known as implantation. Even at this early stage, before the formation of the umbilical cord or placenta, the tiny baby-to-be gets its nourishment from its mother's uterus.

A few days after implantation, the conceptus starts to make the hormone hCG (human chorionic gonadotropin), to tell the woman's body that she is pregnant. Normally the menstrual period begins when the ovary stops making progesterone. But if the ovary detects hCG, it continues to make the hormone progesterone and the menstrual flow is prevented. HCG is what pregnancy tests detect.

Why Doesn't Every Cycle Lead to Pregnancy?

Chance plays a major role in how long it takes to conceive. A young fertile couple having sex regularly has a 20 to 30 percent likelihood of getting pregnant in any given month. More than 70 percent of the time either the sperm doesn't reach the egg, the conceptus fails to implant, or after implantation the cells don't divide properly. This is normal. Over the course of a year, 85 percent of couples will conceive, and 15 percent will still be waiting for the good news.

It took us nine months to get pregnant. It never occurred to me that it wouldn't happen easily. After four to six months I was getting very upset. I got the book **Taking Charge of Your Fertility.** ***Once I felt I was doing my part I relaxed a bit and wasn't as upset. (Heather H., real estate attorney)***

Myths about fertility date back to ancient times. People may offer you some strange ideas about how to speed up conception.

It took me about a year to get pregnant both times. A woman from the Philippines told me that if you're trying to get pregnant, you have to elevate your butt with a pillow and then you can't get up or go to the bathroom after sex—you have to stay on that pillow all night. So, I tried it and I got pregnant that month. I didn't care if it had anything to do with it or not—I was just happy to be pregnant! (Anne O., director, nonprofit organization)

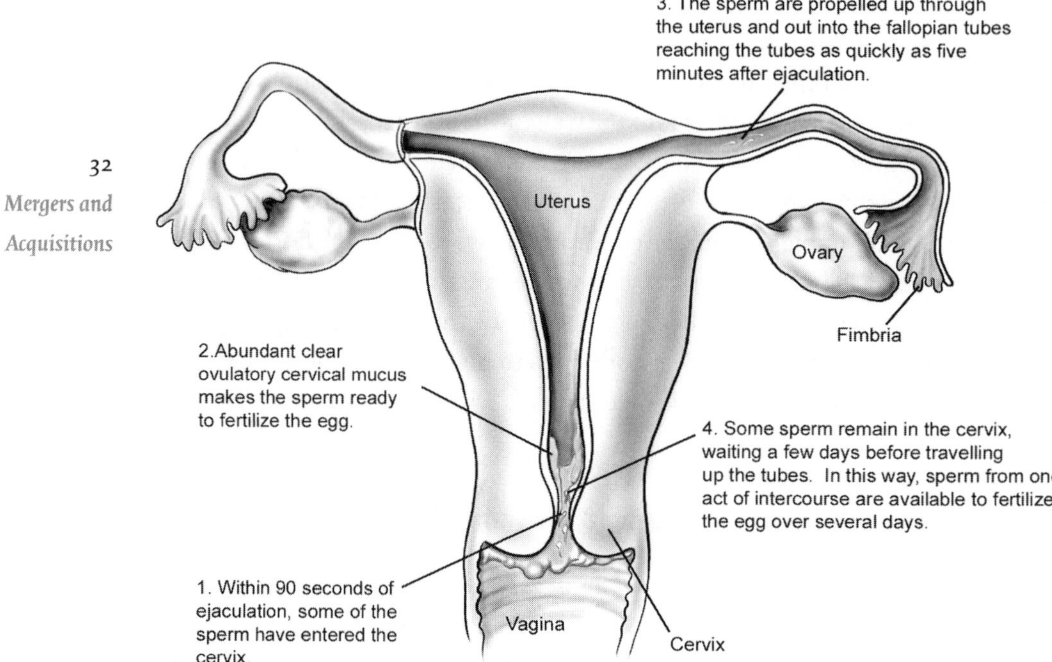

Events of conception. You probably have a pretty good idea of how the sperm get into the vagina, but you may not know what happens next. Just follow the numbers for a tour of events.

It is true, though, that some lifestyle factors—for both the man and the woman—may play a role in a couple's ability to start a pregnancy. Factors that can impair fertility for women include:

- Cigarettes. Smoking cigarettes interferes with fertility and increases the chance of miscarrying. Although some smokers become pregnant without difficulty, overall, being a nonsmoker improves your odds of having a baby.
- Substance use and medications. Avoiding alcohol, marijuana, and other drugs may also help you achieve pregnancy. Moderate alcohol intake (even just a drink or two a day) can impair conception and may cause birth defects. There is also some evidence that medication, including over-the-counter pain medicines like ibuprofen, can interfere with fertility in women. Check with your doctor to find out if any medications you take might affect fertility or pregnancy.

- Caffeine. Caffeine may increase the chance of miscarriage and hinder fertility, so while you are trying to conceive, limit your intake of caffeinated drinks and foods (including coffee, caffeinated teas and soft drinks, chocolate, and medications containing caffeine).
- Occupational exposures. Chemical exposures at work or home can potentially interfere with fertility. If you are exposed to pesticides or other chemicals, learn about the possible reproductive effects either through your doctor or, if the substances are at work, from your employer (see Chapter 2 for more information about potentially toxic exposures at work).

- Being overweight, underweight, or exercising too much. Normal body weight is best. Having an eating disorder, being underweight, or being overweight can all interfere with getting pregnant, especially if your menstrual periods are irregular or absent. And although regular exercise is good for overall health and weight control, exercising more than an hour a day may interfere with ovulation.
- Age. The per-month chance of getting pregnant declines with age. Fertility is highest for women in their twenties, and starts to fall markedly by the late thirties.
- Irregular cycles. If your periods are absent or very irregular, pregnancy is less likely. If you have irregular periods, medical attention should be sought if you aren't pregnant within a few months.

Tips on getting pregnant (at age forty): Don't wait for a year of not getting pregnant to go to a fertility specialist. You may as well find out all the information as soon as possible. (Peggy L., nurse-administrator)

Lifestyle factors can impair a man's fertility as well.

- Overheating. Sperm do best in a slightly cool environment, which is why the testes are located in the scrotum, slightly away from the heat of the body. A hot bath or a soak in the hot tub immediately before sex may temporarily interfere with sperm function. Even excessive bicycling can affect the sperm. When trying for pregnancy, men who bike should wear padded bike shorts, take frequent breaks, and be sure that the bicycle seat doesn't put a lot of pressure on the testicles. Working in a very warm environment may also pose a problem. Yet contrary to popular belief, wearing tight pants, briefs, or athletic supporters, even every day, has not been shown to interfere with male fertility.

- Cigarettes. Men who smoke may have poorer quality sperm; they also have lower sex drives and (perhaps as a result) have sex less frequently. Although it isn't clear how bad smoking is for male fertility, quitting may help the woman to quit and may reduce her exposure to second-hand smoke, both of which could improve fertility and the health of the baby-to-be.
- Substance use and medications. Anabolic steroids, the kind taken by athletes, can contribute to infertility. Alcohol doesn't affect fertility in men unless it is so abused that is causes liver changes, diminished sex drive, or sexual difficulties. Cocaine or heavy marijuana use, in contrast, can temporarily reduce the number and quality of sperm by as much as 50 percent.
- Occupational exposures. It isn't known if chemical exposures from work or hobbies interfere directly with male fertility, but it may be wise for your male partner to avoid exposures to substances with potential health risks, just to be sure that his sperm are not affected.
- An inadequate diet. Although a man's body weight probably isn't as important as the female partner's body weight when it comes to fertility, deficiencies of vitamin C, zinc, or folic acid can lead to problems with sperm production. If a man's diet is lacking, a daily multivitamin should supply the necessary vitamins and minerals.

I don't remember how long I was trying with Isabel, maybe five months, but it is true that we didn't get pregnant until we were on vacation and not going into the hot tub every night. (Jan R., state attorney)

THE FREQUENCY AND TIMING OF SEX

Sperm counts are best when ejaculation occurs every day to every other day. There is no need, and even some harm, in "saving up" for your fertile time. Sex every one to two days around ovulation provides the best chance for pregnancy. While it might be a fun idea, it isn't necessary to run home during the day for a "quickie" to try to hit that most fertile moment: the window of opportunity lasts a few days. If you or your partner travel a lot for work, though, timing can be a challenge. If you are in a hurry to get pregnant, consider traveling together or avoiding trips mid-cycle, when you are most fertile.

FACT AND FICTION

After sex, many women notice that some semen leaks out of the vagina. By that time, however, millions of sperm have already made their way to the cervix and beyond. There is no evidence that lying still after sex, or keeping the legs or hips raised, will improve your chances of conceiving. Couples who have sexual difficulties and can't achieve ejaculation during intercourse should talk to the doctor about techniques to help with conception. And some lubricants used for sex can be mildly toxic to sperm, as can douching after sex. Research has shown that KY Jelly, Astroglide, Replens, olive oil, and saliva all interfere with sperm motility. If you need a lubricant, you may want to try baby oil or canola oil, which are reported not to interfere with the sperm; a sexual lubricant called Pre-seed also advertises that it is nontoxic to sperm.

If you tell friends and family that you are trying to get pregnant, you will no doubt get lots of recommendations, some of which are pure superstition, on how to improve fertility. Rather than turning your life upside down trying to go along with them all, check with your practitioner for accurate advice. And remember that most couples can get pregnant without "trying"—just by discontinuing birth control and letting nature take its course.

The pregnancy seat—there was one computer station in my office in which all the women who sat there got pregnant. (Andrea R., graphic artist)

Discontinuing Birth Control

So how exactly do you go off of your birth control method? Easy, if you have been using a barrier like condoms or a spermicide—just stop. If you have been using an intrauterine contraceptive (IUD), like the progestin intrauterine system (Mirena) or a ten-year copper intrauterine device (Paraguard), your practitioner will need to remove it.

Hormonal methods like the Pill, the Patch, and the Ring should be discontinued at the end of a cycle. Most physicians recommend waiting to conceive until you have had two or three normal periods off of birth control, since menstrual cycles can be irregular for a few months after discontinuing hormonal contraceptives. Why do irregular cycles matter? Your due date will be calculated more accurately if you wait until your cycles have become regular before you get pregnant. Another problem with the irregular cycles you may have after using hormonal contraception is your own emotional state: it can be frustrating to always wonder if your period is delayed because you are pregnant or if you are just having a late ovulation. Conversely, you may assume you aren't pregnant and take chances you shouldn't take during pregnancy, like using medications or drinking alcohol. But if you absolutely can't wait, you will be glad to know that there is no evidence that birth control pills (or the Patch or Ring) cause birth defects, even for those who get pregnant while using their contraceptive. In fact, no risk of miscarriage or any other pregnancy complication has been linked to the Pill. The main reason to use a simple method like condoms or spermicide for a few months after stopping hormonal contraceptives is to avoid the frustration and confusion of trying to get pregnant while having irregular periods.

Long-acting injectable contraceptives like Depo-Provera (depot medroxyprogesterone acetate, or DMPA) take a long time to leave your system; the return of fertility can't be hurried. Women on Depo should consider using another method for about a year before they want to get pregnant, since it can take that long for the effects to wear off. Like the Pill, getting pregnant immediately after stopping the Depo shot doesn't cause birth defects or miscarriage, but since menstrual cycles are notoriously irregular or absent after Depo, you may not realize you have conceived, or you may wonder every day if you are pregnant. You also won't be able to use the day of your last period to calculate an accurate due date.

After years of trying NOT to get pregnant, you have NO idea how long it'll take TO get pregnant! (Edie U., school psychologist)

I was thirty-five when I got pregnant, and I didn't have a whole lot of confidence in my fertility. Other than knowing that I should take prenatal vitamins, I didn't do anything to prepare. I just went off the Pill, waited one month, then started trying. I got pregnant on the second try. (Linda S., creative director)

Overthinking

Those of us who are used to planning our lives and feeling in control most of the time can feel stressed from the uncertainties of trying to become pregnant. Some people handle this stress by turning the conception process into their own little science experiment—complete with urine testing and sex on a schedule. Unless you have reasons that you must conceive quickly, such as being in your late thirties or older, I recommend trying your best to be patient during this time, so as not to turn your sex life into a job for you and your partner. Most couples will be pregnant within a year as long as they have sex fairly regularly—and having fun while you wait for the big news will make it easier for both of you. Don't just pass the time working on becoming pregnant and hoping for a result; enjoy the process. After your baby arrives, when you're immersed in the day-to-day demands of parenting, you'll be happy you learned to cherish life as it happens.

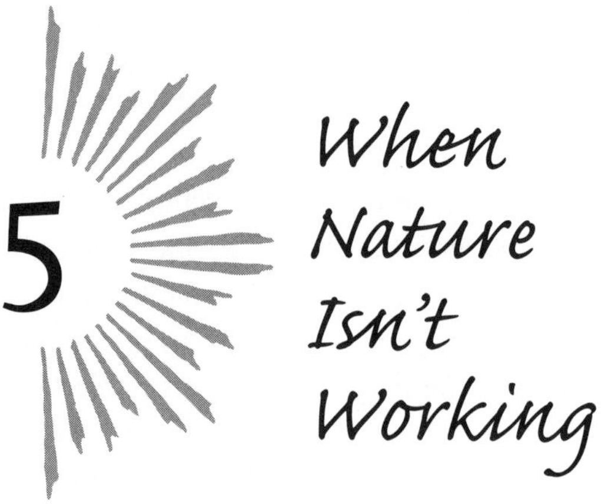

5 When Nature Isn't Working

You probably know people who have struggled to get pregnant; maybe you are having difficulties yourself. Stories about the infertility "epidemic" are all over the news. The statistics are dramatic: in vitro fertilization, the most complex type of fertility treatment, is responsible for the conception of more than one in every hundred babies born in the United States today, and many other pregnancies were undoubtedly helped along by less elaborate procedures. But you can take heart knowing that although about 15 percent of couples have trouble getting pregnant, infertility is often really "subfertility"—that is, with time or treatment most of these couples can conceive.

When Should You Seek Help Getting Pregnant?

You should talk to a doctor if you have not conceived after twelve months of regular sex without birth control. Sometimes the resolution is as simple as skipping the trip to the hot tub or learning when in the month is your most fertile time.

As you get older, fertility diminishes, and the window of opportunity for successful treatment narrows. Most experts recommend seeking help after six months of trying if the female partner is age thirty-five to thirty-nine, and after just three months if the woman is over forty.

Here I was forty years old, always wanting children. After being married for six months, I freaked out and went to a fertility doctor, and they told me that the chances of getting pregnant on my own were grim, based on my age. They sent me home with a cup for my husband to check his sperm

count, and sent me down to the lab that day for a progesterone level test, gave me a prescription for Clomid, and scheduled me for IUI (artificial insemination) for fifteen days later. Two days later, I missed my period; I was already pregnant. (Peggy L., nurse-administrator)

A big part of getting pregnant is simply playing the odds—the possibility of conceiving in any month varies by age and circumstance, but in general, the more months you try, the more likely you are to make a baby. For example, two fertile young people may have a 20 to 30 percent chance per cycle of conceiving naturally, so their odds of getting pregnant in a year are very high. In contrast, some couples that seem infertile may still have a 5 percent chance each month—so that after a year of trying, their number just hasn't come up yet. Even as their fertility workup starts, they still have that 5 percent per month chance—and many people do get pregnant before (or long after) fertility therapy. The goal of treatment is simply to improve those odds each month. Since most therapies will not make the odds better than 30 percent per month, you need to take a long-term view as you start treatment—one cycle of therapy is statistically unlikely to get you pregnant, but over time you are more than likely to succeed.

Causes of Infertility

Most fertility problems are caused by trouble with the sperm, problems with ovulation, obstruction of the fallopian tubes, an abnormally shaped uterus, endometriosis, or sexual difficulties that prevent ejaculation into the vagina, but a significant number of couples have unexplained infertility—that is, testing is done, and nothing is found to explain why they aren't getting pregnant. Luckily, modern fertility treatments are often successful even when a specific cause is not identified.

Doctors Who Treat Fertility Problems

Most obstetrician-gynecologists (ob-gyns) have training in fertility assessment and can start the process. If you are not progressing after a few months, or if you prefer to do so from the outset, you can go to a reproductive endocrinology-infertility specialist. Reproductive endocrinologists, or RE's, have completed a

INFERTILITY: AN EQUAL OPPORTUNITY CONDITION

- 40 percent of infertility situations can be attributed to the woman
- 40 percent can be attributed to the man
- 10–15 percent are due to both partners
- 5–10 percent are unexplained

residency in obstetrics and gynecology and then three years of specialized fellowship training. Many work in programs that provide high-tech assisted reproductive care, such as in vitro fertilization (IVF). The woman's doctor can start the evaluation for both male and female fertility factors, and then refer the man to a urologist if necessary.

The Fertility Workup

The fertility evaluation can vary from fairly simple to quite complex. You can see from the causes of infertility that to optimize treatment both partners must be evaluated. Most of the time, three initial tests help the fertility team assess the problem:

1. A semen sample is collected from the man by masturbation, then viewed under a microscope to check sperm number, shape (morphology), and swimming ability (motility).
2. Ovulation is assessed using a blood progesterone level or basal body temperature charting. A progesterone level drawn the week before the period is due is the easiest way to document that ovulation has occurred, but graphing your daily morning temperature can also help establish if and when you are ovulating.
3. A hysterosalpingogram (HSG) is performed to see that the fallopian tubes are open. During the HSG, a doctor will insert a speculum to see into the vagina, then instill X-ray dye through the cervix up into the uterus. Next, X-rays are taken to see the shape of the uterine cavity and the flow of dye out of the fallopian tubes.

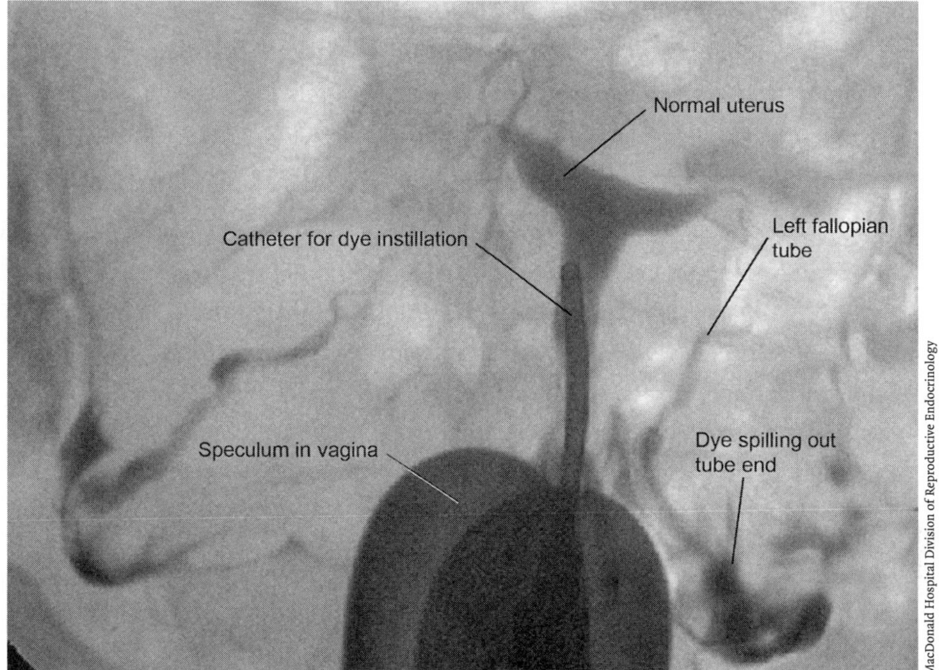

Hysterosalpingogram

Fertility Treatments

Treatments to boost fertility fall into four general categories: lifestyle modifications, medications, assisted reproductive techniques (including IVF), and surgery. Most treatments suggested by your doctor will improve your current chances of pregnancy, but only IVF has the potential (under some circumstances) to push the odds over 30 percent in a cycle; for many treatments, the pregnancy rate per cycle is significantly lower. Your doctor should be able to tell you the likelihood of success with any regimen, based on your age and other individual factors. Typically one approach is tried for a few months, followed by a more expensive or demanding treatment if the first doesn't work. Sometimes a couple with many factors going against them will beat the odds; other times, a seemingly fertile couple just won't conceive. Many of the new treatments are remarkable, but a successful pregnancy can't be guaranteed.

I have polycystic ovaries, so I went on Clomid to get pregnant. I had been on it for two months when I got hospitalized for a ruptured ovarian cyst. They

had me follow up with fertility specialists, but by the time I got there I was pregnant. When my husband and I wanted to have another baby, they said I would need drugs again, so I went to the same fertility clinic. When I got there, they did blood tests, and said, "You're already pregnant." So twice I went to the fertility clinic for treatment and was already pregnant. I hope they're not using my statistics in their success rates! (Janet G., attorney)

I was postmenopausal, but I was on the Pill so I didn't realize it until I went off to try to get pregnant, and there I was having hot flashes. The hard part of IVF was that I couldn't use my eggs because I was forty-five years old at the start of the process, so I went through the shared egg program. I decided to do it this way because I felt uncomfortable asking young friends or relatives to be egg donors; so I went with someone who had already chosen to be a donor. (Juanita G., research scientist)

After my fourth in vitro fertilization procedure I finally got pregnant! I was so happy to finally be pregnant . . . it was truly amazing . . . there are no words to describe the joyous feeling! (Cindy M., supermodel)

Financing Fertility Treatment

Although some states require insurance companies to cover fertility treatment, many states have no regulations. Fertility may be an excluded service, so check your insurance booklet or the company's website, then follow up with a call to your insurer if you're still uncertain. If you and your spouse are both eligible for health insurance through your employers, compare products during the next open enrollment. If one has the option of better fertility coverage, it may make sense to switch. To check the laws in your state, log on to the website of the American Society for Reproductive Medicine at www.asrm.org.

Fertility teams have a lot of experience with insurance issues and should know what may or may not be covered. Parts of the workup that aren't specifically related to fertility, like assessing irregular periods with blood hormone levels, may be included even if "fertility treatment" is denied. Some plans, too, cover the *evaluation* of infertility but not its *treatment.*

Fertility specialists are accustomed to taking costs into account when making treatment plans. The choices you make will depend in part on your financial re-

ALL IVF PROGRAMS ARE NOT CREATED EQUAL

If you are going to need in vitro fertilization, be informed. Statistics on IVF success rates can be confusing and misleading. Check out your local program's success rate at the CDC website: www.cdc.gov/reproductivehealth/ART/index.htm. If a number of programs are available in your area, shop around. Ask about the take-home-baby rate for people in your age group with your cause of infertility, and about the chances of twins or more. Many programs have been able to decrease the number of multiple pregnancies without compromising the chances of having a baby. IVF is a very expensive proposition, so you will want to do your homework and choose a program that will meet your personal, financial, and reproductive needs.

sources and your projected out-of-pocket costs. Most fertility practices require cash up front, because of insurance exclusions and a history of people not paying their bills. Some families finance their fertility charges, to spread the costs over time.

As you sort through the likely expenses, keep in mind that having children costs a lot after conception too—the amount required to treat infertility may be proportionally small over the lifetime of a child. Of course, if you could know for sure that you'd get pregnant, it would be easier to sink a lot of money into this endeavor. Some fertility programs are experimenting with IVF guarantees, in which you pay a certain amount up front, and if you don't become pregnant after a predetermined number of cycles, your money is returned. Talk to your doctor or nurse about your financial concerns to see what options are available to you.

Fertility Treatment and Your Work Schedule

Treatment with injectable fertility drugs can require four to six appointments each month, sometimes three days in a row, for examinations, ultrasounds, blood work, and inseminations. If you are under a lot of pressure not to miss work, ask for an appointment at the beginning of an office session; the schedule will be less likely to be running behind then. Keep in mind, too, that many of the steps in fertility evaluation and treatment are cycle-day dependent. If you travel for work, you may need to restrict traveling for awhile, or stretch your treatments over several months so that you will be in town during the critical part of your cycle.

When I was being treated with intrauterine inseminations, I had to come up with a variety of creative excuses on a moment's notice, once my ovulation test stick turned pink, in order to explain coming in way late for work over the next several days. (Andrea R., graphic artist)

Fertility treatment was very time-consuming. I was fortunate that my boss at the time had been through even more extreme infertility treatments than we were going through, so he was very understanding. (Jane J., advertising executive)

Dealing with Stress

Trying to get pregnant after a problem is identified may be far from relaxing, but new research indicates that fertility patients who feel less stressed get pregnant more quickly. So what can you do to minimize stress, both because it may help you get pregnant and because it makes treatment more bearable?

- Think of your fertility treatment as a project. Map out a strategy with your partner and your fertility doctor, and stick to it. Decide in advance how many and what kind of procedures will be emotionally and financially acceptable, and attempt to determine a final limit. Try to get in a long-term mindset—hope to be pregnant within a year, rather than obsessing each day.
- Write down questions to bring to your doctor, so you will remember to ask.
- Consider what you will do if you don't conceive. Having an alternate plan such as adoption, not having children, or using donor eggs can minimize stress and anxiety.
- Consider taking a break from fertility treatments every few months.
- Communicate with your partner, and expect your partner to have diffi-

culties too. Don't expect him to always feel the same way that you do, though—each person responds differently to the strains of infertility.

- Fertility treatment can be hard on every aspect of a marriage. Try to do things together that you both enjoy and that are unrelated to getting pregnant. And have sex just for fun during some "non-fertile" times of the cycle.
- Don't be surprised at your negative reaction when someone else becomes pregnant—even someone you love. It is hard to be happy for others while you are struggling to become a mother yourself.
- Expect to feel emotional during this process. Fertility treatment often leads to a roller coaster of feelings, including anxiety, excitement, and frustration. Many professional women have never experienced this sort of loss of control over their lives, having always been able to get what they wanted if they worked hard enough. Studies indicate that fertility treatment can be more stressful than cancer therapy, with similar reactions of anger, grief, shame, damaged self-esteem, jealousy, isolation, and loss of control.
- Relaxation techniques can help you to cope. Some couples find yoga, meditation, guided imagery, reiki, massage therapy, and/or exercise helpful. Also consider getting counseling or joining a support group—it can be reassuring to know that you're not alone. Resolve is one of several national organizations that provide information and support to families dealing with fertility issues. For more information, check out the website at www.resolve.org.

After I got pregnant I became a fertility consultant to those who "came out of the closet" to me about their infertility. (Andrea R., graphic artist)

Take Control

Fertility treatment may be tough for different people in different ways. One person may want to avoid surgery, another may want to do whatever is offered to get pregnant quickly, and still another may be limited by the costs. Your fertility team must take your concerns and priorities into account when making a plan for your care.

THE MYTH OF ADOPTION AS A FERTILITY TREATMENT

Once acquaintances learn you are trying to get pregnant, you will get plenty of advice, some of which will be totally inaccurate. One common belief is that adopting a baby makes you more likely to conceive. Although everyone remembers the stories of mothers who became pregnant after they adopted, studies have shown that the reason they conceived has nothing to do with adopting. Instead, since most fertility problems represent subfertility rather than infertility, couples sometimes become pregnant after they are done trying—just because their number finally came up.

Being aware of your fears and communicating them to your treatment team can help ease the process.

> ***Some IVF treatments . . . require you being present for several hours each morning for thirteen out of every thirty days. I can see how many women could lose their jobs this way. We decided that if it got to that point, we would just opt for adoption. (Jane J., advertising executive)***

Many people find fertility treatment terribly difficult, invasive of their formerly private body parts, and distressing to their intimate relationships. Some conclude that it isn't worth it and choose other ways to become parents, or decide to live childfree. Others struggle to find the strength, determination, and financial resources to go through many disruptive interventions for the sake of having a child. To continue to feel in control of the process, periodically rethink what is right for you and how far you are willing to go. Having a plan at the outset, and a backup strategy if fertility treatment doesn't work, can help you get through this difficult time. Good luck!

COMMON CONCERNS AND LIMITING FACTORS IN FERTILITY TREATMENT

- Medical
  - Treatment-related risks
  - Chance of multiple pregnancy
- Social
  - Missing work
  - Inconvenience
  - Lack of privacy
- Financial
  - Costs of different treatments
  - Potential expense of twins or more
- Psychological
  - Stress of the diagnosis
  - Strain on the relationship
  - Emotional ups and downs of treatment

Part 3

Adapting to Change (Through Week 13)

Early pregnancy is a time of transformation: an exciting roller-coaster ride that for many women includes some stomach-flipping surprises. A demanding job can amplify the challenges, but knowing what's ahead can really help. In this section, I will discuss the signs of pregnancy, embryonic development, physical and emotional changes you may be experiencing, how to manage pregnancy symptoms on and off the job, early pregnancy risks (including work-related hazards), and the first prenatal medical appointment. I will also address job-related decisions such as when and how you may want to disclose your pregnancy to others.

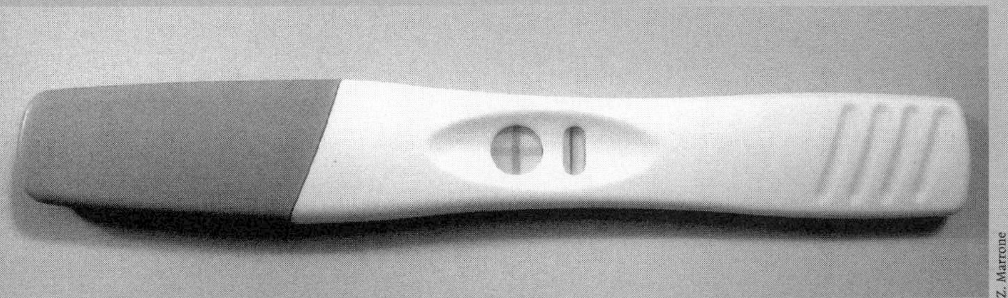

Z. Marrone

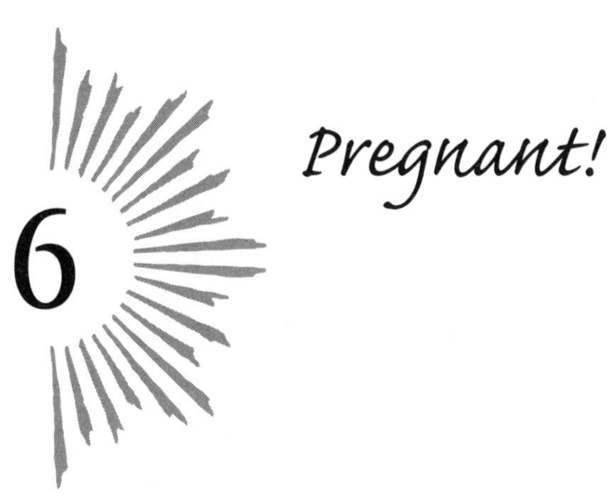

6 Pregnant!

How do you know that you are pregnant? Some women swear that they feel something—an emotional or physical sign—that tells them almost immediately that conception has occurred. Others are oblivious until they throw up a few times or have missed a period or two. For most, the first signs are sore breasts and a late period, followed by some queasiness.

> ***With all of my pregnancies, I knew right away. It sounds bizarre, but the next morning I would tell my husband we were pregnant—each time I was right (this happened four times as I had two losses). The only way I can describe it was that I had this "feeling" that something was going on in my uterus—like a flurry of activity. (Sandy B., social worker)***

> ***We tried the first month, and I didn't get pregnant. So I started reading about it, and I went out and bought a basal thermometer and a chart and started tracking my temperature. My temperature went up and didn't go back down. I was really frustrated with tracking it because it just wouldn't go back down. It turned out I was pregnant. (Heidi R., law professor)***

> ***We had five unsuccessful intrauterine inseminations. It was horrible, month after month, dealing with the disappointment. We eventually decided to adopt, and on the same day of the second meeting with the adoption counselor, I discovered I was pregnant, no drugs or anything. (Jane J., advertising executive)***

Pregnancy Testing

As mentioned earlier, home pregnancy tests measure the hormone human chorionic gonadotropin, or hCG, which is made by the early embryo after implantation and which circulates in the bloodstream until it is excreted in the urine. Blood pregnancy testing usually isn't necessary; under most circumstances a home urine test should be all you need.

I was very tired, and my boobs got enormous so I knew something wasn't right. I had a pretty good feeling that I was pregnant, so I peed on the stick, handed it to my husband (boyfriend at the time), and ran out of the bathroom. He came out and looked at me and said, "I think we're having a baby . . . the stick had two lines on it before you even got out of the bathroom." (Stephanie B., FedEx courier)

I took a home pregnancy test, and it was positive, but I didn't believe it, so I took another one. (This is not necessary, if you've got the hCG in your urine, you're pregnant.) Of course I was happy, but I also had the feeling of uh-oh, there's no turning back now! (Peggy L., nurse-administrator)

With my first baby, I was in graduate school, so I went to the student health center. Usually people coming to a student health center asking for a pregnancy test are undergrads who made a mistake and are very worried. The nurse sat me down and said, "Dear, it's positive." She was very concerned and sympathetic. I remember cracking up. I said, "Oh, that's great, my husband will be thrilled." (Heidi R., law professor)

Neither pregnancy was planned. We were in the kitchen one day and I fixed myself an ice cream bar and a pickle. He looked at me and said, are you ok? And I thought, yeah, this is weird, but I want it. So while we were out, I said let's stop at this Walgreen's and get a pregnancy test. That's how we found out. (Uwimana W., real estate assistant)

How long do you have to wait to run a home pregnancy test? Urine pregnancy tests are most precise if they are done a week *after* the period was due. You may see the advertisement stating that their test is "99 percent accurate" even before the missed period, but this is misleading. Accurate for the purpose of advertising only means that it gives the same results as other available pregnancy tests. Some pregnancies don't start producing measurable amounts of hCG until after the period is late. Conversely, some cycles that are not going to lead to pregnancy can produce small amounts of hCG until a day or two after the period is due. This phenomenon is sometimes called a "chemical pregnancy." Because of these two realities, pregnancy tests can be falsely negative or falsely positive if done too early, leading to unnecessary discouragement and frustration. Unless there is a medical reason to find out extremely early, it is better to force yourself to wait until a full week after you expected your period.

My first urine pregnancy test at the doctor's office was negative but I knew I was pregnant. A few days later it was positive. (Kathy H., software developer)

At the store, the pregnancy test aisle is full of different kits. How do you choose? All home pregnancy tests are easy to use. Three of the kits tested by *Consumer Reports*, "First Response," "Answer Quick & Simple," and "ClearBlue Easy," produced result lines that were darker than others, making them the easiest to read. *Consumer Reports* also found that if you waited for ten minutes before reading the result (instead of the recommended one to five minutes), tests turned positive a few days earlier in pregnancy, when the hCG levels were too low to detect with standard testing procedure. Don't wait longer than ten minutes though: after ten minutes some negative tests start to look faintly positive. (For a charming cautionary tale, check out www.peeonastick.com.) *Consumer Reports* found that even the most ultra-sensitive kit would yield falsely negative results for one in four pregnant women if used before the first missed period. If your home pregnancy test is negative and you still think you might be pregnant, test again in a week—you may be pleasantly surprised.

I was a few days late, so I decided to take a pregnancy test. I'd had a few negative results in the prior two months, so I bought an inexpensive test at the pharmacy. It turned positive almost instantaneously. I made Brad go back and buy a more expensive test just to be sure. Wouldn't you know, positive again. (Jen R., fashion merchandiser)

A few days before I was supposed to start my period I bought a home pregnancy test. I came home and peed on the stick and a very slight second

pink line appeared. I compared it to the unused test in the box and decided there was definitely a slight line, but still didn't know if it was positive. Ben came home and I told him that I thought I was pregnant and showed him the test, but we still didn't know for sure. So the next morning I took the other test. The line was not any darker. I remember in the past laughing at some of the commercials that advertised an easy-to-read test and thought to myself, how hard can it be to tell if there is a line or not? Well, now I knew. I didn't take any more tests, but my period didn't come in a few days so I made an OB appointment and it was confirmed for me. (Christi M., medical student)

Emotions

As your pregnancy test turns positive, your mind will probably start to race. You may not quite believe it. Whether pregnancy is long-planned or a surprise, many parents-to-be describe a jumble of emotions: excitement, disbelief, joy, apprehension, fear, and a sense of the importance of this moment. It is normal to have mixed negative and positive feelings—after all, you are getting on a train that is already in motion and will take you places both wonderful and a little scary. It will probably be a while before reality sinks in. Meanwhile, be sure to take good care of yourself and your baby-to-be. Avoid risky exposures, take your folic acid (or multivitamin), and listen to your body.

Since I wasn't planning for pregnancy and I am not married, I was half excited and half nervous. It was just a shock. (Annette M., store manager)

On the evening of the day I received the good news, I sent him to the grocery store with a list. Of the ten or so items listed, number three was "Pampers." He always goes over the list before he leaves to make sure he has it right. He looked at "Pampers" and started laughing. He figured it out immediately and couldn't stop grinning the entire evening. (Val P., administrative coordinator)

We told our parents at about ten weeks. We asked them not to tell anyone else. Well, this did not work. They told everyone they knew. (Christi M., medical student)

I was feeling very poorly. Tired, washed-out, nauseated, and thought I had an ulcer. I contacted my doctor for an appointment. One of his first questions was, "Could you be pregnant?" He said we should test just to be sure. They had left a message for me to call and like an idiot I called right from my desk in the middle of an office of about five other people. The nurse came on the line and promptly informed me I was pregnant. I was dumbfounded, shocked, terrified, and almost sick to my stomach within seconds. It didn't take long before everyone in the office knew I was pregnant. I had to hurry home and tell my husband before someone else did. (Becky G., administrator)

Keeping It Secret

Is now the time to tell your boss, your co-workers, and the mail carrier that you are going to have a baby? Most women don't want to disclose that they are pregnant this early on. As much as you may want to shout the good news from the rooftops, be thoughtful about whom you tell about your pregnancy. Alternatively, close friends and family who would be involved if the pregnancy ran into trouble might as well get the chance to share your excitement whenever the moment seems right.

I couldn't hide my pregnancy because I was so ill. I told people at five weeks. (Zenia M., nurse's aide)

I told people at work I was pregnant at three months, but really I could have/should have waited longer—until I started showing. Once I told people, they were very interested and, I would say, a bit nosy. My boss, who did not have any kids yet, was especially interested in my pregnancy, doctor appointments, and test results. (Tamika S., web content producer)

I had planned on waiting the full three months to tell them, but before the end of the first trimester, I had bleeding and had to leave work. There was no inconspicuous way of leaving, so I ended up telling a department manager and district manager because they were there. Everyone was really good about keeping it quiet at first. I didn't want to share it at first since there was such a chance I would miscarry. (Zoe B., inventory manager)

When Is the Baby Due?

There are many ways to determine your baby's due date. If you want to calculate it yourself, subtract three months and add seven days to the first day of your last period. If your last period began October 8, for instance, your due date would be July 15. This method assumes regular twenty-eight-day cycles, with conception on day 14. Numerous websites also provide due date calculators, or you can add 266 days to your date of conception, if you know it. Your practitioner will determine your official due date based on whichever parameters are believed to be most accurate: the first day of your last period, your presumed date of conception, and/or the results of ultrasound measurements.

So when will this baby arrive? Only about 5 percent of people deliver on their actual due dates, although a substantial 85 percent give birth sometime between two weeks before and two weeks after. You may be better off focusing on a "due month" so you don't get too attached to just one day. This way, if you are among the 40 percent of moms who go past their due dates, maybe it won't drive you quite as crazy.

HOW DUE DATES ARE CALCULATED

Although it can be a bit confusing, to figure out a due date most obstetricians count forty weeks from the first day of the last period, which means that, on average, they begin counting two weeks before you even conceived. This tradition predates ultrasounds and ovulation detection, when all doctors and midwives had to go on was the date of the last period. So don't be surprised if your practitioner tells you that you are eight weeks pregnant and you know you only conceived six weeks ago—that is just how gestational age is calculated. Ultrasound results are adjusted to this method, too, so if your sonogram says the embryo is eight weeks in size, it means you are six weeks after conception.

Much of the confusion occurs when a pregnant mom wants to figure out which month of pregnancy she is in. How can it be that a pregnancy is forty weeks, and there are about four weeks in a month, yet pregnancy is said to last nine months? You have to remember that a month is more like four and a half weeks. The easiest way to figure out which "month" you are in is to count backward from your due date—for example, if you are due July 15, that will be nine months, then you will have completed eight months on June 15, seven months on May 15, and so on. Traditionally you only get "credit" for time after it has passed, just like your baby will be one year old only after the first birthday. That means you are nine months pregnant on your due date, and "in your ninth month" during the previous thirty days.

A New Identity

Pregnancy often transforms how you see yourself. It's a new responsibility that can't be delegated. During these nine months, your body—and mindset—will change in ways you can't ignore. How will you manage the dual roles of pregnant mom and working woman? In the coming chapters, I offer some advice about how to deal with your pregnancy in the context of your busy, complex life. But first, let's think a little more about your little one.

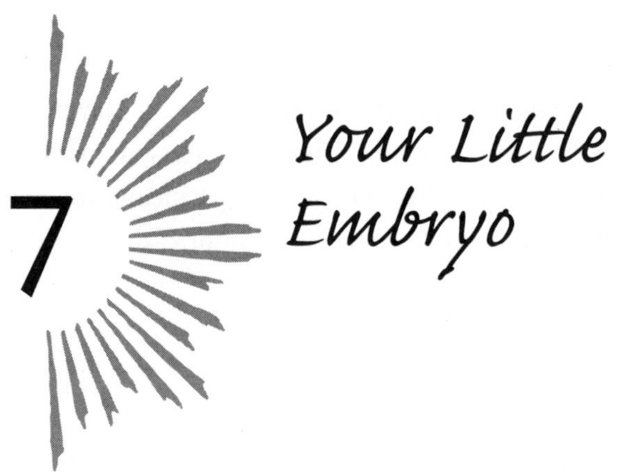

7 Your Little Embryo

While you are at work, in the car, at home, and asleep, your little embryo is growing and changing. In this chapter I will explain these amazing transformations, how you supply oxygen and nutrients to your baby-to-be, and many factors that can affect fetal development and well-being. Throughout, I will count weeks as your own obstetrician will, based on a forty-week pregnancy.

Between the day that the sperm enters the egg and a mere two months later, your little embryo is busy forming all of its organ systems, including the heart, kidneys, intestines, genital system, and brain. This doesn't mean that the organs are ready to function—the baby can't live outside your body for many months—but from ten weeks on, the basic structure is set, and your baby just needs to grow and mature.

Pregnancy Week 4 (Embryo Day 8–14)

By the time your pregnancy test turns positive, your fertilized egg has multiplied its cells, organized into layers, and implanted into the wall of the uterus. At this point it is considered an embryo. The embryonic disc will become the baby, and the outer cell layers will become the membranes and placenta. The yolk sac, which may be visible on ultrasound, helps transfer nutrients from the uterus to the embryo before the more sophisticated placenta and umbilical cord have formed.

Pregnancy Week 5 (Embryo Day 15–21)

During week five, the flat embryonic disc rolls into a tube. Fetal blood cells start to form, and simple tubes arise that will become the heart. By twenty-two

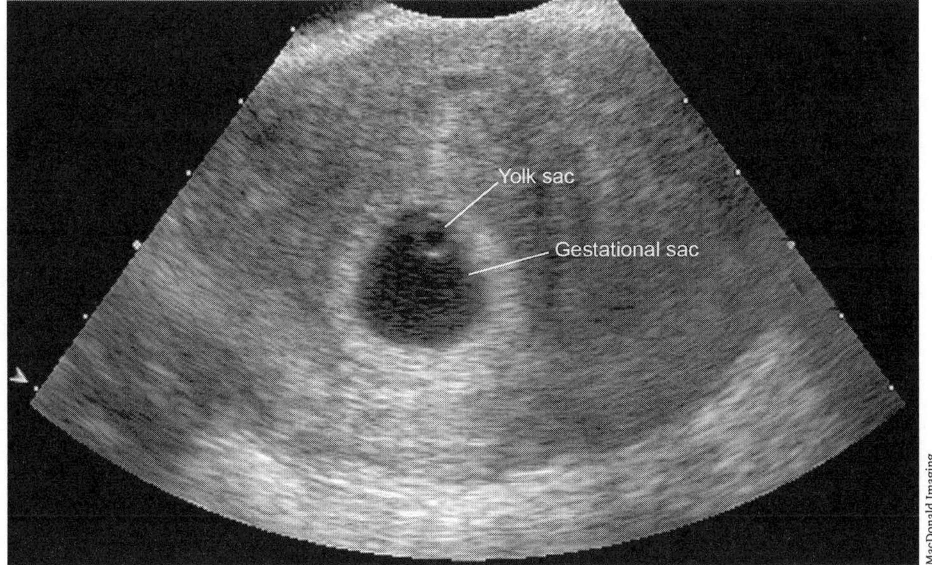

Ultrasound showing a gestational sac. Very early on, all you can see on ultrasound is the amniotic sac and possibly the yolk sac. The embryo is still too small to be visible.

days after conception (just one week after your missed period), your embryo's tiny heart is pumping blood. Although still too small to hear, the flickering of the heartbeat may be visible on ultrasound by your sixth week.

Pregnancy Week 6 (Embryo Day 22–28)

In week six, a head end and a tail end can be recognized as the embryo curls into a "C" shape. From head to bottom (also called crown to rump), your embryo measures about an eighth of an inch. Tiny buds form where the arms and legs will be. For amazing time-lapse embryo images of this development, check out http://embryo.soad.umich.edu/resources/morph.mov.

Pregnancy Week 7 (Embryo Day 29–35)

Sometime during week seven, your embryo's arms and legs grow, but they still look like little paddles. The eyes, ears, and nose start to develop, and the stomach, liver, and intestines begin to form. The brain now has the same three

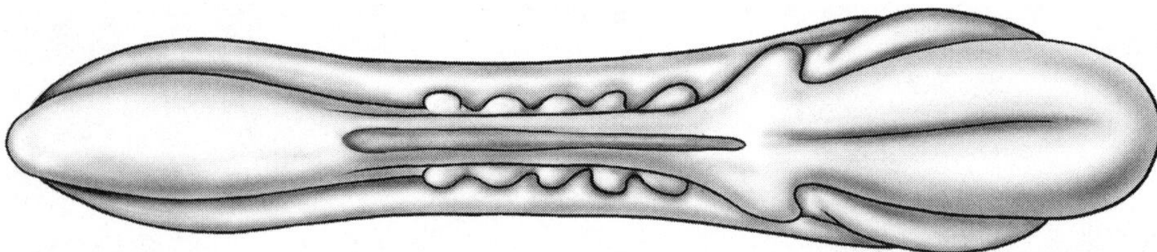

Pregnancy week 5. The tiny bumps on the back, called somites, are destined to become muscles, bones, and skin.

divisions—forebrain, midbrain, and hindbrain—as it does in an adult. Your baby-to-be measures about a quarter of an inch.

Pregnancy Week 8 (Embryo Day 36–42)

During week eight, when your embryo is about half an inch long, the fingers and toes start to form and nerves grow into the limbs; the kidneys are created; and the lens of the eye develops. The brain is rapidly enlarging.

> ***I had a book that went through fetal development week by week. It was really fun to think about. When the eyes were developing, I ate a lot of carrots. (Nancy G., lawyer)***

Pregnancy Week 9 (Embryo Day 43–49)

During week nine, at just three quarters of an inch, the embryo's eyelids cover the eyes, and the tip of the nose becomes more distinct. The upper lip and the inside of the mouth are formed. The arms and legs develop joints. In girls, the uterus and vagina form. In both sexes, the external genitals begin to develop, but haven't yet started down the path to male or female.

> ***The first time around, we sometimes thought about the size of the baby, you know, whether it had arms and legs yet, stuff like that. We would joke around, saying, this week it's the size of a pea . . . this week, a peanut. Later, my husband would say, now it's the size of a watermelon! (Heidi R., law professor)***

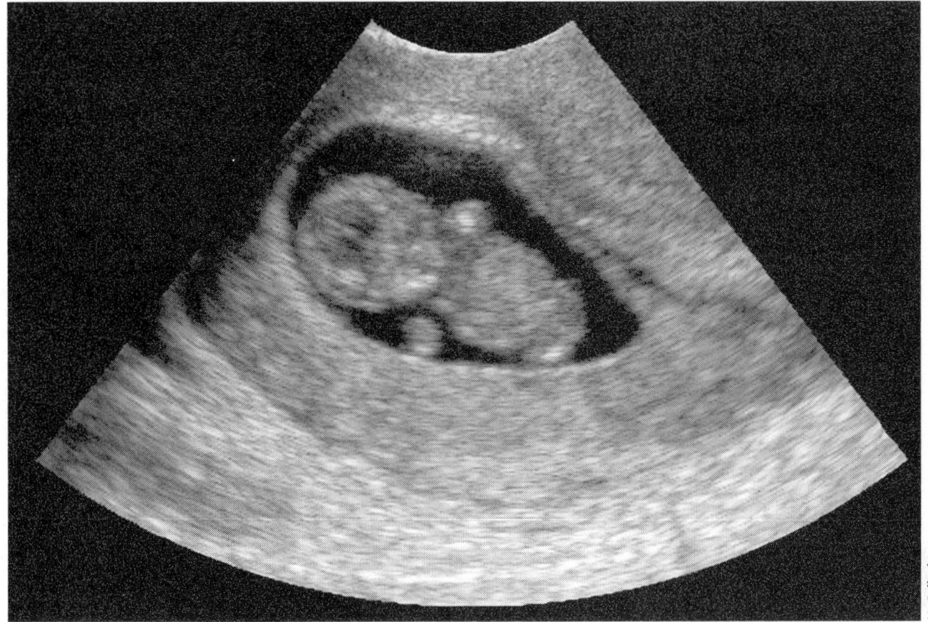

Ultrasound image of a nine-week embryo

Pregnancy week 10 (Embryo Day 50–56)

During week ten your little embryo starts to move its arms and legs. You won't feel these movements yet, but they may be seen on ultrasound. Testes and ovaries become different from each other and start to secrete hormones that will determine the appearance of the genitals. The umbilical cord is formed, and the incredible placenta, which brings the embryo its oxygen and nutrients, is functioning. By the end of this week, at just an inch and a quarter, all essential internal and external structures are present.

I would just go to Barnes and Noble once a week and hang out in the parenting/pregnancy section and read at least five or six different other

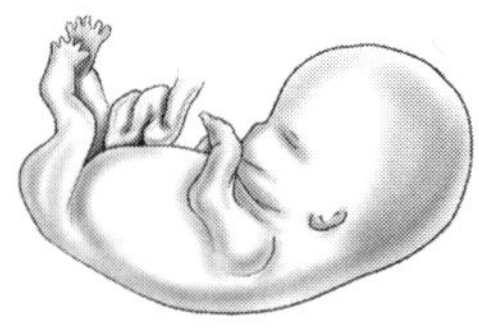

Life-sized drawing of a ten-week embryo

TWINS OR MORE

One of eighty pregnancies is twins. Twins arise either when two eggs are fertilized by two different sperm (fraternal twins) or when one fertilized egg splits before it starts to develop (identical twins). Since the tendency to release two eggs at once is genetic, fraternal twins run in families and are more likely in certain races and ethnicities. Women of African ancestry have the highest rate of spontaneous twins, and women of Asian descent, the lowest. Fertility drugs increase the odds of twinning by causing the release of more than one egg per cycle. Identical twins are random; every pregnancy has about a 1 in 240 chance of being identical twins, although for unknown reasons, identical twinning is also a bit more common in pregnancies conceived with IVF.

random books that would tell you either day by day or week by week how the baby was developing. I was just fascinated with how my baby was growing and changing. (Shani M., student)

Pregnancy Weeks 11–12

After ten weeks, your baby-to-be has graduated from the embryo stage and is considered a fetus. By week twelve, the rapid changes of embryonic life are complete: the face has a human profile, taste buds have developed, and genitals have male or female characteristics. Over the next months, the brain will continue to grow, the respiratory system will mature, the fetus will make its own hormones, the genitals will become more distinctly male or female, and the intestinal tract will begin to function.

How Are You Feeding Your Baby?

Your body supplies the oxygen and nutrients needed for your embryo's exponential growth. At first, when it is very tiny and buried within the uterine wall,

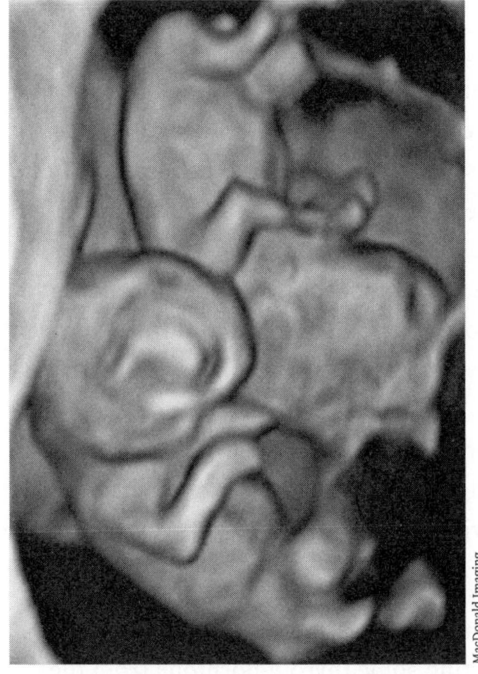

Three-dimensional ultrasound of first trimester twins

everything the embryo needs passes into it directly from your uterus. By the time the embryo is about an eighth of an inch long, a primitive circulatory system has developed to distribute nutrients and oxygen. Over the next few weeks, the outer layers of the fetal membranes organize into the placenta, which used to be called the afterbirth (because it comes out after the baby is born). The blood vessels in the placenta connect to the umbilical cord, which enters the baby through its belly button (umbilicus). The placenta and cord attach the baby to the inside of the uterus, to allow you to feed your baby.

The baby's heart pumps blood through the umbilical cord and into the placenta. Usually the cord has two arteries and a slightly larger vein, so that if you looked at it in cross-section on ultrasound the shape would look like Mickey Mouse's head. The placenta lies tightly against the inside wall of the uterus, and small pools of your blood bathe the placenta's cauliflower-like surface of tiny fetal blood vessels. The close contact of the fetal blood with that of its mother allows the exchange of oxygen, nutrients, and waste products.

The Placenta Isn't a Barrier

Although the purpose of the placenta is all good—to provide nutrition and oxygen and remove waste products—the placenta may allow other substances to pass from mother to infant. Medications, illicit drugs, alcohol, caffeine, cigarette toxins, chemicals, and germs may travel from mother to baby through the placenta. Hazardous exposures can lead to miscarriage, birth defects, or poor fetal growth, depending on the timing of the fetal contact and the type and amount of toxin. The greatest risks are while the organs are beginning to form—fourteen to thirty-five days after conception, or what we call the fifth through eighth gestational weeks.

Some medications are clearly dangerous during pregnancy, while others appear to be safe. The U.S. Food and Drug Administration (FDA) has historically placed all drugs into one of five categories of risk.

- Category A, the clearly safe group, includes thyroid hormone replacement, which is important if your natural thyroid levels are low (hypothyroid). The baby depends on getting some thyroid hormone from the mother at this early stage, and can suffer developmental delay and other problems if a mother with low thyroid function is not treated. Folic acid, another example of a category A medication, actually helps to prevent certain birth defects.
- All medications in class B and higher haven't been *proven* to be safe in studies on pregnant women. Some drugs are so commonly used, though, that their safety seems likely. Insulin for diabetes is in category B, but the benefits of taking it clearly outweigh any theoretical risks, and it should not be stopped during pregnancy.

The key to staying safe with medications during pregnancy is to talk to your doctor before you take any medicine—even over-the-counter drugs or herbal remedies. Your doctor will undoubtedly advise you to avoid taking unnecessary medications, particularly during the most sensitive time of organ development, weeks five through eight of pregnancy (three to five weeks after conception).

Other factors also may affect the developing fetus. Heat and X-rays, for example, don't pass through the placenta, but may have direct effects on the developing fetus.

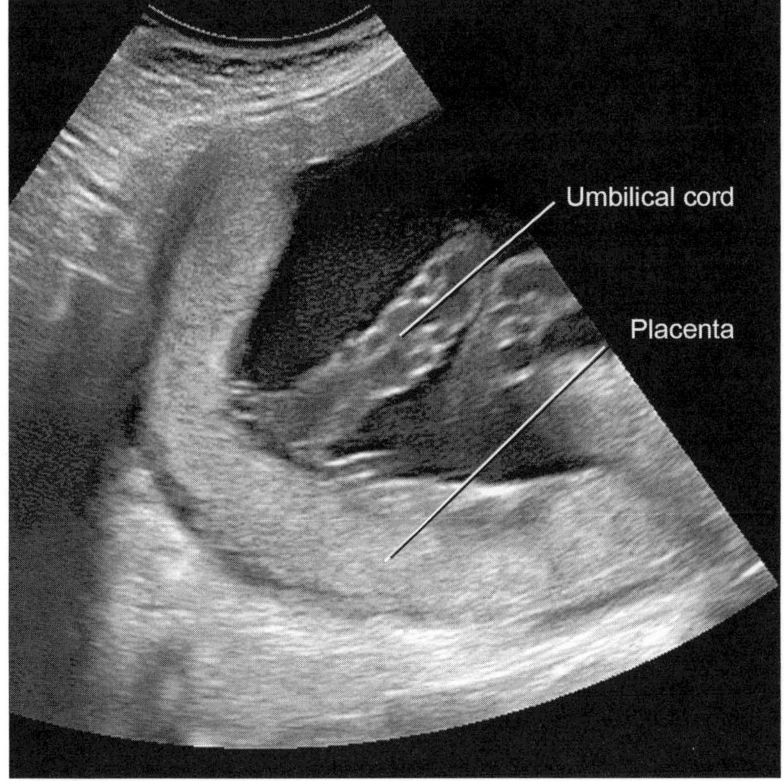

Ultrasound image of placenta and umbilical cord

When you're pregnant, reading about potential problems is always distressing. Although it is your job as the mom-to-be to try to limit dangers whenever possible, keep in mind that these risks are all statistical—contact increases the odds of a problem and protection from exposure diminishes them. About 3 percent of babies are born with some sort of anatomical variation, and 1 percent have a significant birth defect. You don't have total control over how your baby develops, and most babies come out fine, even with some accidental indiscretions on the part of the mother. The best advice is to recognize that many factors play into how your baby is developing: your job is to do your best to be a good mom, protecting your baby from risks that are within your control.

I was worried about the things that I did when I was pregnant but still didn't know. I was worried about that occasional glass of wine, but I realized

that a lot of people get pregnant and don't know until they're a couple of weeks into it. (Amanda O., meeting planner)

I was offered free drinks at a dinner when my period was one day late. I am usually very regular, so I thought I might be pregnant, but I hadn't run a pregnancy test. My friends were like: c'mon, free drinks! I think I had about four drinks that night, and then the positive test the next morning. That was it for alcohol for the next nine months. (Bonnie C., physician)

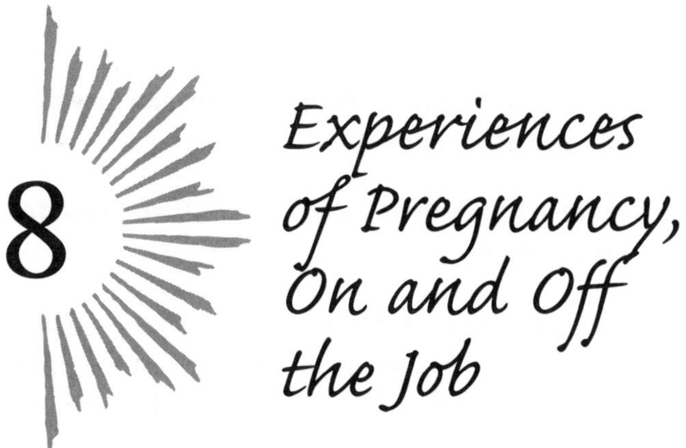

8 Experiences of Pregnancy, On and Off the Job

I don't want this to be one of those books that catalogs every possible pregnancy symptom. It seems unfair to make all newly pregnant moms worry about potential discomforts, when some mothers sail through the nine months feeling terrific. Yet if you are having a hard time, you deserve help. In this chapter, I will explain common, normal pregnancy problems and how to live and work with them, as well as help you determine whether your symptoms could be pointing to a more serious condition.

The symptoms they listed in the pregnancy books were gross and made me afraid. You feel vulnerable in your first pregnancy—reading about symptoms is too depressing. The best thing is to talk to moms and hear about the full variety of experiences. (Annie F., classical violinist)

Fatigue

Even though nausea and vomiting are the most famous signs of early pregnancy, tiredness is the most common one. For the first few months of pregnancy, let's just say that most women aren't as energetic as usual.

I was very tired the first few months; not able to work long hours. I had a one-hour commute and felt unsafe to drive home—too tired. During the first trimester I came home one to two hours earlier than normal, my husband made dinner, and then I fell asleep on the couch. (Heather H., real estate attorney)

During my first pregnancy, I was an intern in pediatrics. We were all very tired, and physically overwhelmed. I could not sort out how much of my

fatigue was due to the demands of my training program, and how much to my pregnancy. (Ilana S., pediatric resident)

I had no problem working in my first trimester. I wasn't that nauseated, just tired. (Karen D., veterinarian)

What can you do about fatigue? For the whole nine months, one good rule to live by is to listen to your body; your pregnancy will tell you what you need to do. If you are tired, you need to rest. But what if your life doesn't leave time to rest? The following list is based on advice from many moms-to-be:

- Accept less of yourself. You may not be able to get anything done in the evenings for a few weeks.
- Say no to extra work until you feel better. Postpone all nonessential extracurricular activities.
- Enlist the help of a few trusted coworkers to lighten your load and get you out earlier. You can do the same for them later.
- Decide which of your home or work responsibilities can be ignored or delegated. For example, if you normally cook dinner, have your partner take over the meal preparation, or eat take-out for a while so you can put your feet up after work.
- Try to figure out what time of day is best for you, and plan the most difficult work for then. For example, if you have energy in the morning but fade by 3:00, see if you can shift your work hours earlier, or bring some work home with you to do later in the evening, after a rest. Women who feel more capable in the morning might also try scheduling their toughest tasks for early in the day, so that their afternoons are less hectic. Sometimes, too, a ten-minute catnap at your desk will revive you.

  I used to put two chairs together in my office and take a nap for twenty minutes once or twice a day. Then I'd get up and eat a Power bar and get back to work. These power naps really refreshed me and made a huge difference in how I got through the day. Walking around helped too. (Kendra F., civil litigator)

  As a professor, I had a great deal of flexibility regarding where and when I worked. When I was feeling terrible in the morning, I didn't work. Instead,

I'd work later in the day when I felt better. Of course, this strategy only works on nonteaching days, but it's certainly better than what most women can manage at their jobs, I'm sure. (Heidi R., law professor)

- Go for a brisk walk when you feel sleepy.

I bought a very comfortable pair of shoes that I could wear for work and also out for walks at lunchtime. (Elizabeth S., online producer)

- Many women find that if they can drag themselves to exercise, it paradoxically improves their energy level. Although forty minutes a day is a good goal, ten minutes of exercise three or four times during the day may be easier to fit into your schedule. Even a little bit may help.

Exercise as much as possible. It helps you feel better, sleep better, and recover faster. It doesn't matter what you do, just move. (Mary Ellen M., pediatric nurse)

- Have a light snack or some herbal tea when you need a few minutes' break. Some women find that a high protein snack like an energy or breakfast bar works best.
- If financially feasible, use money to make your life easier. Pay someone to clean your house, buy prepared foods, or take a cab instead of public transportation.
- Go to sleep early.
- If all else fails, try to reassure yourself that you will feel better in a few weeks.

Nausea

In books and movies, throwing up is often the first sign that a character is expecting. In real life, 70–85 percent of women have some nausea during pregnancy and 50 percent get sick. Although nausea and vomiting during pregnancy are very unpleasant, they generally don't do you or your baby any harm. Nausea is actually a sign you have good levels of pregnancy hormones and are unlikely to miscarry. As long as you can keep down liquids, you don't need to worry (although you still might want help finding ways to cope).

In the first trimester I didn't throw up but I felt queasy—like the afternoon after a bad morning hangover. It was actually shocking how similar the feeling was. I could function fine; it was just uncomfortable, not debilitating. (Kendra F., civil litigator)

Early on I threw up every day—mostly in the evenings. I had a lot of events to attend in the evenings, so I always had to check ahead for acceptable bathrooms. (Jane S., state governor)

Nausea on the air . . . I always kept a garbage can just off camera . . . and I used it during commercials. (Eileen M., weather reporter)

Nausea and vomiting, like most other symptoms, are best treated in a step-wise fashion, starting with the safest nonmedical treatments and resorting to medications if necessary. Once you become dehydrated, though, the condition can escalate, with increasing nausea leading to worse dehydration, leading to more vomiting, and so on. If you think you are going down this path, call your doctor or midwife right away. Sometimes heading off this spiral can save you a few days in the hospital.

AVOID TRIGGERS

- Try to avoid smells that will set you off.
- Some women find that it is easier to eat out than to prepare food at home because cooking makes them sick. Others do best packing lunch for work.
- If your prenatal vitamin makes you sick, take your vitamin during the time of day that you feel best, or talk to your practitioner about just using folic acid or children's chewable vitamins until you feel better.

I made my husband move the rice cooker to the garage. To this day the smell of cooking rice makes me gag. (Margaret M., physician)

For four Saturdays in a row, before finding out I was pregnant, I suddenly found myself dizzy and nauseated every time I would walk through the door to the restaurant. I would be sick and miserable for my whole shift. After finding out the great news of my pregnancy it all made complete

sense. Unfortunately I had to give up my moonlighting. (Jill Ann S., administrative assistant and part-time waitress)

WATCH YOUR DIET

- Eat bland dry foods, multiple times a day.
- Eat crackers (or whatever works) before you get out of bed in the morning.
- Some people do best with high-protein foods, others with starches.
- Drink liquids separately from when you try to eat.
- Keep crackers, or whatever works for you, within reach at all times.

Most women feel worse on an empty stomach—watch the clock if you must, to be sure that you are eating small meals every few hours. Some moms recommend never getting too full or too hungry. Bring snacks to long meetings and when traveling.

Eat light snacks throughout your workday; it keeps you from feeling full and getting more tired. (Mary Ellen M., pediatric nurse)

Keep granola bars in your desk. (Brenda W., lawyer)

I drank a lot of Sprite when I was first pregnant; that helped a lot. (Zoe B., inventory manager)

I used to be able to concentrate at work so intently that I would often miss lunch. Well, when I became pregnant with my first child—I swear I had also been impregnated with my husband's appetite! Every day at twelve sharp I would stand up and stay "I have to eat, NOW!" and practically drag my friend away from her computer to go to lunch with me. As long as I ate with some regularity, I didn't feel queasy. Morning sickness (the ultimate misnomer) is not limited to the mornings. (Ann M., research scientist)

For nausea, ginger hard candies, fresh lemon, or lemonade. An aide would carry a cup of freshly cut lemons (this sounds weird, I know) for me to lick and it would make me feel better. I always carried a toothbrush. (Jane S., state governor)

OTHER HELPFUL IDEAS FOR RELIEVING NAUSEA

- Acupressure bands. Some women find that the elastic wristbands sold for seasickness help with pregnancy nausea. These can be purchased in travel stores, some maternity stores, and over the Internet under the brand name Sea Bands.
- Ginger. Many moms find that ginger, in the form of fresh ginger, ginger ale, ginger tea, or ginger tablets, relieves nausea. The natural forms are preferable because tablets may contain lead or other contaminants.
- Over-the-counter medications. Ten milligrams of vitamin B6 in combination with ten milligrams of an antihistamine called doxylamine was marketed in the United States for many years under the brand name Bendectin. Two tablets (totaling 20 milligrams of each component) were prescribed at bedtime, plus one or two more during the day if necessary. This combination made mothers-to-be a little sleepy, but was proven safe and very effective for nausea and vomiting in pregnancy. Despite its safety, the cost of defending lawsuits closed down U.S. distribution. The same formulation can be purchased in Canada as Diclectin, or can be created by taking vitamin B6 with Unisom, an over-the-counter sleep medication containing doxylamine. Ask your doctor or midwife if this approach would be useful and safe for you.
- Prescription medications. Remember that you and your baby need calories and fluids, so in some cases taking medications poses less risk than avoiding them. If your vomiting is severe, or if your nausea is so bad that you aren't eating, talk to your doctor or midwife about the pros and cons of prescription treatment.

In my first pregnancy I avoided medications for nausea but in the second pregnancy I took them—it was just harder with my schedule and with a toddler at home. (Jane S., state governor)

In my first pregnancy I was sick for two weeks, and it got so bad I had to go into the hospital because I was dehydrated. I got some medicine to help with the vomiting. For my second pregnancy we were able to get on top of the nausea and vomiting sooner so it wasn't as much of a problem. (Stephanie B., FedEx courier)

- Seek help early. Avoid the cycle of dehydration and vomiting. If the vomiting gets so severe that you aren't keeping down fluids, or if you are losing weight, your doctor or midwife will need to see you to decide what to do. Rarely (about 1 percent of the time) vomiting gets so severe that it becomes a danger to mom and baby. (This condition, called hyperemesis gravidarum, requires treatment with medications and sometimes hospitalization.) Generally speaking, the nausea and vomiting of pregnancy peak around nine weeks and then taper off by fourteen to sixteen weeks or so. Most pregnant women feel much better in the second trimester. And no matter how bad you may have it, try to remember that it is for a good cause.

HIDING PREGNANCY SYMPTOMS AT WORK

To be less conspicuous at work:

- Combine trips to the bathroom with other reasons for getting up, such as making copies or putting something in the mail.
- If you are vomiting a lot, try to arrange to do some work at home until you feel better.
- Plan a vacation in your eighth or ninth week, when nausea is often at its peak.
- Sit next to the door at meetings so you can escape more easily when you need to.
- Always have a change of clothing and mouthwash with you.

It was very hard early on when I was rushing off to the bathroom hoping to have it to myself, and not getting as much of my workload done as I had in the past. I was nervous that someone would pick up on my symptoms and ask if I was pregnant before I was ready to tell, and I'm not sure what I would have told them if it had happened. Confiding in one colleague early on was a big relief. (Ellen B., communications manager)

The time when I most needed time off was unfortunately in the first trimester, when I was so tired (catatonic by 1 PM) that I was not very productive. I say unfortunately because of course then it's too early to

EARLY PREGNANCY RELIEF KIT

Consider these items for your briefcase or bag:

- Ginger ale, ginger snaps, or ginger tea
- Saltine crackers or dry cold cereal
- Protein bars and other healthful snacks
- Hard candies (sour flavors or ginger work best)
- Water (freeze half a bottle if you like it cold)
- Sea Bands
- Mylanta or Maalox liquid antacid (more effective than chewables)
- Tylenol
- Wet wipes
- Tissues
- Toothbrush/mouthwash
- Deodorant
- Washcloth for cleaning up or for cooling your face or neck
- Change of clothing
- Plastic bags (for soiled clothes and for use in the car)
- Panty liners or sanitary pads
- Small portable fan
- Comfortable shoes—at least for the trip to and from work
- Doctor's phone number—you can program it into your phone, too
- Insurance information

tell people at work. I had to pretend I had the flu, but if I had known how tired I was going to be I probably would have taken a few weeks off as vacation time (it was my first pregnancy). (Rebecca B., journalist)

The problem with being pregnant at work, especially if you haven't told, is that you're going to the bathroom all the time. I was sneaking to the bathroom all day long. I actually met some really nice coworkers that I hadn't met before. (Peggy L., nurse-administrator)

It can be difficult if you want to keep the pregnancy private at first. Have a plan if someone asks you directly before you feel ready to tell. (Jane S., state governor)

Students pay a little too much attention to what their professors wear. When I was in the early days of my second pregnancy, just when the waist starts to disappear, a student waited for me quietly after class. She said, "Uh, Professor, I drew the short straw and have to be the one to ask you . . . are you pregnant? I mean, we've noticed that you're wearing looser clothes this week." Good grief!!! (Heidi R., law professor)

First Trimester Bleeding

About one in four women has some bleeding before twelve weeks. Technically, any bleeding in the first trimester is defined as a threatened miscarriage. About half of the moms with early bleeding go on to miscarry, and the other half continue on. This may sound cold, but it's important to realize that once first trimester bleeding has started, the outcome of the pregnancy is already determined—and nothing you do, not bed rest, not medications, not any other treatment you can think of, is going to sustain a pregnancy that is destined to miscarry.

We started telling friends after we had an ultrasound that showed everything was okay. I had some spotting early on so we wanted to be sure before we shared with a lot of people. (Christi M., medical student)

My husband came into the lab waving the pregnancy test as soon as it was positive; unfortunately then the miscarriage happened and I had to tell everyone that I was no longer pregnant. This actually turned out to be a good thing; three-quarters of the women had had a miscarriage, and I never knew. I ended up getting such wonderful support from all of the women who shared their experiences. (Juanita G., research scientist)

Bleeding in early pregnancy requires what we euphemistically call "pelvic rest," which really means don't put anything in your vagina—no douching, no tampons, and no intercourse. The purpose of pelvic rest is to avoid introducing germs into the uterus, which could cause a serious infection with loss of the pregnancy.

Anxiety is a miserable feeling, and not knowing the outcome of your pregnancy can be immensely distressing. As much as it may feel like an emergency because you want an answer *now*, the answer won't change the course of events (and may not even be ascertainable yet). A trip to the emergency room is not warranted for a small amount of early pregnancy bleeding in the absence of pain or fever. Instead, call your midwife or doctor the next day so you can get set up for an evaluation, which hopefully will give you the reassurance you are seeking.

I was eight weeks pregnant on vacation in Hawaii and started bleeding. You aren't supposed to use tampons, so I was using pads. I couldn't go in the water because, in addition to everything else, I was worried about attracting sharks. (Maggie P., administrator)

If at any point in your pregnancy you experience severe pain, bleeding heavier than a period, or unexplained fever, seek immediate medical attention. Pain can indicate an ectopic (tubal) pregnancy, and heavy bleeding can lead to excessive blood loss. Fever may indicate infection. All of these complications can become medical emergencies. Ultrasound, physical examination, and blood tests will usually clarify the situation.

Emotions

Most mothers-to-be are very excited to be pregnant. You may find yourself daydreaming about the baby . . . for hours. You may want to spend your work day on the Internet reading articles about pregnancy or stories about new families, or ordering maternity clothes and baby supplies. It can be hard to focus on work.

Dreams during pregnancy are often vivid. A dream journal can be fun to refer back to later on, once you have met the little one who was driving these nighttime travels.

I felt totally normal, except I was distracted thinking about the baby and just felt like going to baby sites on the Internet. (Naomi B., attorney)

Mixed feelings are also quite common in early pregnancy. Even happy, financially secure couples with planned and desired pregnancies can feel dread, anxiety, and ambivalence. Families with money trouble, relationship issues, or work stress may be overwhelmed at the thought of what's to come. Pregnancy and parenting young children affect your personal relationships and your work life. Some negative feelings are normal, and don't harm your growing baby.

There was always a lot of fear in my pregnancy because of that first miscarriage. (Cheryl L., lawyer)

With Layla, we didn't really plan, but we weren't using protection. Will wasn't working, and we were really broke. I was very stressed out. There were many days when I would just cry, thinking about us being homeless. I was constantly worried. (Uwimana W., real estate assistant)

Talking to friends and family can often help you to understand your intense feelings. If you are suffering emotionally or not functioning in your daily life, talk to your doctor or midwife, who can guide you to some professional help. If you are just surprised by this experience, the best advice is to notice and accept what you are feeling, and realize that strong emotions and swings in your mood are normal at this time. After all, you are growing a whole new person inside of you—someone who will affect your life forever.

Don't worry about all of the bad stuff. The second you hold that baby in your arms you forget about all of the aches, pains, nausea and vomiting, and having to go to the bathroom all the time. (Stephanie B., FedEx courier)

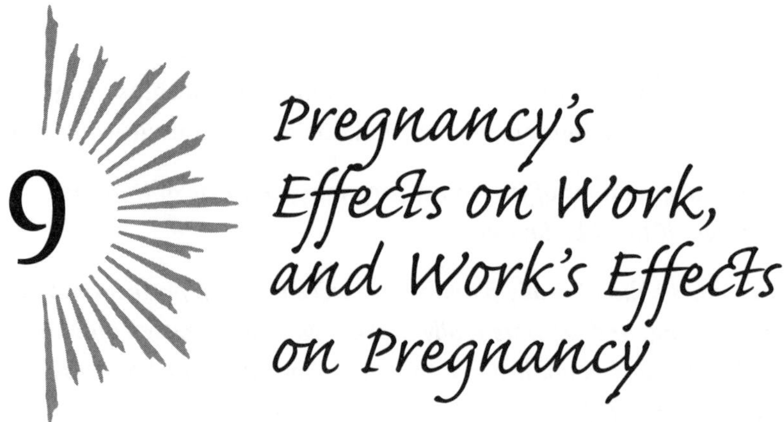

9 Pregnancy's Effects on Work, and Work's Effects on Pregnancy

Some women progress happily through pregnancy, working as if nothing has changed. Others feel differently about their jobs or find that their ability to work is affected by being pregnant. Baby fantasies may encroach on your time, feeling poorly may temporarily affect your day-to-day performance, or you may worry that stress or some other aspect of your job will have a negative effect on the baby. On the other side, employers often believe that pregnancy is an indication that your priorities lie elsewhere. They worry about how your work will get done, and whether you will come back after the baby is born.

> ***Frankly, I had greater concerns over my ability to keep my job than concerns over delivering my child into the world. (Jane J., advertising executive)***

> ***You deserve to be treated seriously at work even if you are pregnant, and you should expect it. But, you need to believe that in your own mind or it will not happen. Women tend to undervalue themselves. (Jenny K., internist)***

> ***At one point my whole office went on a three-day retreat and I spent the time in my hotel room being green and trying to hide it. Everyone thought I was a bit of a stick-in-the-mud because I wasn't hanging out having drinks in the evenings. But once they found out I was pregnant, everyone was supportive and considerate. I felt less like I had to "prove myself" than I did at my previous job, simply because the place was more family-friendly and had more women. (Janet G., attorney)***

Having children is acceptable, even expected, in many careers, especially in traditionally female jobs like teaching and nursing, where women have a track record of balancing career and family. Other jobs have never had a pregnant employee, and haven't established maternity policies—or positive attitudes. No matter which type of situation you are in, it is likely that you, your employer, and your coworkers will have some concerns about how this pregnancy will affect your attendance, your productivity, and your long-term plans. You may also worry about how the job will affect you and your baby.

When Should I Tell My Boss?

Many women wait a while before telling people at work that they are pregnant. In deciding when and how to share the news, mothers-to-be typically take several factors into account:

- Privacy, specifically in case of miscarriage
- Honesty, particularly if someone asks you directly
- Having your bosses hear it from you before someone else tells them
- Safety, if accommodations must be made early on to avoid occupational risk
- Ability to hide it, if you are vomiting at work or otherwise showing signs of pregnancy
- Concerns that you will get less respect once you disclose you are pregnant
- Timing, if you are up for promotion or a special assignment

On the side of disclosure, support from colleagues can be valuable if you are suffering with early pregnancy symptoms, so it can sometimes be advantageous to share your news before you'd planned.

I called my boss right after I took the test and it was positive. I think the earlier you tell, the better. It's good to be honest. (Annette M., store manager)

Disclosing pregnancy in the workplace early on was mutually beneficial. Not having the burden of hiding it made for a healthier, happier pregnancy, and work administrators and colleagues could plan well in advance for my maternity leave. (Anne C., radiologist)

I told my boss at seven weeks because I was so exhausted I was leaving work hours earlier than I used to. It was obvious I wasn't accomplishing as much,

plus I was showing already. Also, I work for a small firm and word travels, and I wanted my bosses to find out from me, not from rumors. They were more sympathetic and flexible once they knew. (Heather H., real estate attorney)

I told my boss I was pregnant at eight weeks—earlier than the end-of-first-trimester they usually recommend. It didn't affect my job—my boss essentially said, "You look fine—here's your work." My job didn't slow down. (Naomi B., attorney)

I wasn't going to tell until I was showing, but Hurricane Charley was coming. I told them I was pregnant because I didn't want to put myself in harm's way. It was a little awkward, but my maternal instincts kicked in and I felt at peace with it. (Monique F., journalist)

No matter what, hide it as long as you can, because after you tell, that's all you are, the pregnant employee. I kept buying bigger and bigger clothes to cover it up. Just larger sizes, not maternity clothes right away . . . because once you start wearing maternity clothes everyone knows you are pregnant. I saved these larger clothes and used them after I delivered, before I lost my weight. (Peggy L., nurse-administrator)

The second time, I began to show right at three months. My belly just kind of popped out one weekend. With the first pregnancy, I had the luxury of waiting to tell people. (Elizabeth S., online producer)

Many women worry that they will be seen as less productive once they disclose that they're expecting. Although some find that pregnancy really slows them down, most mothers-to-be are able to keep at their usual pace, with only minimal accommodations. Remember the 80/20 rule: 20 percent of your effort leads to 80 percent of your productivity. The keys to excellent work performance during pregnancy are luck, in that you aren't hit too hard by nausea or fatigue, and efficiency—finding a way to get your work done despite distractions or discomforts.

Even though I was tired, my work habits were still the same. I worked forty hours per week or more. One week I worked fifty-seven hours. I am just a workaholic. (Annette M., store manager)

I was a little more forgetful than usual—it felt a lot like right before my wedding when I had a lot on my mind—I made lists to stay organized. (Susan G., commercial airline pilot)

Efficiency

Many pregnant and parenting women have told me that being well organized allowed them to keep up even when their lives slowed them down. The suggestions that follow come from a variety of sources—feel free to use what works; you will find your own solutions as you go.

- Make to-do lists. At the end of each day at work, take a few minutes to plan your priorities for the next morning, so you can get right to work.
- Do you hardest jobs when you first get in—or when you are likely to be feeling your best.
- Divide big jobs up into smaller, doable, less overwhelming tasks.
- Prioritize tasks into A, the big important stuff that needs a block of time, through C, the mindless things that you can do when you are working on fewer cylinders.
- Do your "C" tasks at the end of the day or in the waiting room at your OB's office.
- Protect yourself from interruptions. Deal with calls and email in batches, so they don't disrupt productive blocks of time.
- Try to pare down your responsibilities. Say no to extra work until you see how you are doing with the basics.
- Try to touch each piece of paper (at work and at home) only once. Open mail when you have time to read it, open bills when you are ready to pay them. Don't read email or look at phone messages until you have time to deal with them.
- If possible, pay for help at home, or renegotiate the distribution of jobs with your partner. You are the one growing the baby—other tasks may need to be handled by someone else if you are too tired or ill.
- Make copies of a shopping list template with common items in order of the aisles at your grocery store. Circle what you need; when you go shopping you'll remember everything and you won't have to backtrack.

- Lay out your clothes the night before, so you don't have to think when you are getting up and out.
- Schedule exercise and time for yourself into your routine.

A few times, people attributed my forgetting something to the pregnancy and that really bothered me. I was quick to point out that I did not like that, and that my pregnancy didn't make me crazy—just pregnant. (Jane J., advertising executive)

I'm easily distracted normally, but between pregnancy spaciness and being sick, I really feel like I'm not pulling my weight, and that really distresses me, but all I can do is try to do my best each day. (Ellen B., communications manager)

I had a very easy pregnancy. I never was really sick. The only thing I really had to do was adjust to accommodate all of the doctors' visits, so I did have to change my schedule for that. (Amanda O., meeting planner)

In the first trimester, buy a couple of pairs of pants one or two sizes larger than you normally wear. They'll fit well when your normal pants get too tight and yet you feel like a fraud in maternity pants. (Ellen B., communications manager)

Clothing was a big issue for me while I was pregnant and working. It seemed so ridiculous to spend a lot of money, however I had to look presentable. One thing I would encourage is to borrow clothing from friends who have been pregnant, or even women larger than yourself. I borrowed a lot of jacket-type things from my mom who wears things big. (Elizabeth S., online producer)

How Will Working Affect Your Pregnancy?

We have been talking about how pregnancy affects work, but certain aspects of work may complicate your pregnancy as well. Before you start to worry, realize that overall, working women experience a *lower* rate of pregnancy complications than other women do. Compared to those without jobs, women who work have better health habits such as lower rates of smoking and better prenatal care. Most women work in technical, sales, and administrative positions,

YOUR EARLY PREGNANCY WORK WARDROBE

At first, your looser clothing may still fit fine. Eventually, though, the time will come when you're not yet ready for maternity wear, but your clothes don't quite make it around your waist (or breasts) anymore. When this happens to you, try these solutions from experienced moms:

- Buy some larger, soft, loose-fitting clothes. These also will come in handy right after the baby is born, when you aren't quite back to your old shape.
- Borrow clothing from someone a little bigger than you are—male or female.
- Use a rubber band doubled-up through the buttonhole to extend the reach of the top button on your pants, or leave it open and wear a top that covers your waistline.
- If you wear a uniform at work, move into larger sizes before hitting the maternity versions.

types of jobs that don't cause pregnancy problems. Work that only involves normal sorts of activities can usually be continued until labor, provided the mother-to-be is healthy and feeling relatively well.

Three kinds of problems may require changes in the workplace, or temporary leave:

1. Common pregnancy symptoms, like nausea and vomiting, may make certain jobs (like foodservice work) impossible.
2. Pregnancy complications, such as preterm labor, sometimes require time off or special accommodations at work. These sorts of problems don't usually begin until the third trimester, and will be discussed later.
3. Jobs with intense physical demands, long hours, toxic exposures, infection risk, distant travel, and emotional stress may require adaptations to safely accommodate the pregnancy. The Occupational Safety and Health Act states that your employer is responsible for maintaining a safe work environment.

Common Questions—and Answers—about Labor Laws and Pregnancy

- Can my employer require me to go out on disability for safety reasons? If you can do your job and want to work, your employer is not allowed to require you to take time off. The law allows you to choose to work if the risks are acceptable to you.
- What if I don't feel safe in my work environment? Your employer is responsible for maintaining a safe workplace. If you feel unsafe, you can ask for light duty or reassignment to a safer situation. If arrangements are made for other disabled workers, they must be available to women "disabled" by pregnancy. If no light-duty option exists, you may need to go onto disability, but your employer may require a note from your physician before accommodating your needs.

The remainder of this chapter will address aspects of work that may negatively affect pregnancy, and what you, your doctor, and your employer can do to minimize risk. If your job only requires activities that are normally part of daily life, with no special risks to pregnancy, this information is not necessary for you. Feel free to skip on to more relevant sections.

My job is to provide and maintain phone service for our customers. I have to put the ladder up there, slap on the hard hat, the belt, the safety vest, and climb the pole. You have to be cautious, obviously, doing that job. I had already had a two-year-old, so I had been through the whole thing. I waited until four months to tell them I was pregnant. I knew I didn't have to work if I told them, but I didn't want the disability and half pay to start too soon. (Heather M., telephone service technician)

Physical Demands

- Risk of abdominal trauma. Once your uterus has grown so that it is above the protection of the pelvic bones (about twelve weeks), blunt trauma to your abdomen can cause the placenta to separate from the uterine wall, a process called placental abruption, which can lead to miscarriage, preterm labor, or stillbirth. Jobs that may incur abdominal trauma, such as law enforcement work, should be modified. Most police officers obtain light-duty assignments when they find out they are pregnant. Special education teachers, psychiatric nurses, and other personnel who work with unruly individuals may need to make arrangements to avoid abdominal trauma during pregnancy. Contact sports, and jobs that may involve falling or colliding with another person, should also be modified or abandoned during pregnancy.

I was thirteen days pregnant when I found out! When work found out they took me off the road immediately. I was a Field Training Officer and at the time had a rookie with me. I didn't want any harm to my baby, and I think the guys didn't want me out there, either. They switched me to a different job. I had plenty of work to do with the dispatching, and we did a field-training manual. (Tracy G., police officer)

- Heavy lifting. Occasional heavy lifting doesn't pose a risk to the pregnancy, although it's easy to hurt your back. Most women who have physically demanding jobs deliver healthy babies, but repeated lifting of more than about twenty pounds may increase the chance of preterm labor, poor fetal growth, and high blood pressure. Factory jobs with repetitive lifting combined with twisting seem to pose the greatest risk. If your job is very physical, try to modify your activities to avoid repeatedly lifting heavy objects, and use good mechanics when you lift. When possible, explore other options, such as making multiple trips with lighter loads, using a cart or case on wheels, or asking for help.
- Standing. Most women who are on their feet all day have uncomplicated pregnancies, but jobs that require standing more than three hours a shift may increase the likelihood of preterm birth, poor fetal growth and, in late pregnancy, high blood pressure. When possible, modify your job so you are sitting instead of standing, and take frequent breaks. If you are already at risk for complications, or if problems develop during pregnancy, talk to your doctor or midwife. Job modifications or disability leave may become necessary.

I assemble car seats for children. This requires standing for eight hours and a little lifting. I tolerated it well while I was pregnant. I started light

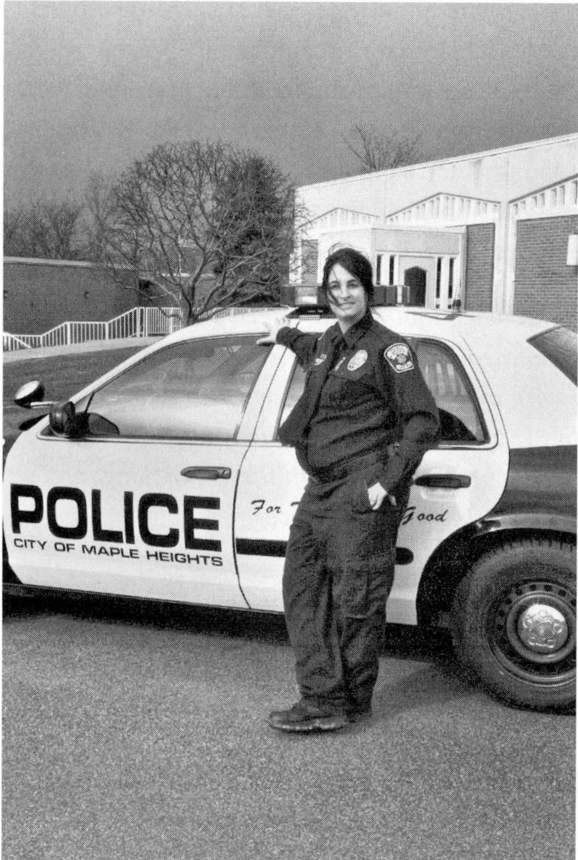

LeRoy Dierker, MD

duty at five months. I would work on the line at times, but usually I would put together things while sitting. I worked from 3 to 11 PM six days a week. (Mihsah B., factory worker)

- Physical activity. Exercise in pregnancy is good for you, shortening labor and actually lowering the risk of premature birth. But exercising more than one to two hours a day, and any exercise at high altitude, may compromise the circulation to your baby and should be avoided. Talk to your doctor or midwife for individualized recommendations.
- Noise. Federal workplace standards allow up to two hours of work a day at one hundred decibels and up to eight hours at ninety decibels. How loud are decibels? A lawn mower at eighty decibels sounds about twice

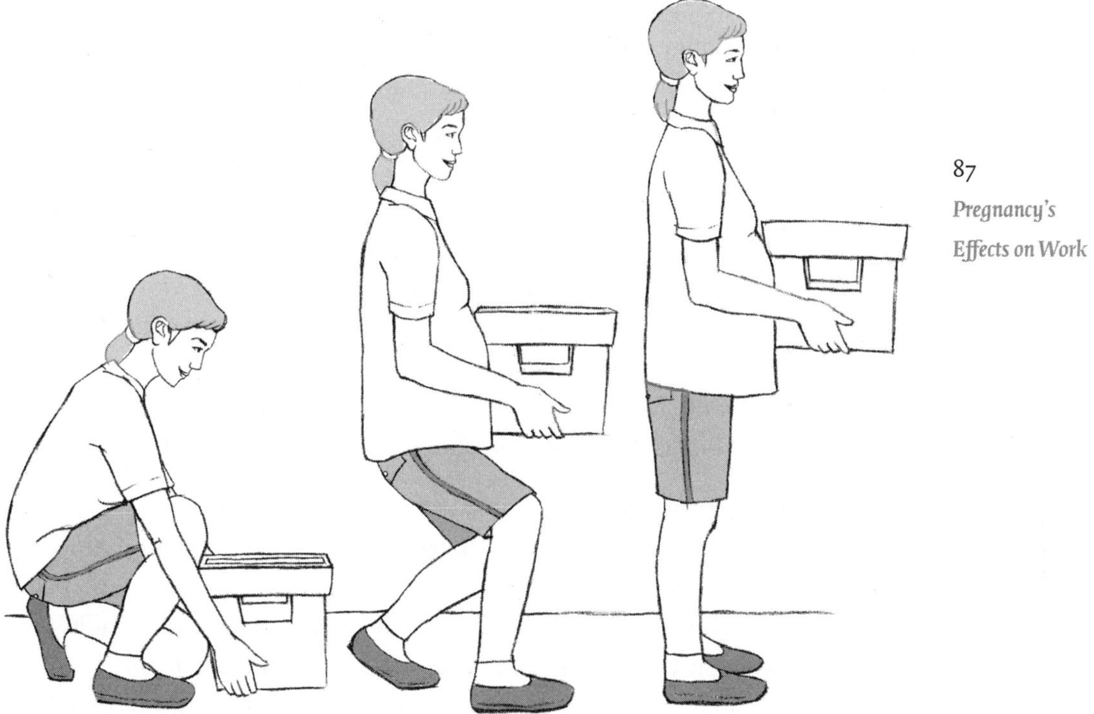

To lift safely, hold the load as close to your body as you can, lift up your head and shoulders, and then use your legs to lift.

as loud as a hairdryer at seventy decibels. Some children of mothers who were exposed to loud noise in pregnancy were found to have high-frequency hearing loss, which makes sense: earplugs worn by the mother would not be expected to dampen the sound that reaches the fetus. Severe noise exposure may also be related to a slight increase in the chance of birth defects.

- Heat. Although hot tubs, saunas, and fever all pose some risk to the fetus, working in a warm environment seems to be safe. It may be particularly unpleasant in pregnancy, though, when you tend to feel warm all the time anyway. Women who work in the heat, for instance in a commercial kitchen, should drink plenty of fluids and dress lightly. A fan or misting spray may help as well.
- Long hours. Research on resident physicians, who often worked from eighty to over one hundred hours a week, showed a rise in preterm labor

requiring treatment, but no increase in actual preterm birth. Poor fetal growth and high blood pressure were also more frequent. For doctors who worked fewer than eighty hours per week, though, the pregnancy outcomes were no worse than for women with more normal working hours. Research on work between forty and eighty hours a week is conflicting, and poor outcomes are more likely tied to fatigue (see later) than to the number of hours logged.

- Night shifts and swing shifts. While most mothers-to-be who work nights or swing shifts do fine, preterm birth is slightly more likely for these women, especially for those who are very tired.
- Fatigue. Severe fatigue in any job is associated with a greater chance of premature birth and a higher likelihood of cesarean delivery.

The bottom line: the working women who have the best pregnancy outcomes have workdays filled with a variety of physical activities—walking, sitting, and standing—and are not exhausted. Although most women have full-term babies regardless of their activity level, doing one thing repetitively, be it standing, sitting, or working on an assembly line, leads to a slightly increased chance of premature birth compared with women who can vary their activities. Try to negotiate with your employer to so that you can alter your position, avoid repetitive heavy lifting, and take breaks when needed. If you are concerned about job-related risks, talk to your doctor or midwife about your options.

Occupational Exposures

- Radiation. Research on radiation exposure in pregnancy, done in Hiroshima and Nagasaki, Japan, after the nuclear bombs, didn't show a problem for fetuses exposed to less than 5 rads (sometimes referred to as 5 rem or 50 milligray). OSHA limits job-related radiation exposure for any employee to under 5 rads a year, and during pregnancy, to 0.5 rads total. If proper procedures are followed when working with radiation, both mother and baby should be safe.

I discussed radioactive exposures with my doctor; I stopped doing many of these experiments while pregnant. It just seemed like common sense to not expose myself to that. (Juanita G., research scientist)

COMPUTER TERMINALS

Years ago, a rumor went around that computer monitors (video display terminals, or VDTs) emitted radiation that was dangerous for pregnant moms. Since that time, however, research has shown that the glass screen absorbs the small amount of radiation produced by the VDT; we now know that exposure to computer monitors during pregnancy is not associated with any increased risks.

- Chemicals. Toxins can enter the body via the lungs, by skin absorption, or through your digestive system. (The table in Appendix B provides information on some of the chemicals commonly found in the workplace.) Your employer is required by law to give you a list of all potentially toxic substances to which you might be exposed. Often, little is known about specific effects. In research on occupational risks, the worst pregnancy outcomes were in mothers who felt dizzy or had headaches from chemical inhalation. Avoid getting chemicals into your system by wearing protective gear and following safety precautions.
- Infections. Your best protection against infection is good hand washing. Healthcare workers are generally well-informed on this topic, but others who care for children or who have physical contact with many people should be just as careful. Antibacterial hand lotions and gels are practical, and safe to use in pregnancy. For details on specific infections, see Appendix B.

I was debating when to tell my principal that I was pregnant. Out of respect I planned to let him know before others found out. My debate was over one Monday morning when a parent came in with her son and announced that he had been sick over the weekend with a "rash from his head to his toes." I immediately went down to the office and told the principal the story, ending it with ". . . and I'm pregnant and prefer to not have him in my classroom today." That certainly wasn't the way I

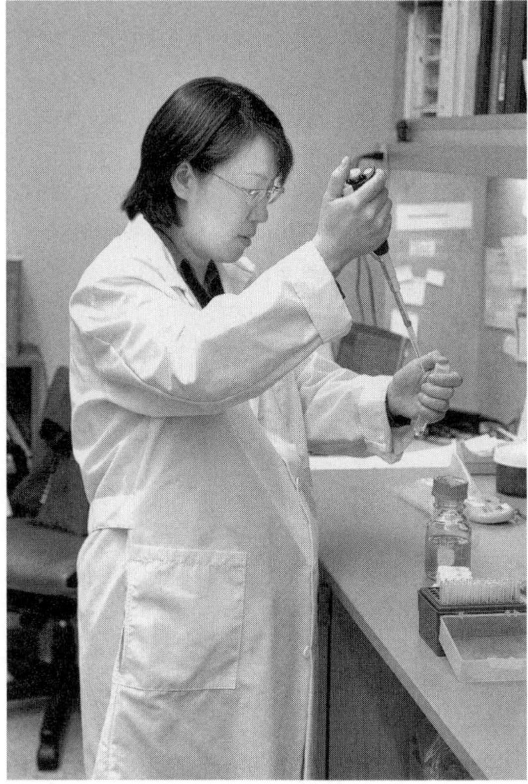
LeRoy Dierker, MD

had imagined breaking the news to him, but I knew that pregnancy and rashes don't mix. (Norma J., teacher) [Note from author: rashes may indicate infections such as chicken pox or fifth disease.]

Hobbies

Although it's great to have outside interests, some hobbies and projects may prove toxic.

- Pottery and jewelry-making can expose you to lead or other metals; furniture stripping exposes you to solvents. Get information and follow safety precautions, including always working in a well-ventilated area, wearing disposable gloves when skin contact is possible, and washing your hands after working.

If you think you or your children have chicken pox, call your practitioner, but please don't go to the office and infect the entire waiting room!

- When gardening, in order to avoid the parasitic infection toxoplasmosis, wear gloves, and wash your hands after contact with the soil. Wash all fruits and vegetables before consuming them, too.
- If you have a sandbox, keep it covered to prevent animals from using it as a litter box. Wash your hands well after touching the sand.
- For outdoor activities in mosquito-prone areas, wear long sleeves, tuck long pants into your socks, and use regular adult DEET spray to protect yourself from mosquitoes and associated diseases. It is probably better to expose yourself to a little DEET than to get Lyme disease or West Nile virus.

Travel during Pregnancy

Most pregnant women can travel safely. From the time you hear or see the heartbeat until early in the third trimester, emergencies are uncommon, and travel is usually fine. But it is always a good idea to check with your doctor or midwife before you go, and women with high-risk pregnancies, such as twins, high blood pressure, premature labor, or poor fetal growth, probably shouldn't travel far.

Because many women travel extensively for work, some issues about travel deserve special attention here.

GENERAL TIPS FOR TRAVELING

- During pregnancy, sitting for long hours increases the chances of blood clots developing in the legs. Walk around every two to three hours in a plane and get out of the car for ten minutes every two hours on long drives.

- Don't forget to wear your seatbelt—it is important for you and for your baby. The lap belt should be placed below your belly, the shoulder strap across your abdomen. You do not need to disable the airbag.
- Traveling can be exhausting. Allow yourself a little extra recovery time, and consider pacing your trips more gently than in the past—you can always ramp them back up if you are doing fine.

TRAVELING SAFELY AND COMFORTABLY BY AIR

- In addition to the slightly increased chance of blood clots, commercial airplane cabins are only pressurized to the equivalent of about eight thousand feet. Healthy women may feel slightly short of breath, but because of differences in fetal blood, the baby will still receive plenty of oxygen. Women with sickle-cell disease and those with complications of pregnancy, however, may experience serious problems with the lower oxygen availability in a plane.
- Airplanes are very dry—pregnant travelers should drink lots of fluids.
- Most U.S. airlines allow travel until thirty-six weeks; international airlines, until thirty-five weeks. Check with your airline ahead of time—documentation of your due date and permission from your doctor may be requested.
- At high altitudes, cosmic radiation exposure is greater than it is on the ground. Although this doesn't amount to much for the sporadic local traveler, it can add up on distant journeys, in which planes fly higher (with consequently less protection from the atmosphere). Flying closer to the poles also slightly increases radiation exposure. Under ordinary flight conditions, in-flight radiation exposure would not be expected to reach harmful levels. One intercontinental trip exposes the fetus to less than 1 percent of the radiation dose thought to pose any risk of miscarriage, birth defects, or growth restriction. Pregnant flight attendants, pilots, and others who fly professionally should follow FAA guidelines.

TRAVELING TO HIGH ALTITUDES

- Oxygen is less available at high altitude. If your body is accustomed to the altitude, this may not be a big problem unless you exercise, but you may notice that you feel more short of breath than usual.

- Some experts recommend that pregnant women stay below eight thousand feet. Ask your midwife or doctor for advice before you travel.

  In my first pregnancy, union policy was to stop flying for three months, then you could fly the middle three months, then off the last three. They felt that women might get sick and shouldn't be responsible for the plane in early pregnancy. I felt fine, so it was frustrating having to be home, plus I didn't get my salary then, just California disability. Next pregnancy I didn't tell them I was pregnant until I was bursting out of my uniform. (Susan G., commercial airline pilot)

MEDICAL CARE AWAY FROM HOME

- One consideration when traveling is the distance from the doctor and hospital you know. To be cautious, carry a copy of your medical records, and, especially late in pregnancy, locate a hospital or practice ahead of time where you can be seen in an emergency.
- Be aware that some insurance plans won't pay for out-of-network delivery if a woman travels later than a certain time in her pregnancy.
- If a problem arises while you are away from home, call your doctor's office; they may be able to help you to decide if you need to go to an emergency room or head home early.

TRAVEL TO DEVELOPING COUNTRIES

Malaria, hepatitis A, typhoid, and tetanus are examples of preventable infections that are more common in the developing world. And if you journey to remote areas, the severity of any pregnancy complication may be made worse by the lack of modern, hygienic medical care. In short, you should think twice about exotic travel in pregnancy. If your trip to a developing area can't be avoided, be sure to talk to your practitioner and if possible a travel medicine specialist before your trip, so you can take proper precautions.

Stress

Most people experience some stress in their daily lives. Pregnancy may increase the strain, as you try to balance your physical and emotional needs with all of the other demands on your time and personal resources.

How does stress affect the baby? Research on the effects of emotional stress is inconclusive. Although some studies show more premature and smaller than expected infants, others show no excess risk. What is known for sure, however, is that crutches like cigarettes, drugs, or alcohol will increase the potential harm to the baby and serve you poorly in the long run. Managing your stress with healthful outlets such as exercise or socializing with friends can help you to deal with difficult times, offset any possible risk, and make you feel better as you navigate the many new experiences and sensations of pregnancy.

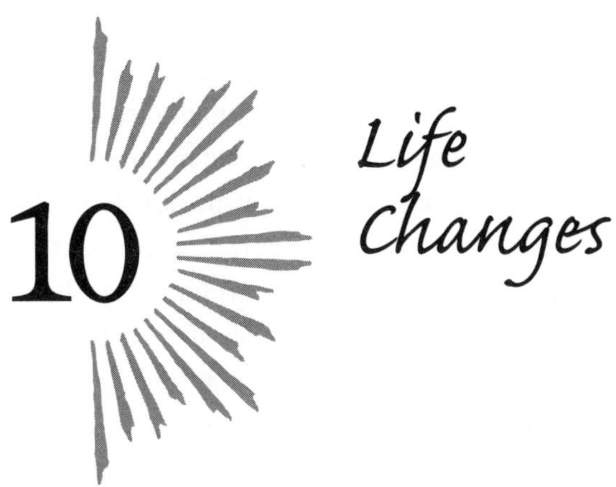

10 Life Changes

Your lifestyle may have changed dramatically since you found out you were expecting, or it might seem much the same as before. But inside you, there is a lot going on, both physically and emotionally: your tiny embryo is developing rapidly, and the reality of your pregnancy is taking hold.

First Trimester Emotions

At this early point in pregnancy, many mothers-to-be—even those with planned and desired pregnancies—feel ambivalent about what they are getting into. No wonder; in addition to feeling sick or exhausted, you are making irrevocable changes in your family and your life. You may feel guilty about any negative feelings, but these emotions are usually temporary and—as long as you continue to take care of yourself—won't hurt the baby in any way. In fact, you can take heart knowing that within a few months, these conflicting emotions usually give way to excited anticipation.

Your Relationship as a Couple

Your connection with your partner may also be in transition. You may feel closer than ever as you plan together for the transformation of your family. Generally, though, the pregnancy is more real to the mother-to-be, who is experiencing physical and emotional changes, than to her partner, who can more easily forget about it.

Women and men often deal with experiences differently (you know—men are from Mars, and women are from Venus), and the response to pregnancy is no exception. Women are more likely to talk about their pregnancies with friends, compare notes, and seek advice; men don't usually focus so much on their inner lives. Meanwhile, some men, whether they recognize it or not, feel left out—jealous of their partner's intimate and seemingly exclusive involvement with the pregnancy. If the man's response to feeling left out is to talk less, the mother may feel that he doesn't care. And if he tries to give advice such as to exercise or take a vitamin when the mom doesn't feel up to it, she may end up feeling that he cares more about their baby than about her. Because of their different approaches to dealing with the new pregnancy, the relationship can stumble. Lesbian couples are not immune to these issues. Regardless of gender, both partners may experience a shift in their relationship and become worried about the changes this pregnancy will bring to their lives individually and together.

To help keep your relationship healthy and growing, you may want to set aside a few minutes each week to take your "relationship pulse"—that is, to see how the pregnancy is affecting each of you. Take turns talking about how you feel, and listen to what the other person is expressing. You may not end up seeing eye-to-eye on every issue, but within a good relationship both partners should feel heard and loved. If you are really struggling together, now is the time to seek help by way of a support group or couples counseling. Having a newborn will almost certainly not make your home life less stressful, and it will be easier to join forces as parents if you are doing well as a couple. Communication and consideration are keys to a healthy relationship and successful co-parenting.

I never thought I was a vain person, but I remember asking my husband early in the pregnancy, "Do I look pregnant or just fat?" His response was "I don't know the right answer to that question." (Peggy L., nurse-administrator)

Your sex life in the first trimester will be influenced by how you are feeling physically and emotionally, by any problems in your relationship, and by what your sex life was like before you conceived. During pregnancy, all sexual activities that don't hurt you are considered safe, with the exception of blowing into the vagina, which can allow air to get into your bloodstream—a potentially fatal situation. First trimester sex can be great: the two of you may be feeling particularly close; you don't have to worry about birth control; and you are no longer timing sex and trying to get pregnant. Conversely, it is also normal for you to have a low sex drive, as you adjust to the physical and emotional experiences of being pregnant.

Your partner's attitude about sex may also change. One father-to-be may feel inhibited about having sex with someone who will soon be a mother or may feel like the fetus is watching; another may be excited by his partner's changing body and how it proves his virility. Both of you may worry about hurting the baby or causing a pregnancy complication. The key with sex, as with other aspects of your relationship, is communication and respect. It is easy to misinterpret disinterest in sex as a lack of caring or attraction. Talking about the situation can help prevent misunderstandings and hurt feelings.

First trimester I was so tired I was always asleep. Maybe we had sex, but I don't remember. (Deb L., writer)

All I used to hear about was the "pregnancy glow." What no one tells you is that I don't think you start to glow for about five or six months. Until then, you just feel thick, which is not cute! All of my pants make me feel like a sausage. (Jen B., dance teacher)

Some relationships have bigger issues than the usual Mars and Venus communication snafus. Abuse can be verbal, such as name-calling, devaluing opinions, or threatening violence; it can be controlling, such as preventing friendships or demanding things be done to earn love; or it can be physical. About one in twelve women experiences violence during pregnancy. Domestic violence crosses all racial, ethnic, sexual orientation, and economic lines, and often escalates during pregnancy, putting the mother and fetus in grave danger. Some women find new strength to get help when pregnant, in order to protect the baby. To see if you are at risk, take the domestic violence quiz on page 98.

Taking Care of Yourself

Although your child likely will be loved by several adults, right now you are the only person who can provide her care. The remainder of this chapter will answer questions you might have about your lifestyle, and what is healthiest

QUIZ: Are you at risk for domestic violence?

Has anyone close to you ever threatened to hurt you?	yes	no
Has anyone close to you ever hit, kicked, choked, or otherwise hurt you physically?	yes	no
Has anyone, including your partner, ever forced you to have sex?	yes	no
Are you ever afraid of your partner?	yes	no

One yes answer puts you at risk. If you marked "yes" to one question or more, talk to your doctor, local women's shelter, or domestic violence support agency, or get more information from the National Coalition against Domestic Violence at www.ncadv.org or 1-800-799-SAFE. If your partner comes to your appointments, you can always telephone your doctor or nurse with your concerns so you can talk privately. Everyone deserves to be safe in her own home.

now that you are pregnant. You also might want to review Chapter 2, which has preconception recommendations about diet, exercise, medications, and other aspects of daily life. But don't worry if you didn't get a healthy start before your baby was conceived. Even if you haven't been "perfect," you have the opportunity now to take care of your baby in the best way possible. Hopefully these suggestions will help to guide you as you accomplish an amazing feat: growing a whole new person inside your body.

Cats and Toxoplasmosis

You may have already heard that you shouldn't change the cat box during pregnancy. Cats can carry toxoplasmosis, a parasitic infection that may infect and harm a developing fetus. Cats catch toxoplasmosis from eating an infected animal or infected meat; they then transmit toxoplasmosis through their feces. If you touch infected feces, such as inadvertently while changing cat litter, and then handle food, you could potentially contaminate you and your baby. Wearing gloves and washing your hands after changing cat litter reduce the potential for transmission. And because the spores don't become infectious until one to five days after being in the litter box, if the cat box is cleaned daily, there is little risk of infection. (Feeding your cat commercial dry or canned cat food and not allowing it outside also help.) Just the same, you will be wise to give someone else cat-box duty until after the baby comes, and to not get a new cat or play with strays while you are pregnant.

Substance Use and Abuse

Cigarettes, alcohol, and drugs should be avoided in pregnancy. For more information about the effects of these substances, how much is too much, and what you can do to quit, see Chapter 2.

I quit smoking after eighteen years when I found out I was pregnant, but other people would still smoke around me. I hated it. (Tracy G., police officer)

Nutrition

In early pregnancy you may not be feeling well enough to focus on good nutrition. Fluids and calories, in any form you can get them down, are the highest priority. Gatorade, milkshakes, Jell-O, bananas, Kool-Aid—whatever works.

How does what you eat become nutrition for your baby? After food enters your mouth, it is digested in your stomach and intestine. Sugars, fats, amino acids (the building blocks of proteins), vitamins, and minerals are absorbed into your bloodstream and travel throughout your body. As your blood flows across the placenta, molecules pass from your blood into the baby's circulation. In other words, if you eat pickles and ice cream, the baby doesn't get pickles and ice cream; she gets vitamins, minerals, sugars, fats, and amino acids from the pickles and ice cream. What does this mean for you? Food that isn't particularly healthful, such as a candy bar, isn't poison; it just substitutes for other fare that might provide more of what you and your baby need. Some women crave substances that aren't food, like laundry starch, chalk, or even dirt. This condition is called pica, and often coexists with anemia (low red blood cell counts). Even if it is embarrassing, it is important to tell your doctor or midwife that you are having these urges.

Frequently Asked Questions about Food in Pregnancy

Every single decision you make about what you eat isn't critical, but once you are feeling well enough, most of what you eat in pregnancy should be healthful for you and your baby. Vegetables and fruits, sources of protein, and whole grains provide the basis for a healthy diet. That said, some foods may contain harmful germs or toxins. Certain infectious agents are particularly dangerous during pregnancy because they can pass through the placenta and infect the baby. Often the mother has few symptoms. Food poisoning that occurs from eating Salmonella, the toxic form of E. coli, and other contaminants doesn't pose a specific risk to pregnant women, but can make anyone very ill; taking simple steps to prevent infection can save you from a bellyache—or worse—later.

ARE SOFT CHEESES SAFE?

Soft, unpasteurized cheese can harbor Listeria, a type of bacteria that can cross the placenta and cause serious problems for a fetus. Hard cheeses are safe, and most cheese that is legally imported into the United States is pasteurized, so infection is rare. The bottom line: Don't eat soft cheeses like brie or the Mexican cheese queso fresco unless you can check the label and see that it was pasteurized.

CAN I EAT FISH?

You may have heard news reports about the dangers of eating fish while pregnant. Certain large fish, including shark, swordfish, tilefish, king mackerel, and tuna, may contain high levels of mercury, which can cause brain or nerve damage when consumed in large quantities. The fetus, which has an immature nervous system, is theoretically at greater risk from exposure to mercury. Ideally, high-mercury fish should be avoided starting three months before conception, because the mercury remains in your body for weeks.

Refrigerated smoked seafood (like lox) can also, rarely, be a source of Listeria. Your safest bet is to eat canned or shelf-stable smoked seafood rather than the kind you find at the deli counter.

It is important to remember, though, that in general, fish are good for you—they provide a great low-fat source of protein. Farm-raised trout and catfish, wild salmon, and fish sticks (which are made from smaller fish) are safe to eat. For more information, check out www.cfsan.fda.gov or call 1–888–SAFEFOOD.

CAN I EAT SUSHI?

Sushi made with cooked fish or with vegetables should be safe. But what if you want to eat raw sushi? Raw fish can carry worms, bacteria, and viruses. The FDA requires that restaurants planning to serve raw fish freeze and thaw it first to kill parasites. Trained sushi chefs know how to buy and handle the fish to avoid contamination; it is very unusual to hear about infection from sushi prepared in a restaurant. But if you want to be totally safe, choose cooked-fish sushi for nine months.

WHAT ABOUT RAW SHELLFISH?

Diseases from mollusk-type shellfish are common; even oysters from approved harvesting sites, where the seafood is bathed in clean water before being sold, carry a 1 percent risk of transmitting a moderately severe intestinal virus. Pregnancy doesn't make stomach viruses more dangerous, but getting one would be unpleasant and could land you in the hospital. To be safe, you may want to avoid eating raw mollusks during your pregnancy. Cooked shrimp, lobster, and other crustacean-type shellfish, though, are not particularly risky.

ARE LUNCHEON MEATS REALLY A PROBLEM?

Refrigerated meat spreads, like pâté, can contain Listeria. During pregnancy, don't eat refrigerated pâté or meat spreads. (Canned or shelf-stable pâté and spreads are okay.) Luncheon meats like bologna and salami only rarely contain Listeria, but if you want to be totally safe, avoid them, or thoroughly heat them (until steaming) before consuming. Cook hot dogs thoroughly.

CAN I DRINK CAFFEINE?

During pregnancy, you should limit your caffeine intake to no more than one or two small cups of coffee a day. Try decaffeinated coffee and sodas, or better yet, water, low-fat milk, and pasteurized juice. For more information on the possible effects of caffeine on your pregnancy, see Chapter 2.

ARE SUGAR AND FAT SUBSTITUTES OKAY TO USE?

Sucralose, the sweetener in Splenda, is made from regular sugar. Although it tastes like sugar, the body doesn't recognize it and not much is absorbed. The FDA reports that sucralose is safe in pregnancy. Aspartame, the sweetener in NutraSweet and Equal, has also been shown to be safe for use in pregnancy. There isn't much information about the fetal effects of saccharine (the sweetener in Sweet'N Low), so most experts recommend avoiding it.

As for fat substitutes, Olestra, used in some snack foods like Wow potato chips, may interfere with the absorption of fat-soluble vitamins, so it is probably best to avoid it during pregnancy, when vitamin intake is particularly important. Simplesse, a fat substitute made from protein, has not been safety-tested for pregnancy and so should not be eaten.

General Food Safety Tips

To help avoid food-borne illnesses, you should

- Rinse fresh fruits and vegetables in running tap water to remove visible dirt and grime. Remove and discard the outermost leaves from lettuce or cabbage.
- Avoid any products made from unpasteurized milk, raw or partially cooked eggs, raw or undercooked meat and poultry, unpasteurized juices, and raw sprouts. Remember that eggnog and Caesar salad dressing are sometimes made with raw eggs. And don't taste that cookie dough until it is a cooked cookie! (If you really want to have something with raw eggs, purchase pasteurized raw eggs, available at many grocery stores.)
- Wash hands, utensils, and cutting boards after they have been in contact with raw meat or poultry and before they touch another food. Put them through the dishwasher, or wash them with one teaspoon of chlorine bleach diluted in a quart of water. Put cooked meat and poultry on a clean platter, rather than back on one that held the raw food, and switch to new utensils for serving.
- Cook meat, poultry, and eggs thoroughly. Use a meat thermometer to be sure ground meat reaches an internal temperature of 160° (steaks should

reach 145° before eating). To prevent salmonella infection, eggs should be cooked until the yolk is firm, or use pasteurized eggs.
- Refrigerate perishable food promptly and defrost foods properly.
- Don't infect yourself or your loved ones! Use soap and warm water to wash your hands thoroughly (palms, backs, and between fingers) after using the bathroom and before preparing food.
- For more information, check out the FDA's food safety website at www.cfsan.fda.gov.

Natural Toxins

Remember that just because something is natural doesn't make it safe. You already know about alcohol and drugs, but herbal supplements and excess vitamins can also be dangerous for your baby. Any herb or vitamin at a higher concentration than what you would find in food may be risky. Check with your practitioner before consuming any herbals or before taking any vitamins at doses greater than the amount in a prenatal multivitamin.

And about those prenatal multivitamins: you may be surprised to learn that the American College of Obstetrics and Gynecology doesn't recommend universal use of prescription-strength prenatal vitamins. For the first trimester they advise that a woman with a healthy, balanced diet take a 400–1000 microgram folic acid supplement, and, later in pregnancy, extra iron. Still, many mothers-to-be choose a prenatal multivitamin as an "insurance policy" to make sure they get all the vitamins and minerals they need. If you are not eating well, a prenatal vitamin, if you can get one down each day, will help to offset any deficiencies in your diet. If your vitamin pill makes you nauseated, though, talk to your practitioner. Some medical professionals recommend just taking a folic acid supplement or daily children's chewables until you feel better.

First Trimester Diet Principles: If It Stays Down, It's Fine

Even if you take a prenatal vitamin, early on it may be impossible to approach what anyone would consider a balanced diet. Some days, you just have to eat whatever will go down—whether that is Jell-O and crackers or Reese's peanut butter cups. Your embryo is tiny at this point, and can absorb from your bloodstream everything that it needs. The best you may be able to do is to stay hydrated and take in some calories. On bad days, try ginger ale or sports drinks; some moms also report that dry saltine crackers can help comfort a sour stomach. (For more ideas, see Chapter 8.) If you can't keep even fluids down for six to twelve hours, call your practitioner, because dehydration and a lack of calories are unhealthy for you and your little embryo.

When you are feeling well enough to try to eat healthfully, make an effort to follow the guidelines suggested by the food pyramid (www.mypyramid.gov), which recommends that everyone eat varied types of fruits and vegetables, lean meat and beans, whole grains, and three or four cups of low-fat milk or milk-equivalents each day. If you are lactose intolerant, consider alternatives to milk or take lactase, the enzyme that helps you digest lactose. Women who have a history of eating disorders, who start off underweight or overweight, or who are vegan vegetarians should ask their practitioners or a licensed dietitian for more individualized information. And while your mother may have told you to eat three square meals a day, you will probably find that during pregnancy eating five or six small meals is more comfortable—and keeps you more energetic—than three big ones.

How to Gain the Right Amount of Weight

Every woman's metabolism is different, and each mother-to-be will put on weight in her own way. But good eating habits will help you to gain the amount of weight that is healthiest for you and your baby-to-be (and help keep you healthy throughout life as well).

- Eat when you are hungry
- Eat small portions
- Choose healthful snacks like vegetables and fruits
- Stop eating when you are full
- Get regular aerobic exercise

On average, pregnancy requires just three hundred extra calories a day—the equivalent of a low-fat fruit yogurt and an apple. As pregnancy progresses, if you listen to your body, your appetite will naturally direct you to take in the right amount of calories for you and your growing baby. If most of the foods you eat

SPECIAL DIETS: VEGETARIAN AND VEGAN

Vegetarian diets can be good for you, as long as you pay attention to taking in enough protein. Vegetarians who eat eggs and milk products can usually meet their protein needs without difficulty. Some people consider themselves vegetarian but eat fish. Fish is good for you, but be sure to avoid large fish—including shark, swordfish, tilefish, and king mackerel—which may contain worrisome amounts of mercury.

Vegan diets exclude all animal products, including milk, cheese, and eggs. Vitamin B12 and vitamin D are missing from the vegan diet, and must be supplemented; in addition, with just grains and nuts as protein sources, it takes careful planning to make sure you eat the recommended sixty-five grams of protein each day. If you follow a vegan or macrobiotic diet, tell your doctor or midwife, and consider consulting with a nutritionist to be sure you are getting all of the nutrients that you and your baby need.

are healthy and you balance what you eat by following the food pyramid guidelines, you will be off to a great start.

Exercise

Nutrition is one aspect of a healthy lifestyle, but exercise is important too—before, during, and after pregnancy. In the old days doctors told pregnant women not to "overdo it," but today we know that aerobic exercise is good for most pregnant women and their offspring, as well as for just about everyone else. Intense weight-bearing exercise throughout pregnancy lowers the chance of going past your due date and of needing a cesarean, and combined with a diet low in processed carbohydrates leads to less weight gain for the mother and significantly leaner (less fat) babies. These children continue to be thinner into childhood—which may mean that exercise during pregnancy offers the baby some protection from obesity later in life. Moderate exercise like walking doesn't provide as many medical benefits, but is still good for the mother's mental and physical health, leading to improved body image, a sense of well-being, and fewer discomforts of pregnancy like low back pain.

Whether you are an elite athlete or a couch potato ready to make a change, you may wonder how safe it is for you to exercise and what activities are best. Talk to your doctor or midwife about specific recommendations. If you have medical problems like high blood pressure or heart disease, or complications of pregnancy that put you at risk for delivering early, exercise might not be for you.

Once you have your doctor or midwife's okay, the next step is to make exercise a part of your regular routine. It may be hard to schedule exercise in with your workday, and right now you may find that napping after work wins out, but once you feel better, it is time to get moving. Your life won't get less complicated after the baby comes, and exercise plays a lifelong role in protecting your health and improving your mood. Most activities are fine, if you can stay within the seven exercise guidelines listed below, as long as you won't bang your belly or fall. Intense aerobic weight-bearing activity, like running, provides the greatest medical benefit. Swimming or water exercise is also good, since you won't get overheated, and as you get bigger the water will support your weight. Unless your doctor or midwife specifically recommends it, the old guideline of keeping your heart rate under 140 is not necessary. The most important thing is to find activities that you enjoy and can do with moderate intensity most days of the week.

The best advice I got was to be active but take it easy. When you stay active, you stay fit. (Annette M., store manager)

SEVEN EXERCISE GUIDELINES

- Find an activity you enjoy (or at least don't hate) so you will do it regularly: a total of at least thirty minutes most days of the week
- Make it fun: listen to music, or team up with a friend
- Keep cool: dress in layers, and take a break if you feel overheated
- Stay hydrated: stop and drink water or sports drinks when you are thirsty
- Avoid lying on your back: after about twenty weeks, lying flat on your back may diminish blood circulation to the baby
- Use the "talk test": your breathing shouldn't be so labored that you can't hold a conversation

- Stop immediately if you get lightheaded or feel awful: this is not a time to "push through the pain"

I had no symptoms—I was one of the lucky ones. I never felt pregnant until toward the end. I actually competed in pentathlon-type events and rode my bike and swam until a month or so before delivery. (Helene L., teacher)

At the Spa

Spa treatments are great for relaxing and rejuvenating. Some therapies are fine, but others will need to wait until after the baby is born. We know that a fever in early pregnancy is bad for the embryo, increasing the chances for miscarriage and birth defects. It isn't totally clear that getting overheated in a hot tub or sauna carries the same risks, but it isn't clearly safe, either, so all treatments that raise your body temperature are off limits. This includes the sauna, steam room, and hot tub, unless you keep the temperature below 100 degrees.

Massage is a great way to unwind tired muscles and pamper yourself. Pregnancy massage tables have a cutout for your belly. If you aren't lucky enough to have access to a specialized table, as you get bigger you can either position yourself with pillows so that you are slightly on your side, or use a massage chair. Massage of the abdomen or breasts can cause contractions. If you notice strong contractions, stop that part of the massage.

Aromatherapy is fine as long as it is pleasant for you; however, essential oils may be absorbed through the skin. Until more is known, it is probably best to use oils that have been tested for safety in pregnancy such as rose, eucalyptus, lemon, mandarin, frankincense, and lavender, and to avoid extensive use of oils on your skin, especially during the first trimester.

Your Skin

Tanning is never good for you—it increases the risk of skin cancer and early aging. During pregnancy, your face may be particularly sensitive to the sun, developing long-lasting pigment changes, called melasma, on your chin, cheeks, and forehead after sun exposure. In short, you shouldn't try to get a suntan while pregnant. What about self-tanning? The active ingredient in sunless tanning

WHICH EXERCISES AND SPORTS ARE SAFE?

Check with your practitioner before exercising to be sure you are choosing the right physical activity for you. In general, the following activities are safe and healthy for pregnant women:

- Swimming, water aerobics, snorkeling
- Low-impact aerobics, step class, prenatal aerobics, dance, walking, or jogging
- Stair climber, elliptical trainer, ski machine, or stationary bike
- Weight machines (but don't lie flat on your back) and hand weights
- Prenatal yoga

Also okay for many women (but again, check with your doctor first):

- Running, bicycling, or cross-country skiing
- High-impact aerobics
- Tennis and other racket sports if played at low intensity
- Yoga
- Free weights
- Scuba diving at depths of less than thirty feet

You should definitely avoid these activities until after delivery:

- Scuba diving requiring decompression (the pressure changes may not be safe for the fetus)
- Exertion at high altitude (over 6,000–8,000 feet—even if you live at that altitude)
- Waterskiing
- Contact sports such as soccer, basketball, or ice hockey
- Surfing, in-line skating or skateboarding, downhill skiing, horseback riding, vigorous racket sports, gymnastics, or other activities that risk falling
- Hot yoga, or other exercise in an overly warm environment

lotions, dihydroxyacetone (DHA), appears to be harmless and is not absorbed into the body. If you want to play it extra safe, wait to use self-tanners until after the first trimester, when the baby's organs have formed.

Hair and Nails

I get asked all the time about the safety of hair treatments; unfortunately, there isn't an easy answer. Hair dye, bleach, perms, and relaxing solutions are all absorbed into the bloodstream to some degree. In animal studies, some of these solutions caused birth defects in the offspring, but only in much higher amounts than you would normally use. There is also no reason to believe that "natural" products are any safer than manmade ones. Most obstetricians, then, recommend that you do not have these hair treatments during your baby's first trimester—this way, the baby's organs will have been formed before exposure. Highlighting, which doesn't touch the scalp, is probably safe throughout pregnancy.

On days when you feel like a blob, a manicure or pedicure can be just the thing. Especially if you need to look professional at work, having your nails done can make you look "put together" when you feel anything but. Some of the chemicals used in nail polish (as well as some food packaging and many other household items) are dibutyl phthalates, or DBPs, which help to keep plastics pliable. Over the past few years, DBPs have been suspected of causing birth defects in animals. Absorption into the bloodstream is probably through food sources or inhalation; they aren't absorbed through the nail. Until more is known, it is sensible to do your nails in a well-ventilated area, and not to chew on polished nails.

I want to treat myself to a pedicure. I can't really even cut my own toenails anymore, much less paint them myself. (Jen B., dance teacher)

Well-Meaning Advice

Once people know that you are expecting, they seem to come out of the woodwork to give you advice on health and safety. Your partner, too, may seem to be counting your calories and watching for hazards around the clock. But although others may see you as a vessel for the care of a fetus, you of course still feel like yourself, with your usual likes and dislikes and busy schedule—possibly combined with first trimester fatigue and nausea. All of the advice may be well meant, but it can feel confining and controlling. Try not to get into power struggles about what you eat, how much you exercise, and if you have a single sip of wine. You are responsible for the baby, but you are also an adult and have the right to make decisions as you see fit. Get accurate information and then look into your heart; if you know that you're on the right track, allow yourself to relax. And if you sense that you should be doing things differently but find it hard to make changes, talk to your doctor or midwife about getting some help.

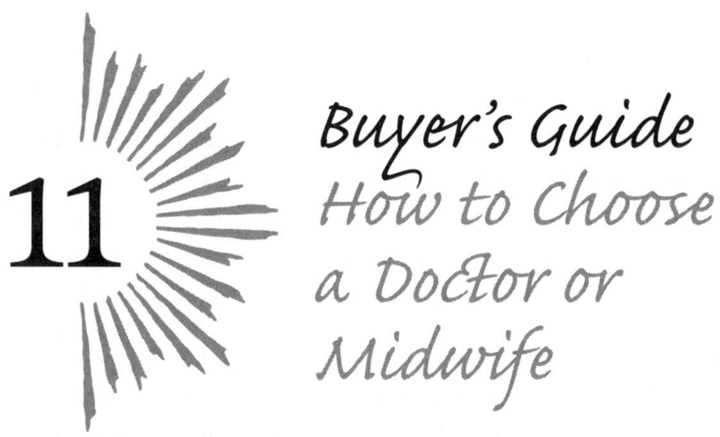

11 Buyer's Guide: How to Choose a Doctor or Midwife

Your birth experience will be shaped in part by where you give birth and who delivers your baby. If you already have a doctor or midwife you like, who is on your insurance plan, and who practices at a convenient location, you're all set. If not, several factors should play into your decision about where to get your prenatal care. Becoming informed about different types of practitioners and practices, the kinds of locations you can choose for childbirth, and the financial costs of having a baby will allow you to understand what the various options might mean for you and your partner. After considering the advice in this chapter, you may find it helpful to use the worksheet at the end as a way of evaluating your options for pregnancy care.

Practitioners Who May Be Involved in Your Care

There are several different kinds of medical professionals who provide care during pregnancy, labor, and delivery. Which one you choose will depend on your personal preferences and circumstances.

OBSTETRICIANS

Obstetrician-gynecologists (ob-gyns or OBs for short) are doctors who have completed medical school followed by four years of residency in gynecology and obstetrics. During this residency training, they receive instruction in gynecologic surgery, women's health care, prenatal care, treatment of complicated pregnancies, vaginal delivery, and cesarean sections. Some ob-gyns limit their practice to gynecology and don't deliver babies, but most do both. The training of ob-gyns is focused on keeping the mother and baby healthy, not on your "birth experience." Obstetricians vary in their philosophy: some are more natural-childbirth oriented, whereas others are more high-tech. Women who choose OBs over other sorts of practitioners cite their high educational level and their ability to handle complications should problems arise. Many women already go to gynecologists they like who can take care of them during pregnancy and afterward.

With my second child, I had found an ob-gyn through several friends. I actually ended up getting an appointment with her partner, and as it turned out, she was the better fit for me anyway. I developed a really great relationship with her, and she was there for the delivery, which was nice. (Shani M., student)

My ob-gyn was the nicest man with such an attentive staff. He had his nurse call all the time because I was vomiting so often. When I was in the office he was like family . . . so excited about the baby and how I was feeling. I think because he is a father of four it makes him a more understanding doc. (Zenia M., nurse's aide)

FAMILY DOCTORS

Family doctors have completed medical school followed by three years of residency training, during which they learn how to provide care for both children and adults, and how to deliver babies. Family doctors who choose to practice obstetrics usually take care of women with uncomplicated pregnancies, and work with an obstetrician who can back them up if problems arise. Your family physician can provide medical care for all members of the family, from before birth through old age.

CERTIFIED NURSE-MIDWIVES

Certified nurse-midwives (CNMs) are advanced-practice nurses, registered nurses who have completed a two- to three-year program of additional training in prenatal care, women's reproductive health, and childbirth. Most have a master's degree, and all have passed national certifying examinations. Nurse-midwives care for women with uncomplicated pregnancies and work with physicians who can collaborate or take over if problems develop. They usually deliver babies in hospitals or birth centers. Many CNMs are interested in natural birth and in helping you to have a satisfying experience.

I remember Joel fought with his parents for a few days about getting a nurse-midwife. His parents thought, "You go to the person with the most education." (Lori G., professor)

My midwife was someone I had selected. She had done all my gynecological care. I just didn't care all that much about the specifics of the birth. I read about birthing plans, and people wanted the lighting a certain way, and I just didn't care about lighting. I just liked my midwife's attitude of let's just see how things go. (Janet G., attorney)

CERTIFIED MIDWIVES

The certified midwife (CM) credential was established by the American College of Nurse Midwives in 1997. CMs complete the same graduate training as nurse-midwives and must pass the same national certifying examinations, but they are not nurses first. They may be physical therapists or physician assistants or others with undergraduate degrees in health-related fields. Just like nurse-midwives, certified midwives typically take care of women with uncomplicated pregnancies and attend mostly hospital births. Currently, only a few states recognize CMs.

DIRECT-ENTRY MIDWIVES

A direct-entry midwife has undergone midwifery training, but is not a nurse. Training for this sort of midwifery varies widely. Direct-entry midwives usually attend births at home or freestanding birth centers and are specialists in the unique characteristics of out-of-hospital births.

There are three kinds of direct-entry midwives:

- Licensed midwife. A licensed midwife has attended a direct-entry midwifery school and passed a state midwifery exam. Not all states provide midwifery licenses, but in those states that do, some of the licensed midwives are established enough to carry malpractice insurance and take payment from your health insurance. Licensed midwives care for uncomplicated pregnancies and attend out-of-hospital births. They have recognized relationships with physicians to consult with if any complications arise prenatally or during labor.

- Lay midwife. A lay midwife is someone who has trained by apprenticing with an experienced midwife. Their profession is not recognized by the state. Lay midwives attend home births, and may or may not have a formal relationship with a backup physician. Because the lay midwife is not regulated or certified, you must do your own research to find out about her skills and experience.

- Certified professional midwife (CPM). In the late 1980s, the Midwives Alliance of North America (MANA) created a standard to provide consistency in the credentialing of midwives. As of 2005, there were nearly nine hundred CPMs in the United States; nineteen states used all or part of the CPM process in their licensing. A CPM may be a licensed or lay midwife; if apprentice-trained, she must go through a lengthy process of establishing her experience and demonstrating her skills. To preserve their certification, CPMs must maintain their credentials, complete continuing education units, and recertify every three years. A registry of CPMs has shown that their safety statistics for home births are comparable to those of low-risk hospital births.

If you are considering a direct-entry midwife, you should research the laws of your state. Some questions to ask the midwife include: What is your background and training? Are you certified or licensed? Where do you attend births? What do you do if complications develop during the pregnancy or birth? For more information see www.mana.org (Midwives Alliance of North America), www.cfmidwifery.org (Citizens for Midwifery), www.narm.org (North American Registry of Midwives), and www.acnm.org (American College of Nurse Midwives).

I didn't intend to have a home birth at first, I just wanted a doula to be with me, since I would be in Alaska and far away from my family. I looked up midwives in the phone book and started talking with Kaye. She gave me books to read and people to talk to who had chosen home births, even the ones that ended up having to be transported to the hospital, so I got a realistic picture. It also helped that my sister had had two home births by then, so it wasn't a foreign concept for my family. (Jan R., state attorney)

REGISTERED NURSES

While you are in labor, your nurse will probably be assigned between one and three patients, depending on staffing and the practices of the institution. She may not stay in the room with you. Hospital nurses vary in their interests, from very supportive of natural childbirth to more comfortable with epidurals and high-tech fetal monitoring.

Laurel, my labor nurse, got to know my husband and me as people. She spoke to us like intelligent, informed consumers—which we were. She showed humor and candor, along with a healthy dose of empathy, from her first words. Given that I had never been through labor before—or any other medical procedure—and given that my primary contact with the medical world for the past eight months, my doctor, was signed out to one of her partners, I needed to be able to trust and to connect with Laurel in order to stay relaxed for what lay ahead. (Rebecca M., senior vice president, financial corporation)

NURSE PRACTITIONERS

An ob-gyn nurse practitioner is an advanced-practice nurse, a registered nurse who has completed a two- to three-year program of additional training in prenatal care and women's reproductive health. Most have a master's degree, and all have passed national certifying examinations. Unlike nurse-midwives, ob-gyn nurse practitioners work only in the office and do not deliver babies.

DOULAS

A doula, also called a professional labor assistant or PLA, is trained in the emotional and physical support of laboring women. Doulas have expertise in comfort measures for labor and often also teach childbirth classes. Doulas don't deliver babies; their primary interest is you and your partner's experience. For more information on doulas, see Chapter 18 and www.dona.org.

MATERNAL-FETAL MEDICINE SPECIALISTS

A maternal-fetal medicine specialist, or MFM, is a fully trained obstetrician-gynecologist who has completed two or three additional years of postresidency fellowship in the care of women with complicated pregnancies. Most MFMs have special expertise in ultrasound as well. Although some MFMs provide prenatal care for healthy, low-risk women, most focus on the care of mothers-to-be who have medical problems, prior obstetric complications, or disorders identified during pregnancy.

Group Practices

Most doctors and midwives practice in groups, so that they can take turns being "on call" and available for delivering babies anytime of the day or night.

- Solo practitioner. Solo practitioners cover their own patients for prenatal care and childbirth. When you have a doctor or midwife who practices alone, you really get to know them, and they get to know you. The downside is that you may have to wait long hours in the office if they are off at a delivery, and if they happen to go out of town when you are due, the practitioner who is covering may not take as much personal interest in you as your own doctor does.

  I live in a really small town. There were three ob-gyns. Two work in the same office; mine was in solo practice. I would see him every time. I really liked the personal attention. (Norma J., teacher)

- Small group practice (two to five doctors or midwives). If you go to a small group practice, you will probably see all the members during your prenatal appointments. For delivery, some groups run strictly by their call schedule: the on-call person will take care of you when you come in to have your baby. In other groups the custom is (when possible) for your primary doctor or midwife to attend your birth.

  I started off with an obstetrician and later switched to a midwife. There were only two midwives in the practice, so I was guaranteed that one of them would be there for the delivery. (Elizabeth S., online producer)

- Large group practice. In larger groups, you might not get to meet the doctor or midwife who will take care of you during labor. It may not be practical to see every practitioner, and if you tried to rotate through them

A Comparison of Practitioners' Certification and Skills

Type of practitioner	*Prenatal care*	*Vaginal delivery*	*Cesarean*	*Stays with woman in labor*	*Graduated from accredited midwifery school*	*Graduated from accredited residency*	*Registered nurse*	*Licensed physician*	*Type of certifying specialty examination*	*To check on certification status of a doctor or midwife*	*For more information on the specialty or to find a practitioner*
Obstetrician	⋆	⋆	⋆			⋆		⋆	American Board of Obstetrics and Gynecology certifying exams	American Board of Obstetrics and Gynecology at www.abog.org	American College of Obstetrics and Gynecology at www.acog.com
Family doctor	⋆	⋆	variable			⋆		⋆	American Board of Family Medicine certifying exams	American Board of Family Medicine at www.theabfm.org	American Academy of Family Physicians at www.aafp.org
Certified nurse-midwife	⋆	⋆		⋆	⋆		⋆		American College of Nurse-Midwives certifying exams	American College of Nurse-Midwives at www.acnm.org	American College of Nurse-Midwives at www.acnm.org

A Comparison of Practitioners' Certification and Skills (Continued)

Type of practitioner	*Prenatal care*	*Vaginal delivery*	*Cesarean*	*Stays with woman in labor*	*Graduated from accredited midwifery school*	*Graduated from accredited residency*	*Registered nurse*	*Licensed physician*	*Type of certifying specialty examination*	*To check on certification status of a doctor or midwife*	*For more information on the specialty or to find a practitioner*
Certified midwife	*	*		*	*				American College of Nurse-Midwives certifying exams	American College of Nurse-Midwives at www.acnm.org	American College of Nurse-Midwives at www.acnm.org
Licensed midwife	*	*		*	*				State-by-state laws listed at www.mana.org	Depends on state regulatory process: see table at www.mana.org	Midwives Alliance of North America at www.mana.org
Certified professional midwife	*	*		*	maybe				North American Registry of Midwives certifying exam	North American Registry of Midwives at www.narm.org	Midwives Alliance of North America at www.mana.org

Lay midwife	varies	*		*				Unregulated		Midwives Alliance of North America at www.mana.org
Registered nurse		in a pinch!		varies		*				
Doula				*				Doulas of North America certification (optional)	Doulas of North America at www.dona.org	Doulas of North America at www.dona.org
Maternal-fetal medicine specialist	*	*	*		*		*	American Board of Obstetrics and Gynecology certifying exams	American College of Obstetrics and Gynecology at www.acog.com	Society for Maternal-Fetal Medicine at www.smfm.org

all for your prenatal visits, no one would get to know you well. Some large groups deliver by a strict call schedule, while in others your primary practitioner will try to attend your birth.

My friend had used a midwife and really liked her, and that midwife was actually covered by my insurance, and so I switched to her. I liked that much better than the big OB practice where you see a different doctor every time; that was very impersonal. (Kafi P., teacher)

- Hospitalists. In the United Kingdom, women obtain prenatal care from midwives in the office, and have their babies with a different set of midwives who practice only in the hospital. American obstetrics may be shifting toward this style of practice as well, assigning some doctors to staff the labor unit and just deliver babies—which frees up their office-based counterparts to provide prenatal care uninterrupted by long nights and daytime calls to the hospital.

  Hospital care of ill patients has already been divided this way in the United States, with many medical doctors handing their sickest patients over to "hospitalists" who take care of them while they are inpatients and send them back to the primary doctor when they go home. Although this is a less personal system, many experts believe that hospitalists take better care of sick medical patients; it is possible that, if the practice catches on, obstetric hospitalists will make deliveries safer as well.

Birth Locations

Most births in the United States take place in hospitals. Many hospitals have made an effort to be more homelike, with combined labor, delivery, and recovery rooms that allow the mother to stay in one place instead of moving to an operating room for the birth. Birth centers are structured to be less formal and far more homelike than the hospital, but are available only in limited locations. Few U.S. births take place at home.

How far away from home can your birthing place be for a safe delivery? First babies usually take their time, so a forty-five- to sixty-minute drive, while not ideal, doesn't usually pose a problem. For subsequent babies, the pace of your first labor can help you decide if you should plan to give birth closer to home.

NEWBORN MEDICAL CARE

Some families choose their hospital by its ability to handle a problem with the baby after birth, just in case. Although most hospitals encourage the mother to keep her baby with her in her room, newborn nurseries are assigned levels depending on the intensity of care they can provide.

- Level I facilities offer care for healthy babies beyond thirty-five weeks' gestation.
- Level II nurseries can support babies with some complications and premature babies older than thirty-two weeks.
- Level III nurseries (newborn intensive care units) can provide continuous life support and comprehensive care for extremely high-risk infants and those with complex and critical illnesses. Newborns with serious problems are usually transferred to a level IIIb or IIIc nursery at a teaching hospital, where the most sophisticated intensive care is available.

Your practitioner or hospital will be able to tell you the level of their nursery. In an emergency, any hospital should be able to stabilize a newborn and call for an ambulance to transport the baby to a Level III facility.

Depending on your geographic area, you may have several choices of where to have your baby.

TEACHING HOSPITALS

Teaching hospitals are large multispecialty medical centers with major responsibilities for patient care, research, and teaching.

- Advantages:

  Teaching hospitals are the most up-to-date kind of facility, providing innovative medical equipment and techniques. Your doctor has access to many colleagues, who can provide consultation in difficult cases; specialists are available to help with medical and obstetrical problems

All kinds of anesthesia are available
All staff are experienced with complications of labor and birth

- Disadvantages:
  More people will be involved in your care, probably including students and residents
  May seem impersonal compared with a smaller setting
  May be farther from home
- Nursery: Usually a level II or III nursery is available. At most modern hospitals, if all is well, the baby can stay with you after birth.
- Notes: Teaching hospitals are the safest settings for dealing with obstetric or medical complications.

COMMUNITY HOSPITALS

Community hospitals tend to be smaller than teaching hospitals, and are staffed by nurses and a "house doctor" in case of an emergency before your doctor arrives. Some community hospitals teach residents and students.

- Advantages:
  Depending on the location, community hospitals may employ high-risk OB doctors and newborn specialists, and/or offer twenty-four-hour in-house anesthesia
  Most community hospitals keep up with the latest news and treatments
  They may have suites in which you can labor, deliver, recover, and rest with your baby postpartum; this way, you won't have to move to a different room after you give birth
- Disadvantages:
  Often have higher cesarean rates than teaching hospitals
  Fewer specialists are available than at teaching hospitals, and some practitioners' knowledge or attitudes may be out-of-date
  Vaginal birth after cesarean (VBAC) is less likely to be offered at smaller community hospitals, especially if they can't provide 24/7 emergency anesthesia and surgical teams
- Nursery: Anything from a level I to a level IIIa nursery may be available.

At most modern hospitals, the baby can stay with you after birth unless problems arise.

- Note: Most U.S. babies are born in community hospitals.

Breastfeeding is very important to me. I fully understand the medical benefits of breastfeeding and I believe in it. I chose to deliver at a hospital where all of the OB nurses are trained by the lactation consultant, and the lactation consultant sees you every day. (Melissa Z., emergency medicine)

We only have one anesthesiologist in our small town, and he works 8–5 PM only. He doesn't come back to the hospital except in an emergency. So you won't get an epidural if you go into labor naturally in the middle of the night. (Norma J., teacher)

BIRTH CENTERS

Birth centers are small low-tech units just for having a baby; they may be free-standing or physically attached to a hospital.

- Advantages:
  Homelike and informal; supportive of your autonomy
  Oriented toward natural childbirth
  Very low rates of cesarean delivery
- Disadvantages:
  Anesthesia is not available
  About 10 percent of women need to be transferred to a hospital during labor, which can be emotionally and physically difficult.
- Nursery: Level I capabilities, but the baby normally stays with you.
- Notes: For a birth center near you, check out the National Association of Childbearing Centers at www.birthcenters.org.

It really wasn't until my labor classes that I really began to focus and consider what I wanted out of the pregnancy, and I decided that I was sort of uncomfortable with the medicalization of what seemed to me like a natural process. Since I was having a very normal pregnancy up to that point, I didn't see why there needed to be all these interventions during

the labor and delivery. Eventually I switched to a midwife practice and arranged to give birth at a birth center. (Linda S., creative director)

I planned to have the baby in a birthing center, which was in the basement of the hospital. I wanted to avoid an epidural, but I was ok with anything else that happened. When I was in the birthing center, the baby's heart rate was decelerating every time I pushed. And my uterus wasn't un-contracting. So they took me up to the hospital for the birth. (Elizabeth S., online producer)

HOME

Like it has been done for thousands of years.

- Advantages:
  No hospital rules or procedures
  Most births go well
  Very low rate of cesareans and other medical interventions
- Disadvantages:
  Anesthesia not available
  Lack of emergency equipment may require that the mother or baby be transferred to the hospital, and this lack of support can make a minor situation life-threatening
  Most doctors (and many parents) believe that home birth is more dangerous than having your baby in a birth center or hospital. One study indicated that infant mortality for home births, though rare, was double that of births in the hospital. In 2005, the records of planned home births by North American certified professional midwives were analyzed in the *British Medical Journal*, and outcomes were found to be similar to low-risk hospital births.
- No nursery
- Notes: Most home births are attended by direct-entry midwives. Doctors and nurse-midwives usually can't get malpractice insurance to cover home births, so they are generally unwilling to attend. For information on lay midwives and home birth, see www.mana.org.

The home birth for Megan was not easy, but it worked out and was so empowering. Since I don't have a hospital birth for comparison, I don't know what that would have been like; all I know is that it gave our little family a great start. Isabel's home birth was a relative breeze, and it was wonderful to be at home, with Megan sleeping in the next room and woken up just as Isabel was being born. The two of them are so close and loving; no doubt their bond began at that moment (if not before). ***(Jan R., state attorney)***

Birth Philosophy

I can't state this strongly enough—if you have a clear picture of what you are looking for, choose your practitioner, practice, and birth location based on your philosophy. It is a lot easier and more effective to make this choice now, than to create an elaborate "birth plan" that conflicts with the norms of the hospital or your OB's practice.

In this spirit, now is the best time to do some research on natural childbirth, epidural, common birth procedures, and cesarean section. For example, if you want a waterbirth, you'll need to choose a practitioner with waterbirth experience, and a birth location with a birthing tub or that can accommodate a rented tub. If you have a strong desire for minimal intervention, or alternatively if you think that you'll want the earliest possible epidural, knowing the philosophy of your practitioner and hospital will help you get the birth experience that is right for you. For more information on childbirth options, read ahead to Chapter 24.

My OB was kind, supportive, and very nurturing throughout my entire pregnancy. When I started contractions one night at about 11 PM, I called him and he met us at the hospital at midnight with his guitar in hand. It was a tiny rural hospital so we were the only ones there in the labor and delivery ward. He stayed with us the entire time, playing his guitar and singing. I had a completely natural childbirth (no drugs of any kind) and Aron was born a short (and very intense!) two hours later. Dr. M was right there with me the entire time, coaching and encouraging me. He stayed until about 4 AM just to make sure everything was ok, then went home

COSTS OF PREGNANCY CARE

The costs of your medical care during pregnancy will vary depending on your health insurance and where you live. HMOs tend to be the most comprehensive, with the fewest hidden costs. Generally, prenatal care is billed as a bundle—the office appointments and the doctor's delivery charge are grouped together, and any extra visits are included in the global fee. Deductibles would still apply, but co-pays would only be charged for emergency room or after-hours visits. Tests and ultrasounds are billed separately, as are hospital charges. Be aware that your insurance may not cover some genetic testing, extra ultrasounds, or other tests that you or your practitioner may want; if you are concerned about these or other expenses, ask your health insurance company and your practitioner for more information.

and slept for a couple of hours before going back to work the next morning. (Lisa H., community planner)

At one of my first prenatal appointments I asked the doctor what he used for pain during childbirth, and he said, "Oh, are you going to be a baby?" I walked out and never went back to him. (Sonya G., secretary)

We interviewed a couple of nurse-midwives. We didn't want too much medical intervention. It wasn't that we were all that spiritual or earthy, but just didn't see any reason to get it all doctored up. (Lori G., professor)

I lucked out. I didn't plan it this way, but it turned out that my OB had the perfect personality for me. We are nothing alike. She was always calm and competent. She didn't panic or preach—she always seemed to know what was happening to me when I called her with questions or problems, and she would be calm and efficient in her response. (Jane S., state governor)

Decision Points Worksheet

Making a plan for where and with whom to have your baby takes some careful thought and research. The worksheet provided here is designed to guide your reflections about which elements of the experience are most important to you. Information to help you answer these questions may be obtained from the Internet, from materials provided by your insurance plan, from the practitioner you are considering, or by word of mouth. If you are looking at a few different practices, you may want to create a worksheet for each one to help you compare.

Try to find a practitioner, practice, and birth location with which you are comfortable, and then stay with this plan through the birth of your baby. Although of course you can change practices if you are very dissatisfied, doctor- (or midwife-) shopping disrupts the continuity of care that helps assure the health and well-being of you and your baby.

I really liked her office, because in the exam room, she had a small but nice dressing room, where you could change, and store your clothes. There was even a hanger to hang up your stuff. It made you feel a little less exposed, and a lot more comfortable. (Shani M., student)

WORKSHEET: CARE OPTIONS FOR PREGNANCY AND BIRTH

PERSONAL BELIEFS

Which type of practitioner do you want? Obstetrician / Family doctor / Midwife / Unsure

Where do you want to give birth? Most practitioners go to only one or two sites to deliver babies. If you have a specific hospital or birth center in mind, choose a practitioner who delivers there. The hospital's website may list all of the admitting physicians.

If you are planning natural childbirth, does waterbirth sound appealing? Yes / No

If yes, be sure to ask any potential practitioner if the option of waterbirth will be available to you.

What philosophy of practice are you seeking? Natural / Undecided / Epidural / Cesarean

Some practitioners are more oriented to natural childbirth, while others offer a more high-tech approach. If you know what you are hoping for in a birth experience, you can pick a practice that is likely to support your wishes. If you don't have strong feelings about your labor and delivery experience, pick a practitioner whose personality and approach feel right to you. And if you have a serious medical condition or a prior pregnancy complication, be sure to choose an obstetrician experienced with problem pregnancies.

How does the practice work? Will you receive prenatal care from different members of a group or from one person?

Who might deliver your baby if your doctor or midwife isn't available?

QUALIFICATIONS

Which practitioners are most highly recommended by your friends, family members, or other doctors?

If you are new to a community, it may help to call the labor and delivery unit of the local hospital and ask the nurses for recommendations. You can check a doctor or nurse-midwife's board certification status with the relevant organization; your state medical board will have documentation of active complaints and disciplinary actions.

If you will see a family doctor or midwife, how will he or she manage any complications during delivery? What kind of backup support is available for you and your baby?

If you are choosing a direct-entry midwife, ask about her credentials, her experience, where she attends birth, and if she works with a physician.

What level is the nursery? Level I / Level II / Level III

Having an onsite nursery that can provide intensive medical support to your newborn is especially important if you have medical problems or other risk factors for premature birth.

FINANCES

Which practitioners and hospitals that you are interested in accept your health insurance plan?

Be aware that the booklet or website of your insurance company often has out-of-date lists of participating doctors: if you really want to go to a particular practice, call the office itself and ask if that practice will take your insurance.

Which practices and hospitals will keep your out-of-pocket costs lowest?

If your insurance doesn't cover well, or you choose to go out of network, you can be out a lot of money. Depending on where you live, charges for prenatal care, delivery, and hospitalization range from six to eight thousand dollars for a normal vaginal delivery to as much as fourteen thousand for a cesarean. Often, midwives charge less for delivery than doctors do, and birth centers in general are less expensive than hospitals. Although home birth may be the least expensive option, the medical drawbacks may outweigh the financial benefits.

LOGISTICS

Location, location, location. Where are the offices located?

If you plan to go to your appointments during your workday, a location near your job may be more valuable than a location near home. Easy access (via public transportation or close-in parking) can save valuable time, though doctors' offices located at a hospital may not provide free parking. Be aware, too, that if your employer is required to comply with the Family and Medical Leave Act (FMLA), by law you will be given time (although not necessarily with pay) to go to medical appointments.

How does the office flow? Does your practitioner usually run on time or will you have to wait long hours? Keep in mind that practitioners who spend time talking with their patients may be more likely to run behind.

Can the office notify you if they are behind schedule?

To minimize the disruption of your schedule, can you be seen on weekends or evenings? And if not, can you get appointments at the beginning or end of your workday?

How pleasant is the office staff? Do they make you feel welcome and comfortable, or do they seem distracted or antagonistic?

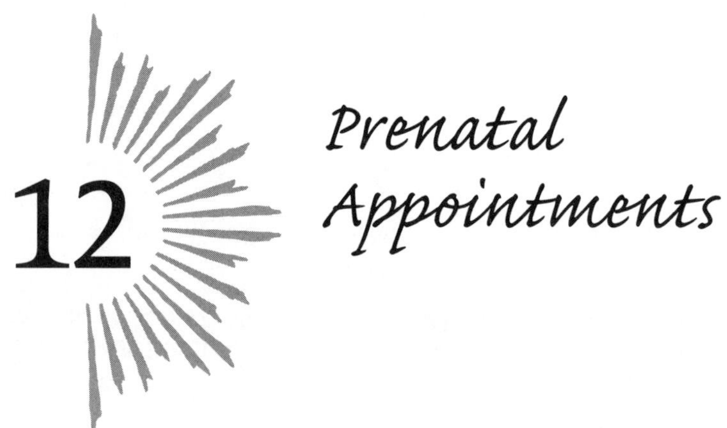

12 Prenatal Appointments

Although your body accomplishes the true work of pregnancy, prenatal care is an important and effective way to prevent and treat pregnancy complications, and to guide you in taking care of yourself and your baby. Prenatal visits can be fun; your pregnancy is the center of attention, and you will be able to ask a lot of questions and (except for the earliest visits) hear the baby's heartbeat. Your partner should feel welcome at your prenatal visits. It is an opportunity for both parents to learn about the pregnancy and to have their questions answered.

Your First Prenatal Visit

The first prenatal appointment, which typically occurs eight to ten weeks into the pregnancy, is much like the preconception visit described in Chapter 3. You will be asked about your personal health, your partner's health, and each of your family histories (with careful attention to genetic conditions). The first prenatal visit and ultrasound appointments are the best ones to have your partner come to, if he can come to some but not all of them. He can provide his side of the family history, become more informed, and bond with the baby.

The prenatal visits were all very routine. My husband came with me to them when there was some big thing, like for the ultrasounds. (Heidi R., law professor)

At the first visit you will probably have a physical examination, routine blood work, urine testing, and a check for sexually transmitted infections. If you are due for a Pap test you may have it that day, and you can obtain health advice. HIV

YOUR BABY BOOK

Pregnancy is an exciting time of life, but with all you have to manage, your memories of it may soon disappear. To remember all about your pregnancy, consider keeping a record of the important events. A calendar for writing milestones like feeling the baby move or hearing the heartbeat can even include other aspects of your life such as travel, meetings, and when and how you tell your boss. When you have a moment later to look back on this remarkable stage, you'll no doubt marvel at the complexity of your full and interesting pregnant life.

testing is routine, and is mandatory in some states. One good reason for getting tested is that a mother who is HIV positive can take steps to prevent her baby from becoming infected during birth. If you don't get tested, you won't have this opportunity to protect your little one.

Your doctor or midwife will ask about your last period and will estimate how far along you are. If you have pregnancy symptoms, your practitioner can assess the severity and offer you suggestions or treatment. The most exciting part of the first visit may be hearing the baby's heartbeat. You can expect to first hear the heartbeat, using an amplifying device called a Doppler, between nine and twelve weeks; how early depends on the position of your uterus and how thin you are.

I loved hearing the heartbeat. It's pretty amazing to contemplate the tiny human being growing within! (Edie U., school psychologist)

By the time you hear the heartbeat, the risk of miscarriage has declined to about 1 percent. If you were waiting to tell everyone until the likelihood of miscarriage had diminished, you are there. The only other obstetrical reason to wait is if you are concerned about finding a problem during first or second trimester ultrasounds or genetic testing. For this reason, some families hold off telling casual acquaintances until they have completed fetal screening.

Many practitioners routinely perform an ultrasound at the first appointment to double-check how far along you are; others do so only if there is a medical reason, like vaginal bleeding or pelvic pain. A woman who has previously miscarried may want the reassurance of hearing her baby's heartbeat or seeing it on ultrasound as early as possible.

Ultrasound

Ultrasound (sometimes referred to as sonography) uses sound waves to make images of internal structures. Ultrasound can be transabdominal, which creates an image through the lower abdomen, or transvaginal, in which a condom-covered probe is placed into the vagina for a closer view. Although ultrasound has never been shown to be dangerous to human fetuses, it can't be assumed to be totally innocuous. Health experts agree that ultrasound should not be used excessively if no medical benefit is anticipated, and they debate whether any ultrasound is necessary for most expectant mothers. In the United States, more than 65 percent of pregnant women have at least one ultrasound.

Decision Points

At your OB visits you will probably have some decisions to make about what types of testing you want. Most tests are routine and don't have personal or social implications; but other tests, particularly genetic ones, are optional and can be declined or sought after. Your values and beliefs play a role in whether to get this sort of fetal assessment, so your doctor or midwife can't really decide for you.

Some genetic conditions are more common in certain ethnic groups. For a list, see Appendix A. Parental testing, like checking to see if you carry the gene for the lung disease cystic fibrosis, can be done before conception, although many women don't get tested until they are pregnant. Other tests check the fetus, either indirectly through the mother's blood or ultrasound, or directly, with chorionic villus sampling (CVS) or amniocentesis. Fetal evaluation is done between ten and twenty weeks, depending on the test.

The purpose of screening the fetus for genetic findings is to provide the family with information, and to allow time for termination of pregnancy should the parents choose that option. Sometimes knowing about a condition ahead of

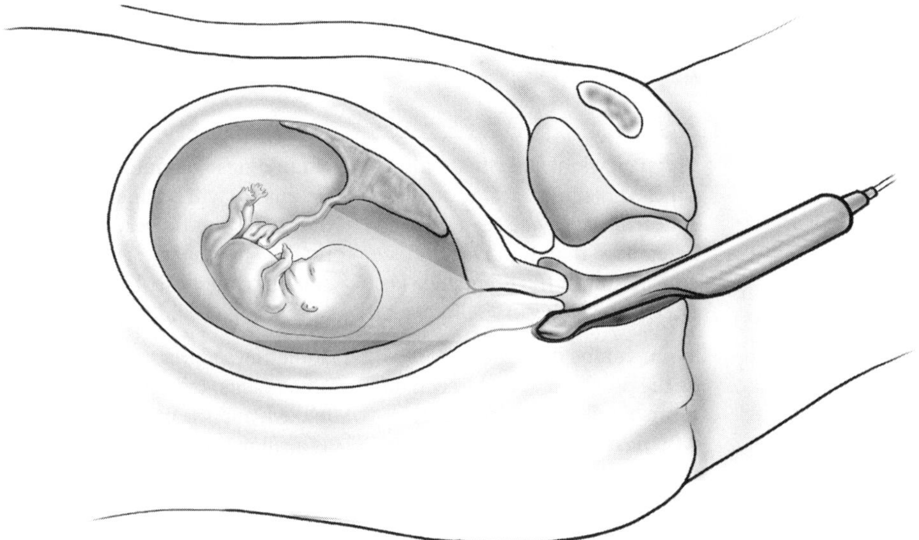

Transvaginal ultrasound uses sound waves to see the uterus through the back of the vagina.

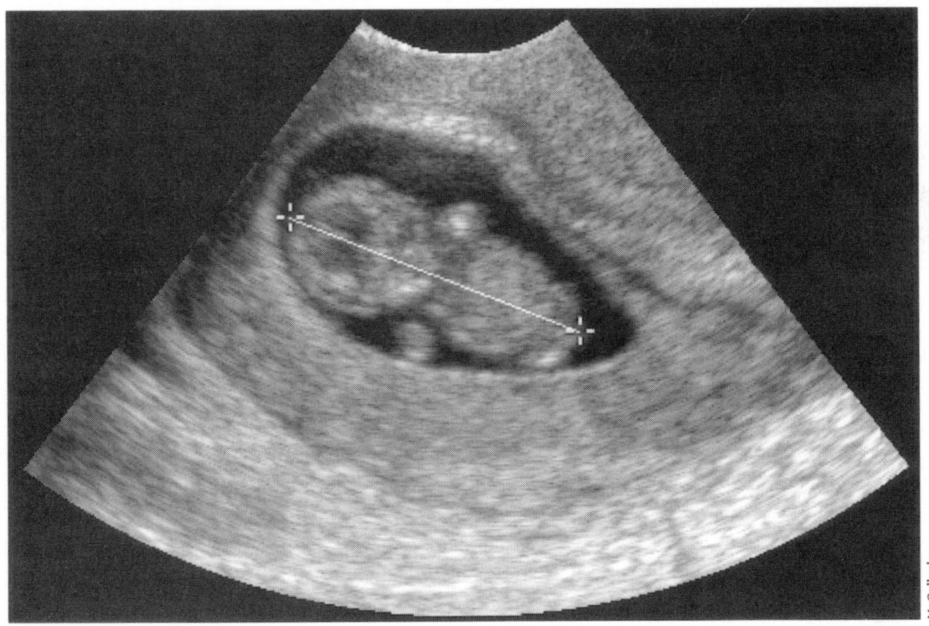

M. Gallogly

The first trimester embryo is measured from head to bottom; the measurement is called the crown-rump length.

Common Ultrasound Findings in the First Trimester

First trimester ultrasound finding	*Description*	*What does it mean?*
Normal pregnancy	Pregnancy looks like it should for the presumed gestational age. A heartbeat may be seen if it has been more than four weeks since conception (if the pregnancy is later than week six)	No findings guarantee that the pregnancy will be fine, but a normal ultrasound is very reassuring that the pregnancy is where it should be (not tubal) and that miscarriage is unlikely
Twins	Twins can be detected as soon as the pregnancy can be seen on ultrasound. Once two fetuses with heartbeats are seen, the pregnancy is likely to continue to be twins. Two babies in the same sac are always identical twins. Most identical twins, however, and all fraternal twins, have their own amniotic sacs, a much safer situation that avoids the risk of the babies' becoming tangled in each other's umbilical cords	Sometimes a pregnancy starts off as twins, but one doesn't make it and the other continues as a singleton. If early ultrasound weren't done, the family would not have to deal with this disturbing knowledge. Most twins identified by ultrasound, however, continue as twin pregnancies. If an early ultrasound isn't done, twins will show themselves later on, either during a routine ultrasound, or during prenatal visits when the uterus is found to be bigger than expected
Date discrepancy: more advanced than expected	The gestational sac or crown-rump length of the embryo measures larger than expected	A larger than expected pregnancy in the first trimester means that you are further along than the age that was calculated by your last period
Date discrepancy: less advanced than expected	The gestational sac or crown-rump length of the embryo measures smaller than expected	A smaller than expected pregnancy in the first trimester may indicate that the pregnancy is younger than the age that was calculated by the last period. If no heartbeat is seen, however, the embryo may have stopped growing and be destined to miscarry

Sometimes ultrasound indicates miscarriage or finds an abnormality. For more information on these and other complications, see Appendix B.

time can help the doctors and the family prepare for a baby with special needs. But not all parents want all this information. It is really important to understand what tests are being done and what an abnormal result might mean.

First Trimester Genetic Screening

No one wants to think about the possibility that her baby might have a birth defect. Yet about 3 percent of newborns have some sort of anatomical or genetic variation, and 1 percent have significant alterations. Some of these can be identified during pregnancy if the right tests are done. The two most common types of conditions that may be diagnosed during pregnancy are:

1. Structural disorders, such as spina bifida (incomplete coverings over the spinal cord) and congenital heart defects.
2. Conditions involving extra chromosomes—such as Down syndrome (DS), which is associated with mild to moderate mental retardation and possible anatomical birth defects.

Often *screening* tests are done first, and if the findings are suspicious, more definitive *diagnostic* tests are performed.

The Difference between Screening Tests and Diagnostic Tests

Screening tests identify those who might be at a higher risk than expected, but such tests don't diagnose a specific problem. That is, an abnormal result on a screening test such as a blood sample or ultrasound measurement doesn't tell us for certain that a baby has a particular condition; it is simply an indicator of risk. Many women have "false positive" screening test results and after further evaluation (and a few sleepless nights) they discover their baby is fine. From the doctor's perspective, the purpose of screening is to sort patients into two groups: those who require more testing and those who don't. About 5 percent of women who undergo screening will receive an abnormal result, but *most mothers with abnormal test results are carrying normal, healthy babies.*

Knowing what you would do with an abnormal result can help to guide your decisions. For instance, if you would terminate a Down syndrome pregnancy, you need to know if your fetus has Down syndrome in order to make that decision.

Even though Down syndrome is more common in older moms, any age mother can have a baby with Down's. If you don't have the testing done and the fetus does have Down syndrome, your life will be changed, because you won't have the opportunity to terminate. But if you would continue a pregnancy with Down syndrome, the value in testing is only to be prepared when the baby comes; your life overall probably won't be much different if you decline screening. For this reason, many of my patients who wouldn't terminate under any circumstances decline most of the available screening tests.

If you do take a screening test, you have to be prepared for a positive result because these occur in about one of every twenty women tested. Think of screening as a two-step process in which the first test might get you off the hook from having to do the second test. If you receive a message from the office saying you need further testing, don't panic—just call in and set up your diagnostic test, to clarify whether there really is a problem. If you are unsure what to do, your doctor or a genetic counselor can help guide you.

First Trimester Fetal Screening Tests

Many different strategies incorporating ultrasound and/or blood work can be used to screen for Down syndrome and other fetal conditions during the first trimester, if testing is desired. Not all tests are available in all areas; your practitioner can tell you what tests are available to you.

- Ultrasound. From ten weeks until the sixth day of the thirteenth week, prenatal ultrasound can identify anatomical changes, including a neck measurement called nuchal translucency, that are associated with Down syndrome and several other conditions. If this scan is available in your area your practitioner might refer you to a specialist to have it done; many OBs have been trained in basic ultrasound but lack the specialized skills necessary to distinguish subtle differences in fetal anatomy. Unfortunately, even in expert hands, first trimester ultrasound findings aren't very specific—they can be abnormal and the baby is fine, or normal and the baby is affected by a chromosomal condition. Ultrasound markers like nuchal translucency just lean us toward or away from further testing. For example, if the findings are suspicious, your doctors might recommend CVS at eleven weeks, and if they are borderline, they might counsel you to wait until sixteen weeks for a quad screen (blood tests that recalculate risk level) or amniocentesis. The strategy you develop with your practitioner for how to manage abnormal results will depend on what tests are available in your area, as well as your and your doctor's assessment of the risks and benefits of the different options.

- First trimester maternal serum (blood) screening. New blood tests that are similar to the traditional second trimester quad screen test (but used earlier in pregnancy) have been developed to help estimate the risk of Down syndrome. These approaches involve measuring pregnancy-associated plasma protein A, or PAPP-A, and a version of the pregnancy hormone called free beta hCG in your blood. First trimester screening is already routine at some centers, and will probably become more widespread as the accuracy improves and practitioners become convinced of its advantages.

We were on tour and our second violinist got results of her screening test and it was positive for Down syndrome. We couldn't go home for five days. It was really hard. Eventually she and her husband decided they would continue the pregnancy anyway. And then they had the amnio and it was fine. (Annie F., classical violinist)

Diagnostic Testing

Diagnostic tests are taken to find out for sure whether a fetus has a serious abnormality. They are done when the risk of having a significant genetic condition is high, and when the parents want to know (perhaps because they are trying to figure out whether to continue the pregnancy). The risk assessment that determines whether a diagnostic test is the right next step may be based on a screening test result, or other factors such as maternal age.

In the future, techniques will probably be developed to isolate fetal cells from the mother's circulation. These cells will be obtained simply by drawing blood from the mom; laboratory testing will avoid the risks associated with amniocentesis and CVS. Until this is available, however, obtaining fetal cells requires "invasive" testing.

- CVS

  During chorionic villus sampling (CVS), a tiny piece of placenta is removed for testing. A needle is placed either through the mother's abdomen or up through the vagina and cervix, and a pinch of the placenta is obtained (all while watching with ultrasound to keep the fetus out of harm's way). Chromosomes can be grown from this tissue and evaluated for Down syndrome and other conditions. The best thing about CVS is that the results are available much sooner than from amniocentesis, allowing earlier decisions about pregnancy termination. CVS is done by doctors specially trained in this technique. The risk of miscarriage caused by the procedure, usually estimated to be 1 percent, may be higher than the risk from amniocentesis. As centers gain experience, their success rates improve. If CVS is available in your area, the team will be able to give you their statistics on miscarriage and other potential complications.

- Amniocentesis

  In amniocentesis, often called amnio, a sample of the fluid around the baby is drawn out with a needle, and then tested for evidence of genetic abnormalities. Amniocentesis typically isn't done until about sixteen weeks. For more information, skip ahead to Chapter 17.

Proceeding Directly to Diagnostic Testing

The chance of Down syndrome increases with maternal age (see the table in Chapter 17). First or second trimester screening test results, which take age into account, recalculate the odds specifically for that pregnancy—for better or worse. But blood tests and ultrasounds will not detect every case of Down syndrome—they just help to recalculate the chances. Depending on which tests are used, screening actually misses between 5 and 30 percent of all cases of Down's. If 100 percent detection is very important to you, you may not want to bother with screening, since you will need amniocentesis or CVS for definitive results.

These concepts are complex and confusing. Many families find the decision-making easier after they talk to their practitioner or consult with a genetic counselor, particularly if age or test results put them at elevated risk.

Genetic Counseling

Genetic counseling can be immensely helpful in sorting through the ever-expanding list of available tests. Genetic counselors have two sets of skills: they provide accurate information about genetic conditions, and they are true counselors in that they help you understand and sort through your options based on your own values and beliefs. Health insurance typically pays for genetic counseling if you are over thirty-five years old, have risk factors for genetic problems (such as multiple miscarriages or a previous baby with a birth defect), or receive an abnormal screening test result during this pregnancy. Lower-risk couples may also benefit from genetic counseling, although they may have to pay for the consultation. A genetic counselor can help you understand your risks and decide on the approach that's right for you.

Remember, many options and strategies are available, but testing isn't for everyone. *Before any genetic investigation, be sure to think through what you would do with an abnormal result.* Use your prenatal visits to get all your questions answered.

Scheduling Prenatal Appointments

Appointments are typically scheduled monthly until 28–32 weeks, then every two weeks, and in the ninth month, every week. If you have medical problems or complications of pregnancy, you may be seen more often. If you are low risk, fewer appointments may be necessary. The first visit is usually the most time-consuming because it involves taking a medical history, getting a physical exam, and having a Pap smear if you are due. Until the last month, routine appointments will consist of checking your blood pressure, weight, and urine, measuring how big your uterus is getting, and listening to the baby's heartbeat. Your practitioner will ask you how you are doing and guide you with what to expect over the next few weeks, but feel free to bring a list of questions. You will probably get a lot of advice from friends and acquaintances; this is your chance to get health advice from a professional.

Even though I was an OB nurse I found that when I became the patient I knew nothing. I frequently worried about things that as a nurse I would not

have worried about. I asked questions that I knew the answer to but just felt so unsure about everything. (Susan H., nurse)

Hints for Managing Prenatal Appointments

- Compose a list of questions so you don't forget what you—or your partner—wanted to ask.
- Although the first appointments in the morning or right after lunch usually run more on time, waiting in doctors' offices is almost inevitable. Bring work or pleasure reading with you, or do some minor task for your work, to help prevent frustration. If the doctor's office often runs late, it may help to call ahead to see how things are flowing.
- Try hard to avoid scheduling an appointment for before you have a meeting or other important timed obligation. You never know when there will be a delay, or if your doctor will send you for an ultrasound or some other test right from your visit.
- If possible, scheduling your next few prenatal appointments all at once may help you to get times that are convenient, and allow you to arrange work obligations around your prenatal care.

Doctor's appointments were time-consuming because I always had to wait. I would be typing on my Blackberry or editing briefs balanced on my knees. My doctor was only a few blocks from work, which shortened the time I had to be away. (Kendra F., civil litigator)

Sometimes OBs run late—but think when you are waiting how some woman may be waiting there when the doctor is out delivering your baby—so it all comes around. (Jane S., state governor)

Part 4

Going Public (Weeks 14–26)

Most women experience a renewed sense of energy during the second trimester, and feel more comfortable in their bodies and with the concept that a baby is on the way. Pregnancy also becomes a more visible and public event, a transformation that brings new pleasures and an occasional challenge. This section will review normal physical and emotional transitions, how your baby and placenta are developing, and second trimester fetal testing. Employer and coworker reactions to the pregnancy, making accommodations at work, and the complex legal issues related to maternity leave will all be addressed. And finally, I'll give you some guidelines for diet, exercise, and travel, as well as advice to help you start preparing for labor and birth.

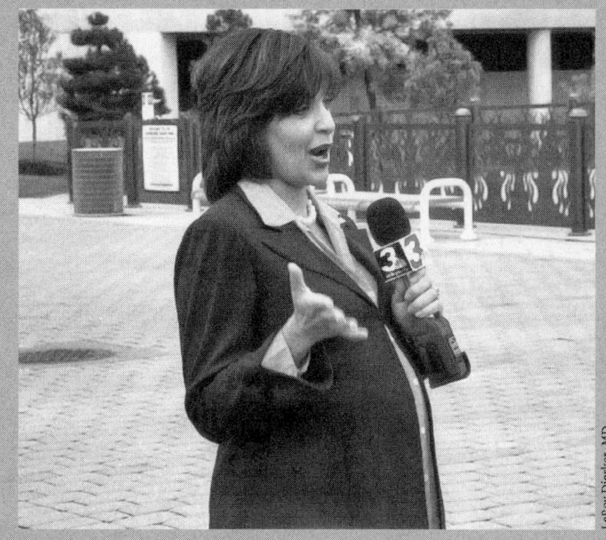

LeRoy Dierker, MD

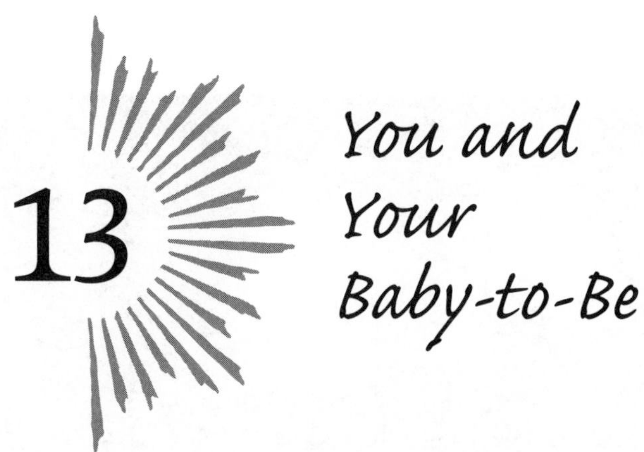

13 You and Your Baby-to-Be

The second trimester is sometimes called the "honeymoon" phase of pregnancy. The exhaustion and queasiness of the first trimester usually start to resolve, and most women don't feel uncomfortably big. Although some women still have nausea, and others experience new discomforts, for many moms-to-be, this part of pregnancy is an enjoyable time to settle into a new identity and begin planning for the baby's arrival.

The fatigue and nausea subsided and the second trimester was lovely. (Zoe B., inventory manager)

I loved being pregnant. I felt healthy and strong, like I was glowing. I could be a baby-making machine. (Jan R., state attorney)

Your little one is growing at a rapid rate. During the second trimester, he matures from being the size of a gerbil, totally dependent on your oxygen and nutrients, to a functioning twenty-six-week baby who, with the help of modern medical care, could potentially survive outside the womb.

The Placenta, Cord, Membranes, and Amniotic Fluid

The fetus floats in a sac of warm amniotic fluid. The placenta, attached to the wall of your uterus, comes in close contact with your blood. In this way, the fetal blood, which is pumped to the convoluted surface of the placenta, obtains oxygen and nutrients and eliminates waste. The refreshed fetal blood then flows back through the umbilical cord into the baby.

From this point on, amniotic fluid is primarily made up of fetal urine. That

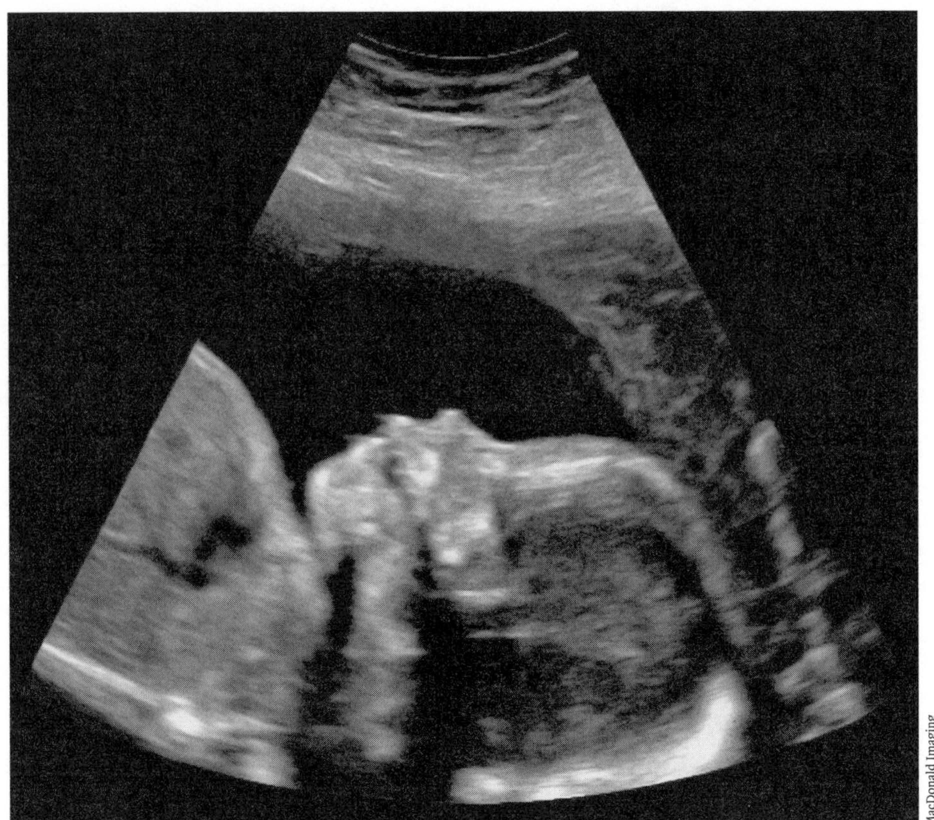

MacDonald Imaging

Sometimes ultrasound catches the baby's face in profile

may sound strange, but remember that the baby eliminates waste through the umbilical cord, not in urine and feces, so the amniotic fluid is just a sterile solution of water, salts, and some fetal cells. The body systems need practice for their roles after birth; the fetus swallows amniotic fluid, and then excretes fluid through the kidneys, recycling. Fetal breathing movements also carry amniotic fluid in and out of the lungs, a process important for lung development.

The absolute earliest that babies can survive is twenty-three to twenty-five weeks, when the tiny air sacs of the lungs start to form. Until then, the fetus is dependent on oxygen that comes from the mother through the umbilical cord and placenta. Under most circumstances, the baby is better off inside its mother until after thirty-seven weeks; the temperature, oxygen, nutrients, sounds, and light in the womb are just what a baby needs.

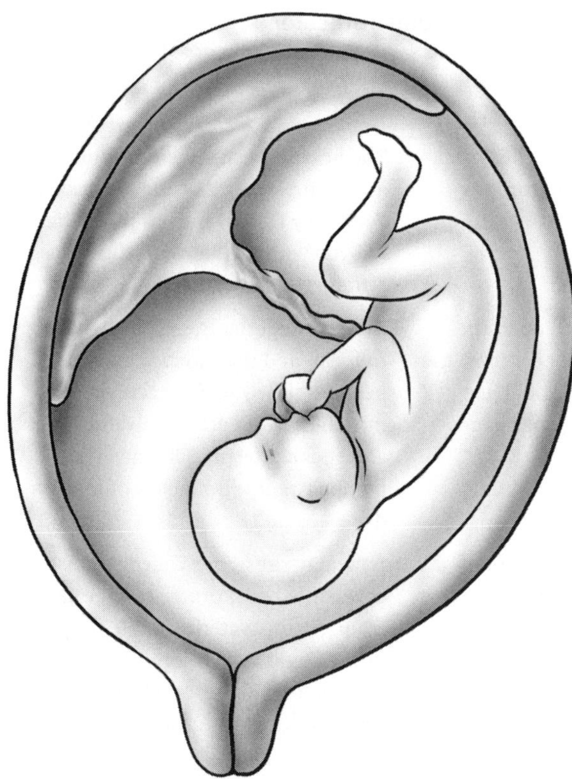

The fetus floats in a sac of warm amniotic fluid. The placenta, attached to the wall of the uterus, comes in close contact with the mother's blood so that the fetal blood, which is pumped to the convoluted surface of the placenta, can obtain oxygen and nutrients from the mother and eliminate waste. The refreshed fetal blood then flows back through the umbilical cord into the baby.

Interacting with Your Baby

Hearing the heartbeat during a prenatal visit is often your first objective experience of your little one. Some parents record the heart sounds, to play back for family and friends, or maybe to save for a multimedia "baby book." After about twenty weeks, the heartbeat may be heard with a simple stethoscope by pressing firmly with the concave "bell" side. It's always easier to hear if the mother is slim, and if the placenta isn't right in front of the baby. The fetal heart rate is usually between 110 and 160 beats per minute—a lot faster than an adult's. Contrary to rumors, the heart rate doesn't foretell the baby's sex. A heart rate slower than 100 beats a minute is usually the mom's. Entrepreneurial companies sell amplification instruments for home use, but you don't need to listen to the baby's heartbeat at home. Soon you will have flutters and kicks reassuring you that all is well.

Fetal Growth and Development in the Second Trimester

Gestation	*Weight*	*Size*	*Highlights of Development*
14 wks	Over an ounce	Three inches from head to rump	The heart, intestines, arms, and legs are all in place, maturing and growing. Your baby already moves quite a bit—but you won't feel it until the kicks get stronger
16 wks	Four ounces	Curled up in the "fetal position," the baby would just fit along your hand	Eyelids, fingernails, and toenails begin to form, and the external genitals become clearly male or female. Eye movements, breathing, swallowing, and sucking begin. The tiny heart pumps twenty-five quarts of blood a day
18 wks	Just over six ounces, the same as a tin of tuna fish	Six inches long (The placenta is almost the same size as the baby)	A creamy substance called vernix now covers the body, protecting the skin from getting waterlogged. Fingerprints begin to develop. The baby is starting to take in sounds and light, so while you are trying to feel your baby move, your baby also is starting to perceive you
20 wks	Ten ounces (about the size of a can of soup)	About seven inches	Girls' ovaries already have all their eggs; boys' testes, although still located in the abdomen, have begun to descend toward the scrotum. The fetal nerves are becoming coated with myelin, a fatty material that speeds nerve signal transmission. The fetus has periods of sleep and wakefulness, and on ultrasound may be seen sucking his thumb
22 wks	Just under a pound	About nine inches long	A fine hair called lanugo, which helps to hold the creamy vernix on the skin, now covers the head and body. Brain growth accelerates—and continues at a rapid pace until age five

Fetal Growth and Development in the Second Trimester (Continued)

Gestation	*Weight*	*Size*	*Highlights of Development*
24 wks	About one pound, five ounces.	Almost a foot from head to toe	Calcium hardens the fetal bones. The three tiny bones of the ear—the hammer, anvil, and stirrup—are now rigid enough to transmit sound. Your baby can hear your breathing, heartbeat, and voice, as well as stomach gurgles. The eyelids, which were protectively fused closed for the past few months, can now open. The fetus may blink when startled by a noise. Some babies born at twenty-four weeks survive
26 wks	Just under two pounds	Thirteen inches from head to toe	Twenty-six-week babies have a good chance of survival—with months of neonatal intensive care. Some (but not all) of these very early preemies have normal physical and intellectual development

Fetal Movement

First-time moms usually start to sense fetal movement, a moment called quickening, between weeks eighteen and twenty-two; experienced mothers have these sensations as early as fifteen weeks, and almost always by twenty weeks. Why do repeat moms feel movement sooner? No one knows for sure, but it may be that mothers who have previously experienced these sensations, which can feel like flutters or tiny pokes, recognize them earlier. Until about twenty-four weeks, it is normal not to feel the baby move every day.

We had our twenty-week ultrasound done on Monday. I've started to feel little flutters here and there (usually after I eat too much), but not anything too strong. (Jen B., dance teacher)

TWINS

You probably know by now if you are having twins. Between prenatal examinations and the almost universal use of ultrasound, surprise twin pregnancies are very unusual today.

Since twins tend to be a little smaller, you may wonder whether these fourteen- to twenty-six-week weights are accurate for multiples. Yes! Twins typically grow and develop at the same rate as singletons until about thirty-two weeks. After that point, the two babies pretty much share the normal amount of weight gain. At birth, then, twins are usually smaller than their single counterparts, both because they tend to be born earlier, and because those last few pounds have been distributed between them. For this reason, your weight gain is especially important for helping your twins grow to their potential.

When I was pregnant with my first, we went to see* Stomp. *The baby was kicking the whole time, and I was cracking up. I thought, this kid's got rhythm. (Heidi R., law professor)

Over time, you will find that your baby's movements become predictable. As he gets bigger, he may even push back if you poke at him. Noise or music may cause changes in activity. By twenty-two to twenty-three weeks a fetus will startle upon hearing a loud noise, but then become accustomed to it. A different pitch noise will again trigger a startle response. This is one of the earliest examples of learning.

Fetal Learning

Speaking of learning—you may have heard that babies recognize music and speech that they heard during fetal life. It's true! In numerous scientific experiments, mothers either read aloud a passage from Dr. Seuss's *Cat in the Hat* or played the same music each day. Then, when the baby was between a few

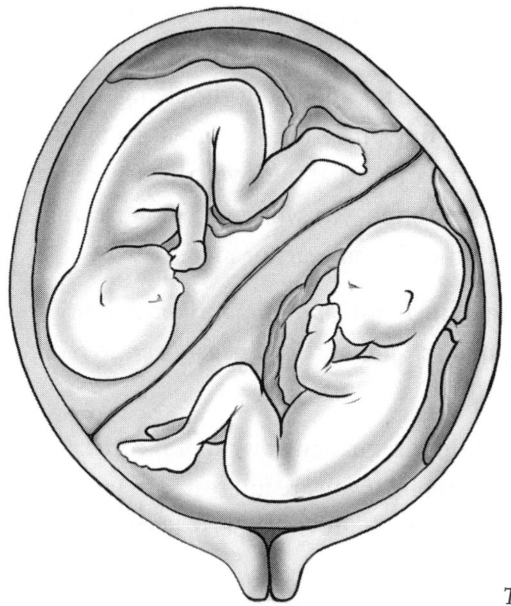

Twins at twenty weeks

days and a year old, the music or passage was repeated. Babies responded to the known sounds differently than they did to unfamiliar music or words; in contrast, control-group babies who didn't have the repeated stimulation in utero didn't differentiate between different works. This learning didn't occur until after thirty weeks of gestation. Although fetuses begin to hear in the second trimester, learning to recognize sounds doesn't begin until later. For fun, you can decide now what you want your baby to remember from his fetal life, and about ten weeks before your due date get started with your own experiments.

During my last few months of pregnancy, my husband would read to the baby—something he still enjoys doing with both kids. (Sandy B., social worker)

Your Inner World

As the baby grows more real to you, your fantasy life may become pretty active. You will probably want to talk about the baby and your pregnancy and may feel drawn to other mothers. Websites and books about pregnancy are suddenly more interesting, as you find yourself daydreaming about this new life inside of you.

It is normal to have fears, too, about the baby and about the changes in your life. Women who tend to obsess about things may find themselves convinced that the baby will be malformed or ill. Remember that these worries are common and not a sign or premonition. If you ask around, you will find that most women worry during pregnancy (and for the next eighteen years or more).

For me, being pregnant was a time of such anticipation, optimism, and dreaming . . . and fear, insecurity, and self-doubt. I had never been so scared or so happy! (Cindy M., supermodel)

Dreams and nightmares may be wild in pregnancy. A written record of your dreams will make your baby book truly unique. If you are interested in pregnancy dreams, check out the book *Dreaming for Two* by Sindy Greenberg, Elyse Kroll, and Hillary Grill.

I had a dream I left her in the car unloading groceries. In the dream I couldn't get used to having a baby and I forgot about her. (Danielle R., trust analyst)

I dreamt I gave birth to a small kitten—in the dream it was a practice run for the real thing. I was glad it was so small and soft. (Marge G., obstetrician)

"Pregnancy Brain"

Many women feel scatterbrained during pregnancy. Reseach on this subject has been unconvincing; nevertheless, forgetfulness is a shared perception of many mothers-to-be. It could be caused by distraction from the changes in your body or thoughts about the baby, or it could be biochemical, if it is true. Staying organized and making lists seem to help most women remain competent at work and at home. Keeping your sense of humor helps, too—remember that this condition is temporary and will resolve over time.

Toward the end of the pregnancy, I was scatter-brained. I would work on a project and forget why I was doing what I was doing. We were all laughing at it. (Annette M., store manager)

I was very forgetful during pregnancy. Sometimes I put the kids' shoes on the wrong feet. I'd forget my lunch, my purse . . . I think it was hormones. Now my baby is four weeks old and despite the sleep deprivation I am more organized and less forgetful. (Jennifer A., secretary)

Stress

You may find that pregnancy makes you more emotionally sensitive, which can affect your stress level at work and at home. Several stress-management techniques are safe and beneficial for pregnant women:

DEAL WITH THE STRESS CONSTRUCTIVELY

- Take a minute for you. Excuse yourself from a volatile situation and go to a private place to calm down. Take slow deep breaths and clear your mind.
- Call a good friend to vent.
- Read *Getting to Yes*, an excellent book about negotiating and a terrific resource for dealing with stressful interactions.

SOOTHE YOURSELF

- Schedule daily aerobic exercise into your life.
- Start to practice the calming techniques you plan to use for labor—Lamaze breathing, self-hypnosis, or deep relaxation.
- Stretch gently at your desk. Each of the stretches on pages 152–153 can be held for five seconds, in sets of five or ten unless otherwise specified, and repeated throughout the day.
- Listen to music (take a ten-minute MP3 break—while you take a walk—or play music as you work).
- Sink into a warm bath when you get home.
- Try yoga classes, or tapes for home use.
- Knit, play a musical instrument, fill in a crossword puzzle, or do any hobby that takes your full attention.
- Meditate (Belleruth Naparstek has created some terrific guided-imagery CDs that can be found in your local bookstore or ordered over the Internet).
- Get a massage.

STRETCHES YOU CAN DO AT YOUR DESK

Neck retractions
Shoulder rolls
Shoulder shrugs
Shoulder blade pinch
Arm extensions
Touch the sky

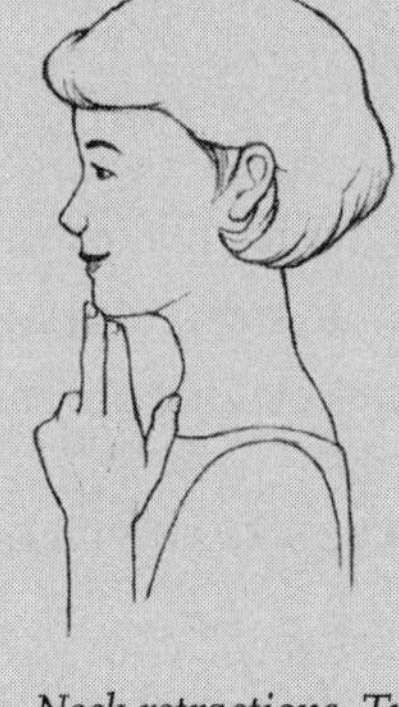
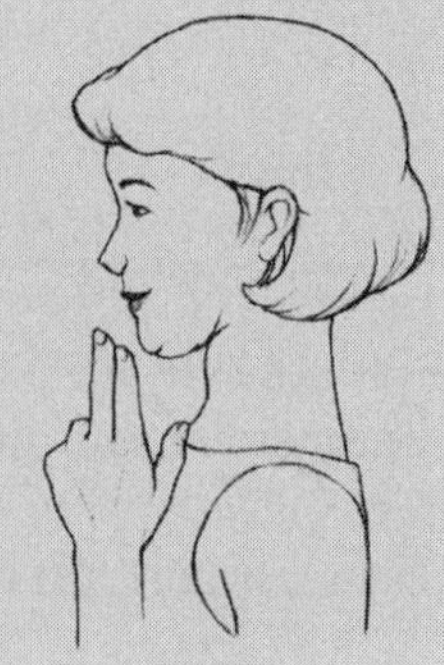

Neck retractions. Tuck your chin down and move your head back. Don't tilt your head—look straight in front of you. Hold for five seconds, then release slowly, without letting your head protrude forward.

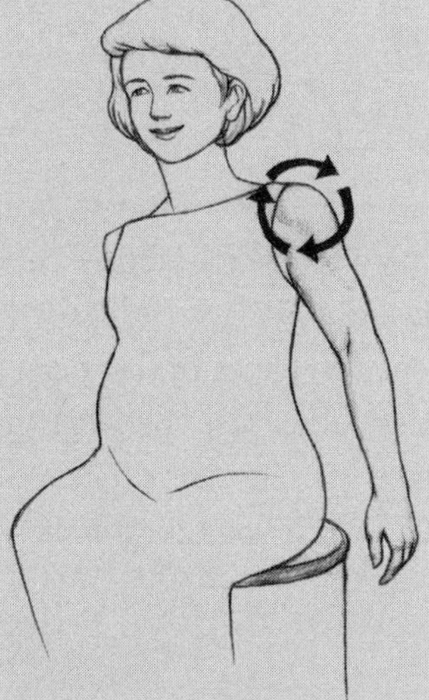

Shoulder rolls. Roll your shoulders forward and up, then backward and down. Always circle in a front to back direction. Make ten circles.

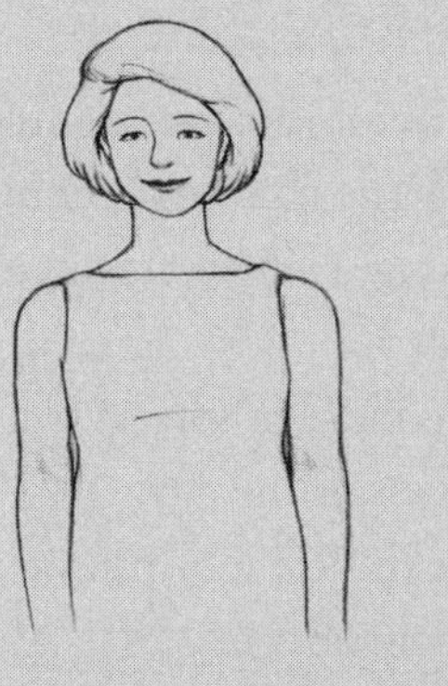
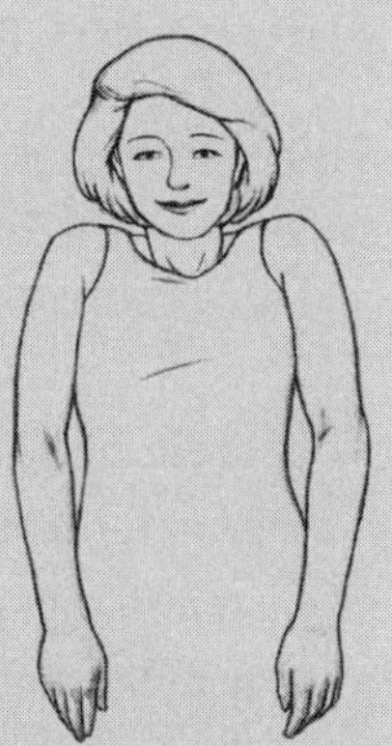

Shoulder shrugs. Bring your shoulders up toward your ears, hold for five seconds, and release.

Shoulder blade pinches. Sit up straight with upper arms at your sides and elbows bent. Keep your shoulders down—don't shrug. Pinch your shoulder blades together, keeping your upper arms at your sides, hold for five seconds, then release.

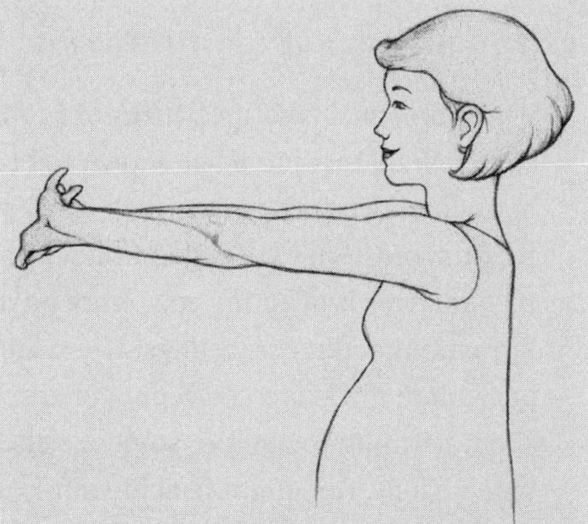

Arm extensions. Sit up straight, and reach your arms out in front of you. Lock your fingers together, then invert your hands so your palms face away. Hold that stretch for a count of ten, then reverse the steps and release. Repeat once.

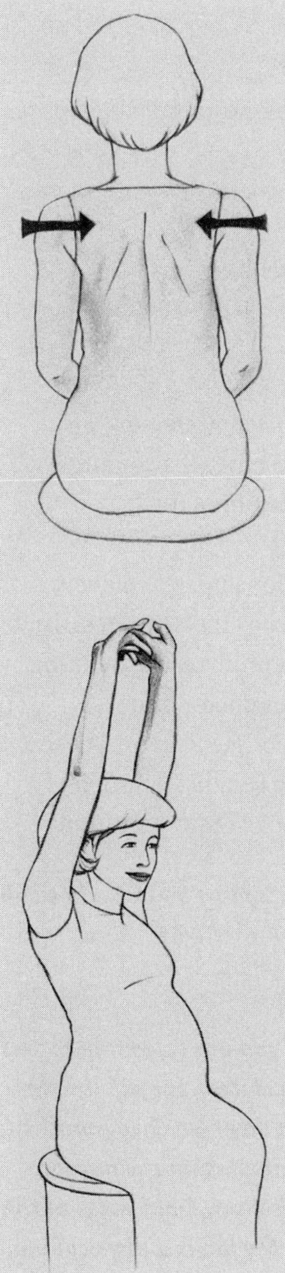

Touch the sky. Sit up straight. Reach above your head, clasp your hands, and invert your hands so your palms face up. Be careful not to arch your back. Hold for a count of ten, then reverse the steps and release. Repeat once.

DE-STRESS YOUR LIFE

- Get more organized.
- Delegate some work.
- Don't seek stress (for example, by taking on excess work, moving houses, changing jobs, or starting major projects).
- Learn to say no to requests that don't serve your goals.
- Get enough sleep—or at least rest.
- Remember to have fun—schedule time for yourself.

IF YOU ARE REALLY STRUGGLING

- Find a therapist who specializes in cognitive-behavioral therapy, an approach that research has shown to be most effective. If a cognitive-behavioral therapist isn't available, ask your practitioner for a recommendation for any good therapist.
- If your stress is affecting your work or your relationships; if you have intrusive thoughts or feelings; if you are falling back on cigarettes, drugs, or alcohol; if you aren't sleeping or aren't eating; or if you are thinking about harming yourself or someone else, call your doctor or nurse immediately. You might benefit from counseling or medication. Although medicines aren't the first-line choice, they can be beneficial during pregnancy, and may spare you and your loved ones needless suffering.

I went to work, went home, ate, and I was in the bed by 7 PM. So basically that was nine months of sleeping and working. (Annette M., store manager)

I believe your attitude affects your experience. If you are expecting to feel poorly you will; if you feel strong and expect to feel like yourself, it helps. I tried to keep my life as normal as possible. One day I was five months pregnant and found myself pulling two heavy suitcases up the outdoor jetway stairs in 100-degree heat thinking, "This is crazy," but most of the time I felt fine doing things I was used to doing. My job is a physical job, but it was really fine. (Susan G., commercial airline pilot)

Seek out people you know that will be supportive, so that they can help create an environment in which you feel like "everyone is behind you." I felt like everyone was my cheerleader. (Mary O., vice president, financial services corporation)

My mom had ten kids and gave me the best advice—don't worry so much. The things that stress you out will pass, and if you spend all your time worrying you can forget to enjoy it. (Eileen M., weather reporter)

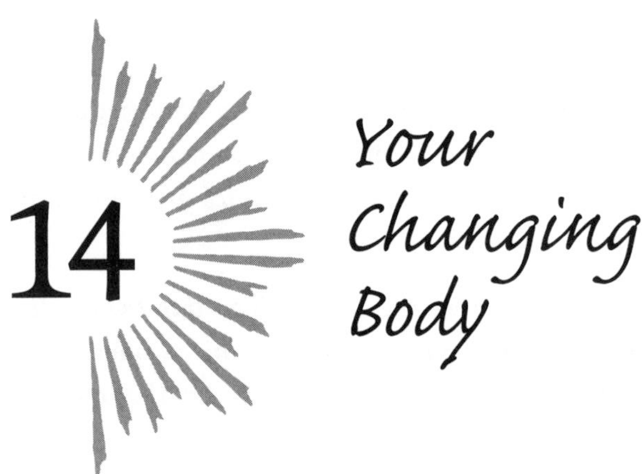

14 Your Changing Body

Your pregnancy becomes visible in the second trimester—on the earlier side for women who have had babies before, and maybe as late as the third trimester for some first-time moms. But everybody "shows" a little bit differently, depending on how fast your baby is growing, how much weight you've added overall, and how you dress and carry yourself. Sometimes it can be frustrating to look as though only your waistline is enlarging, when actually your whole life is expanding.

I was working in the cardiac intensive care unit when I was pregnant the first time (at the young age of twenty-three and horrified at what was happening to my youthful figure) when my head nurse, a rather blunt loudmouth, said to me one day as I was walking into a patient's room, "You know, Wendy, you're starting to look pregnant from behind." Amazing . . . (Wendy C., registered nurse)

People kept asking me if I was still running since I gained weight that first six months while I was hiding the pregnancy; they were relieved when I finally told them I was pregnant. One said, "Oh good, I thought you let yourself go." (Peggy L., nurse-administrator)

Getting Bigger

Many factors play into how you feel about your changing body shape: your body image before pregnancy, your overall well-being, how you feel about a baby growing inside you, and your outlook on becoming a mom. The reaction of your partner and others around you also has its effects.

At seventeen weeks, I've only gained a pound and a half so far. I find that hard to believe since it seems like my boobs weigh at least five pounds each. (Jen B., dance teacher)

When you're very pregnant, it's obvious and you can enjoy it. But earlier you don't feel pregnant, you just feel fat, and it makes you uncomfortable and insecure in your appearance. Here I was forty years old, always wanting children and feeling bad about the way I was looking. (Peggy L., nurse-administrator)

With my first baby (at twenty-two weeks, ten pounds of weight gain, and just barely into maternity clothes), a nurse at work came up behind me and loudly proclaimed, "Wow, Dr. H, you are carrying that baby all in your butt!" This resulted in a tunic shopping spree and weeks of self-consciousness. (Jill H., gynecologist)

I'm starting to look ridiculous when I teach my classes—my ballet skirt barely fits! (Jen B., dance teacher)

Optimal weight gain guidelines are pretty clear: twenty-five to thirty-five pounds for average-sized women, more if you are underweight or carrying twins, and less if you start off heavy. But you may know women who gained much more or less and had healthy pregnancies.

I gained forty-seven pounds with both pregnancies and lost it by a month. I think it was just what my body needed. (Jan R., state attorney)

We were vacationing near the world headquarters of Ben & Jerry's. At the time, they still sold seconds out of the factory, which we brought back to the condo. At my prenatal visit following that vacation, I'd gained nine pounds, and the doctor was concerned I might be carrying twins. I assured him that the only twins I had were my thighs, Ben & Jerry. (Deb L., writer)

THE PROBLEM WITH INADEQUATE WEIGHT GAIN

We women have been conditioned to watch our weight, so it may be hard to allow yourself to gain as you should. But babies need nutrition to grow, and sometimes if the mother doesn't gain enough weight, the baby's growth is restricted. Smaller babies may be easier to push out, but they are at risk for distress

WEIGHT GAIN FOR TWINS

Mothers carrying twins or more need to put on extra weight, and to be even more careful to get the needed calories, protein, vitamins, and minerals, so that the babies gain and grow to their potential. Research has shown that weight gain early in pregnancy is particularly important for good growth of twins—roughly a pound a week, for a total of about forty pounds.

during labor, learning problems in childhood, and possibly diabetes, hypertension, heart disease, and obesity later in life. One way to help your baby get enough nutrition is to get good nutrition yourself. Women who start off underweight are at the greatest risk for fetal growth restriction and may need to put on as much as forty pounds to help their babies thrive.

THE PROBLEM WITH EXCESS WEIGHT GAIN

It is also possible to gain too much weight. One problem with putting on a lot of weight is how distressing and difficult it can be to lose those pounds after the baby comes. It turns out that women who aren't back to their prepregnancy weight by two years postpartum are more likely to be heavier later in life.

I gained sixty pounds, and still have forty-five to lose three years later. (Zenia M., nurse's aide)

Some pregnancy complications are more common in women who gain excess weight—including gestational diabetes, unsuccessful induction of labor, lacerations of the birth canal, and cesarean section. Excess weight gain can be hard on the baby, too. Mothers who start off overweight or who gain excess weight are more likely to have larger babies, which can lead to difficult births. And overly plump newborns are more likely to struggle with weight later in life. (Although scientific evidence is still unclear whether this association is directly cause and effect: family eating habits, for example, may independently lead to both excess pregnancy weight gain and weight problems in children).

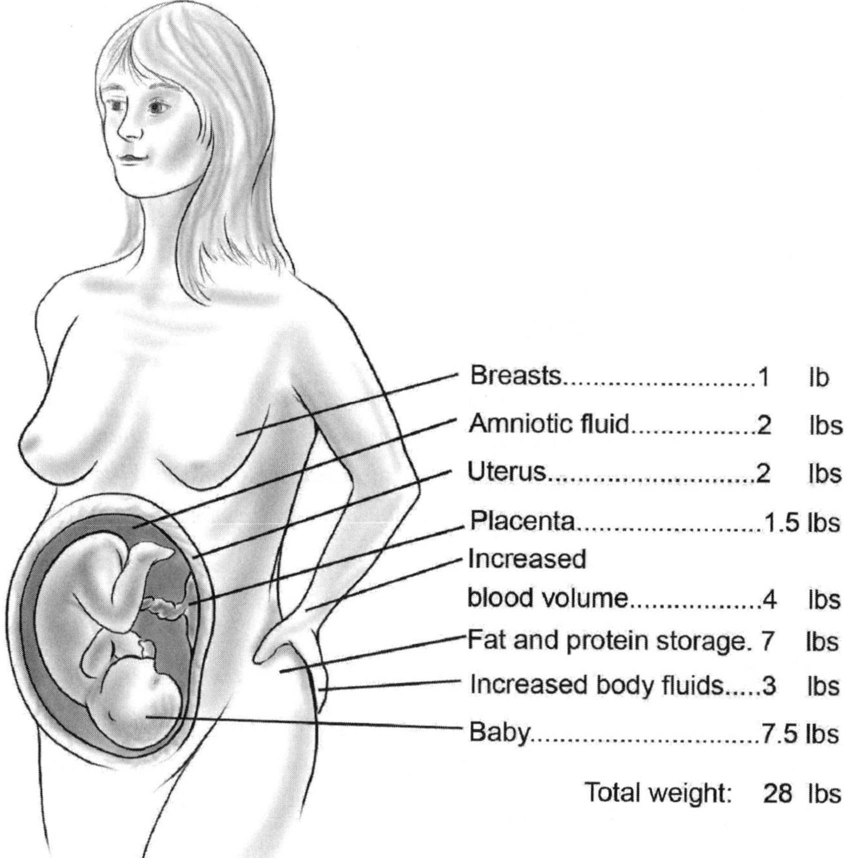

Weight gain in pregnancy: where does it go?

Sometimes excess weight gain is all water retention. You can tell you're retaining water if your hands and feet feel swollen, or if you gain more than five pounds in a week. If you are retaining water, it is not because you ate too much, and the swelling itself won't hurt your fetus; in fact, you will "pee out" excess fluid within a few weeks after birth. But severe water retention can be a sign of a serious pregnancy complication called pre-eclampsia, which occurs in late pregnancy. For this reason, you should *call your practitioner if you have rapid weight gain or severe swelling, particularly after twenty weeks; pre-eclampsia requires immediate medical evaluation.*

A gain of ten pounds during the first half of the pregnancy followed by a half a pound to a pound each week is optimal for most women. If you find you are gaining too much, look at your balance between exercise and diet. You can either ramp up your calorie expenditure through exercise, or dial down your calorie intake by eating lighter foods. Pregnancy is not a time to skip meals or go on a diet. You have to eat when you are hungry, but try for smaller portions and foods with fewer calories (like grapes instead of raisins, and skim milk instead of 2 percent). If you aren't gaining enough, add healthful snacks or small meals, or consider foods with a higher calorie density, like Boost or Ensure (milkshake-like supplements), or even real milkshakes every day.

Be comfortable. I bought regular clothing in bigger sizes. I found the pregnancy clothing horrendous (WHY do they make the stretch panels on pants a different color than the pants???) and unprofessional looking. I am a plus size and that just made it that much harder to find decent-looking clothing. (Jane J., advertising executive)

Clothing

Outfitting your changing body can be frustrating. Most women find that at some point their regular clothes don't fit any more, yet maternity wear doesn't feel—or fit—right. It's time to buy or borrow bigger clothes. (And don't give these clothes away when you outgrow them—you will need them again for a few months after the baby, before you fit back into your favorite jeans.) Some women find that "queen-size" underwear and pantyhose are less expensive and more comfortable than those marketed as maternity wear. If you need new bras after the seventh month and plan to breastfeed, it makes sense to purchase nursing bras, although they may be too small by the time the baby arrives.

I never liked maternity clothes. Period. Instead of buying the run-of-the-mill boring clothes, I simply purchased bigger clothes from a plus size store. It worked well. I was able to be stylish and comfortable. (Val P., administrative coordinator)

As my belly quickly grew, my figure-flattering polyester uniform pants didn't fit so well. I started wearing street clothes, which posed a problem. With no waist to hang a gun on, where does one carry her sidearm? A shoulder

PLUS-SIZE AND PREGNANT

If you started off pregnancy overweight, you are not alone. About 40 percent of women in their childbearing years weigh more than the ideal. Does being heavy cause complications of pregnancy? The extent of the risk depends on how overweight you are.

In order to take height into account, body mass index, or BMI, is used to assess for overweight. To calculate your BMI, use the table in Appendix A. But to give you a general idea, a five-foot tall woman weighing 155 pounds; a five-foot, four-inch woman weighing 175 pounds; and a five-foot, eight-inch woman weighing 200 pounds all have a BMI of thirty—and women with a BMI of thirty or more are at greater risk for:

- Gestational diabetes
- Having an overly large baby
- Needing a cesarean
- Developing blood clots in the legs or lungs
- Difficulties assessing the baby's well-being during prenatal care and throughout labor

Limiting your weight gain to about fifteen pounds with exercise and prudent eating (as well as getting tested for diabetes) will prevent some of these problems.

holster would have been an option but another female officer said how uncomfortable it was for her with her breasts growing, so I chose to wear an ankle holster with an Airweight .38 caliber revolver. Problem was, I was out of qualification with that particular weapon. I had to go to range. Well, the nurse was stumped when I posed the question, "Is it okay to go to the shooting range while pregnant?" (Tracy G., police officer)

Once you really need maternity clothes, you may want to try borrowing from relatives or friends; many mothers are happy to share, especially because these clothes are only useful for a short time. Just keep a list so you can return the (cleaned) items after your baby is born. When buying maternity outfits, be aware of the seasons. A navy blue wool dress purchased in winter when you are early in the second trimester may not work by the time the baby is due in late spring.

For six months I hid my first pregnancy. I just bought bigger clothes, and wore skirts with the zipper unzipped a couple of inches. After six months, I showed up in maternity clothes, which really make you look pregnant. (Peggy L., nurse-administrator)

Unbuttoned blazers from your regular wardrobe will continue to look okay as they dress up your pregnancy pants. (Ellen B., communications manager)

I was really lucky—I had a friend who had a nice collection of working maternity clothes that she lent to me. We passed a lot of things around the neighborhood—maternity clothes, baby clothes, baby car seats. (Anne O., director, nonprofit organization)

My company had a whole wardrobe of maternity uniforms that were available for me to order which were horrible. I ordered a maternity shirt, and it was the worst fit ever. It was perfectly straight, and came down past my knees. The maternity pants weren't much better. What I ended up doing was borrowing shirts and pants from larger guys for the last three months of the pregnancy. They were all very supportive and would let me borrow their extra uniforms. (Stephanie B., FedEx courier)

Trying to look professional during pregnancy can be an adventure. Many working women recommend trying to keep your overall look the same. A blazer over a maternity jumper can be comfortable, yet look polished. A few catalog companies cater to working women, offering clothes with a more professional look. Two maternity clothing websites with options for professional attire are www.maternitymall.com and www.lizlange.com. Also check out Lauren Sara's gorgeous book, *Expecting Style*.

My friends warned me that I'd be so sick of my maternity clothes that I'd never want to see them again. Boy, were they right! I splurged on a nice dress, a pair of jeans, and a couple of shirts for work. Otherwise, I tried not to spend too much money on clothes. I was thrilled to send all of my

maternity clothes to my sister-in-law when she found out she was pregnant. (Elizabeth S., online producer)

Common Second Trimester Symptoms

Although the second trimester is often a time when mothers feel pretty comfortable, some pregnancy symptoms can be a nuisance.

LIGHTHEADEDNESS

Dizziness and lightheadedness are usually caused by one of two common problems: low blood pressure or low blood sugar. Your blood sugar may drop if you haven't eaten in a while; the kind of food you choose also makes a difference. High protein foods will keep your sugar up, whereas high sugar foods and simple carbs will give you an initial boost, followed by a drop in energy a few hours later. If you notice that you feel unwell at the same time of day, have a snack so that you feel better, but consider what you have been eating, and when. If you have a midday lull, for example, it may help to move some protein to your breakfast—for instance, toast with peanut butter, or eggs, and to avoid that sugary pastry. Low blood sugar is not a sign of diabetes—it is normal in pregnancy and just means you need to eat differently.

Lightheadedness from low blood pressure occurs because blood collects in your legs or in the placenta and doesn't reach your brain quickly enough. Symptoms are most common when you just get up from lying down, when you stand still for a while, or when you are warm. *When you feel lightheaded, you must sit down right where you are, even if it is embarrassing.* Many mothers-to-be, in trying to find a discreet place to rest while feeling lightheaded, have fainted and fallen, risking head injury, abdominal trauma, and almost certainly more embarrassment.

ROUND LIGAMENT PAIN

The round ligaments are muscular bands that run from each side of the uterus to the groin area. Many pregnant women feel pain in their round ligaments when they change position quickly, such as when they turn over in bed. The pain is usually sharp, localized on one side or the other, and quick to resolve, especially after resting. Usually round ligament pain doesn't require treatment, but Tylenol

STEPS TO PREVENT LIGHTHEADEDNESS

- Get out of bed slowly—sit at the side of the bed for a few moments before you stand up
- Keep cool—dress in layers that you can shed if you feel warm
- Take cooler showers
- Wear support hose. The squeeze on your legs helps keep the blood circulating. If regular maternity support pantyhose aren't enough, talk to your doctor about a prescription for maternity compression hose
- Drink a lot of fluids—don't let yourself feel dehydrated or thirsty
- Eat regularly—generally five to six small meals a day, or three meals and a few snacks
- Try to shift your weight from leg to leg if standing, and walk around periodically
- If your job requires you to stand, see if you can instead sit on a high stool to do your work, and be sure to take frequent breaks

is generally okay if needed. If the pain lasts more than an hour or two or doesn't resolve with rest, call your doctor.

BACK AND LIMB PAIN

Pregnancy is a time when your body may be particularly sensitive to positioning. Carpal tunnel syndrome (a painful tingling of the hands) and low back pain can both be worsened by your work environment. If you sit for long periods, try to find a chair with good back support; a lumbar pillow roll can make all the difference to your back. Don't sit for more than thirty to forty-five minutes at a time—set a timer if necessary. For keyboard work, arm and wrist supports may prevent carpal tunnel syndrome, which is worsened when your wrists are flexed back. If your job has good health services, you may be able to get help with ergonomics at your workstation. A physical or occupational therapist can also offer suggestions to keep you comfortable at work as your body changes.

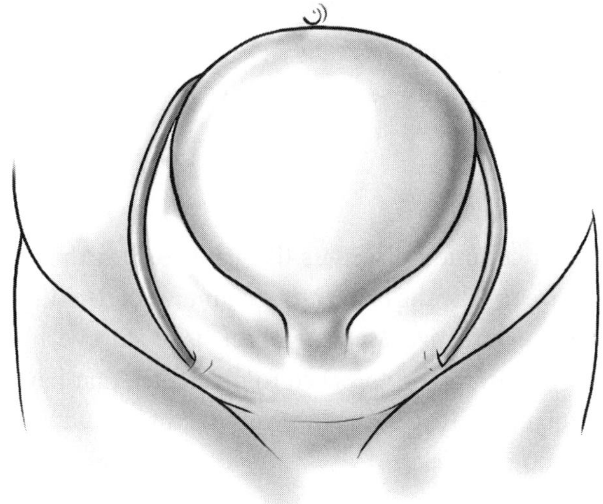

The round ligaments extend from each side of the top of the uterus and connect to the groin.

SHORTNESS OF BREATH

Mild shortness of breath is normal in pregnancy. You might notice it when speaking, walking briskly or climbing stairs, or being in a plane. Severe or sudden shortness of breath should be reported to your practitioner.

At a meeting the other day I just had to tell the clients, "I get out of breath so just bear with me." Sometimes I sound like my grandmother, who is on oxygen! (Kristen S., public relations)

BLURRY VISION

Your prescription for glasses may change during pregnancy. Spots before your eyes or sudden changes in your vision, though, should be reported immediately to your doctor or midwife.

INFECTIONS "DOWN BELOW"

Vaginal discharge is common in pregnancy, but if you develop itching or an odor, tell your practitioner; a yeast or bacterial infection might be to blame. Bladder infections may be diagnosed by routine urine testing, or by your symptoms. Since urinating frequently is normal in pregnancy, it can be hard to tell if you are getting a bladder infection, but diagnosis and treatment are important to prevent a kidney infection, which can make you really sick. For more information about urinary tract and vaginal infections, see Appendix B.

Common Ailments

Most of us treat ourselves for common disorders like colds or heartburn. During pregnancy, though, you have to take the baby into account when deciding what treatment will be safe as well as effective. My general rule is to start with a nonmedical approach, and if that doesn't work proceed to medicines that have been used extensively and are probably safe. Check with your doctor or midwife if simple firstline measures don't do the trick.

ALLERGIES

First: Avoid triggers. If you are battling hayfever, seek out air-conditioned rooms at work and home. If pet dander has you sneezing, steer clear of animals for a while.

If those measures don't work: Try Claritin, Chlortrimeton, or a prescription cromolyn or steroid nasal spray.

Call your doctor if . . . you develop wheezing, hives, or shortness of breath.

CONSTIPATION

First: Drink plenty of liquids, exercise, and eat fiber-rich foods like high-fiber breakfast cereals and fruits (prunes are especially helpful). Fiber laxatives like Metamucil or Citrucel are safe in pregnancy and can be used on a daily basis, but they work better for *preventing* constipation than as a treatment for obstruction.

If those measures don't work: Milk of Magnesia is safe in pregnancy and can be used as often as twice a day. Stimulant laxatives, even the over-the-counter ones like Correctol or Ex-lax, and herbals like senna, should not be used unless specifically recommended by your doctor or midwife. Colace, a stool softener, may help.

Call your doctor if . . . the problem doesn't respond to first treatment within a day or two, or if you develop abdominal pain.

DIARRHEA

First: Hydrate with clear liquids like water, sports drinks, or Kool Aid; try the "BRAT" diet (bananas, rice, applesauce, and toast); or use the over-the-counter liquid, Kaopectate.

If those measures don't work: Imodium is safe in some circumstances—check with your doctor or midwife.

Call your doctor if . . . you see blood in your stools, if your diarrhea persists beyond a few days, or if you can't keep even liquids down.

FEVER

(Note that fever puts stress on the baby; this is one situation in which medications are preferable to just bucking up.)

First: Try Tylenol, the treatment of choice for fever in pregnancy, and drinking more fluids to help prevent dehydration.

If those measures don't work: Take a cool bath or shower.

Call your doctor if . . . the fever doesn't respond to Tylenol, or if you feel very ill. Fever can be a sign of a serious infection—if no obvious simple cause is apparent, talk to your doctor.

HEADACHE

First: Avoid triggers, rest in a quiet dark room, use an ice pack on your head, or ask your partner or a friend to give you a gentle head massage.

If those measures don't work: Tylenol or a small amount of caffeine may help. Ibuprofen (found in Motrin and Advil, for instance) is probably safe between twelve and thirty weeks, but check with your doctor. Prescription pain medications are sometimes necessary.

Call your doctor if . . . your headache doesn't respond to Tylenol, particularly if it is more severe or different from headaches you have had in the past.

HEAD COLD

First: Try a vaporizer, saline nose drops or spray, and Tylenol for fever.

If those measures don't work: Use Sudafed or Afrin nasal spray (if you don't have high blood pressure), and Robitussin for cough.

Call your doctor if . . . you develop wheezing, shortness of breath, or symptoms that persist beyond a few days.

HEARTBURN AND INDIGESTION

First: Avoid spicy and fatty foods, caffeine, and alcohol; allow a few hours between eating and lying down; don't smoke; elevate the head of your bed with cinder blocks or sleep with your head raised; or try liquid antacids like Mylanta or Maalox. Calcium-based chewables like Tums are good sources of calcium and effective in the short term but lead to increased acid production.

If those measures don't work: Zantac, Pepcid, and Tagamet are probably safe. A prescription liquid, Carafate, coats the stomach and esophagus (food tube) and isn't absorbed into your system, so should be totally safe, except a bit constipating. Other prescription antacids may also be safe and effective.

Call your doctor if . . . indigestion or chest pain doesn't at least temporarily respond to liquid antacids. This may be a sign of a more serious condition.

I had a lot of heartburn with my first child. My husband put bricks under the headboard of our bed per the doctor's instructions trying to help. I had trouble staying in the bed. I would wake up and have to crawl back up to keep from sliding down onto the floor. (Becky G., administrator)

They say that heartburn is a sign that the baby has a lot of hair—but my first was totally bald. I had just as much heartburn in my second pregnancy and she had a head full of hair the day she was born. (Eileen M., weather reporter)

SNORING

First: Try adhesive breathing strips that attach across your nose.

If that doesn't work: Have those who are bothered by it sleep apart from you.

Call your doctor if . . . you have severe snoring with irregular breathing, which may represent sleep apnea. Sleep apnea may lead to hypertension in the mother and low fetal oxygen levels.

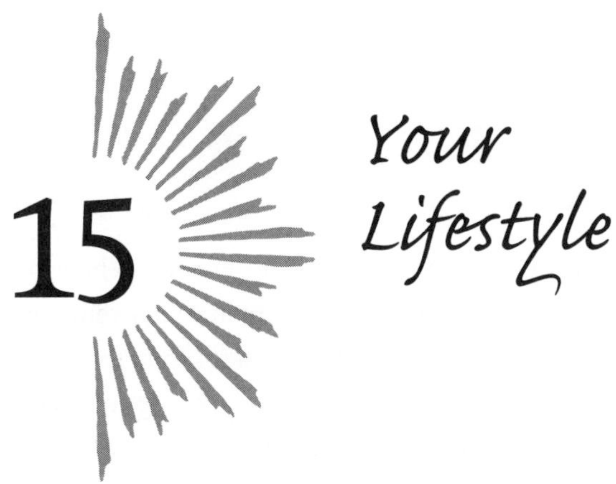

15 Your Lifestyle

Pregnancy is a time when most of us want to be physically healthy—we try to make thoughtful choices, exercise, and eat right. During the first trimester, it can be difficult to be "good" all the time—you may feel tired and nauseated and barely able to get through the day. But now you are in the second trimester; you're probably feeling better, and ready to get on a good health kick.

> ***During pregnancy was the best I ever took care of myself—I ate well and exercised—I wanted to know that I had done everything within my power to have a healthy baby. (Eileen M., weather reporter)***

Exercise

Exercise makes you feel good, energizes you, and helps control weight gain. If you have been pretty sedentary, you may want to start with walking or swimming. If you have been working out, your exercise program will probably evolve as your body changes. Any activity that doesn't cause pain can be continued or initiated in the second trimester. The one exception is that you should no longer lie flat on your back for more than a few minutes at a time. Beyond that, just follow the same guidelines as in the first trimester and listen to your body.

> ***The best advice: Exercise as much as possible. It helps you feel better, sleep better, and recover faster. It doesn't matter what you do, just move. (Mary Ellen M., pediatric nurse)***

"WHY CAN'T I LIE ON MY BACK?"

As the uterus enlarges, it can compress nearby parts of the body. When you lie flat on your back, the weight of the uterus presses against your vena cava, the large vein just to the right of your backbone that brings blood from your legs back to your heart. Compressing the blood vessels can cause your blood pressure to drop, diminishing the flow of blood and oxygen to the placenta and the baby.

To avoid compressing the vena cava:

- Modify your exercise program so that you are on your back for no more than five minutes at a time.
- If you tend to sleep on your back, stuff a pillow under your right hip so you are tipped slightly to the left. As long as you are tipped to the left, or lying all the way over on your right side, the weight of your uterus will not affect your circulation.

Many women wake up flat on their backs and worry that they have hurt the baby. Although we know that lying flat can impair circulation, no scientific studies have shown that sleeping on your back does damage. Just do your best to keep a pillow behind you so that you will be tipped a bit to the left side if you happen to roll onto your back.

I did almost no exercise or sports during my first pregnancy, but worked out religiously in my second full-term pregnancy. I felt much better during the second and my labor was so much easier. (Sandy B., social worker)

Diet

While first trimester eating can be irregular, the second trimester, when you are probably feeling better, is a good time to pay attention to a healthful intake. So when you are ready, go back and read about healthy eating. Planning your meals in advance can help you to get the best nutrition. As extra insurance, continuing your prenatal multivitamin will meet your vitamin and mineral needs. Routine prenatal blood testing for anemia in the early third trimester assures that you are getting enough iron. Your weight change can help you to tell if you are eating too much or too little—in my view, calorie counting isn't realistic, but calorie awareness is a good life skill—so try not to overeat and to avoid excess sweets and junk foods that will fill you up without providing what you and the baby need most. Don't skip meals; just let your appetite and your weight gain be your guides. With this approach, you have the baby covered, although you may still be lacking the calcium that you need for yourself.

> ***I appreciated that my obstetrician didn't panic. But eventually we were six to seven months into it and I couldn't take a vitamin, couldn't eat any whole grains, etc. Not exactly what they tell you to do in pregnancy. And his approach was, "Don't worry, it will all be over once the baby is born." Finally, I just bagged the doctors and went to see the midwives, who seemed to have a more sympathetic ear and had some other suggestions like vitamins that wouldn't make me nauseous, and seeing a dietitian. (Cheryl L., lawyer)***

Pregnant women require 1,500 milligrams of calcium a day. Not getting enough won't hurt the baby, because any calcium that the baby needs will be taken out of your bones. But your bones need that calcium to stay strong and to prevent osteoporosis when you get old. You can get calcium from natural food sources, like milk and other dairy products; enhanced foods like "calcium fortified" juices; and calcium supplements. Keep in mind that supplements can be constipating—food sources may be better. See table and box on pages 174–176.

TIPS FOR GETTING CALCIUM INTO YOUR DIET

- Unless you drink a lot of milk, most mothers-to-be need a calcium supplement to get the whole 1,500 milligrams. Take one 500 or 600 milligram supplement in the morning. Supplements that contain magnesium as well as calcium may be less constipating.

- Have calcium-fortified cold cereal with skim milk for breakfast—and drink the milk when the cereal is gone.
- Drink calcium-fortified juices, and look for other calcium-fortified foods, like frozen waffles, hot cereals, and breads.
- Add milk instead of water when you prepare pancakes, hot cereals, pudding, and hot cocoa. Add nonfat dry milk if you bake bread. Use your imagination for other ways to add milk or nonfat dry milk when cooking.
- Put a lot of milk in your coffee.
- At the end of the day, think about how much calcium you were able to eat or drink. If the amount seems inadequate, take a second calcium supplement.
- Have a glass of warm skim milk at bedtime.
- When reading labels at the store, remember that the recommended daily allowance (RDA) for adults is 1,000 milligrams. That means if one serving has 30 percent of the RDA, it will give you 300 milligrams of calcium in each serving.

PICKLES AND ICE CREAM

Food cravings can start at any time in pregnancy. Unless dangerous to you, any food can be eaten in moderation, even if it is pickles (which, after all, might have some vitamins . . .) and ice cream (calcium!). Cravings make each pregnancy unique; some women even jot down in their journals what foods they sought out in pregnancy, in part to see whether their child likes those foods when he is older. Just keep in mind that a varied diet is the best way to meet all of your nutritional needs.

I was a vegetarian. But with my second, I ate two hamburgers. I was a family therapist in the middle of a session, and all of a sudden, I got a craving for a Big Mac. I hadn't had a hamburger in ten years. I was trying to slyly look at my watch to see if I could end the session five minutes early, and start the next session ten minutes late. (Kathy C., family therapist)

Women hunger after anything from the healthiest foods, to items like ice, dirt, or laundry starch, which have no nutritional value. As I explained earlier, ingesting non-food is called pica, and may lead to constipation and iron-deficiency anemia. If you have a strong urge to eat these sorts of non-food items, tell your doctor or midwife, so you can be checked for anemia and counseled. If you know the risks, you'll be better able to deal with craving substances that aren't helpful to you.

PLANNING MEALS

Most people find it easier to eat healthfully if they plan meals ahead of time. Using your weekend to cook a few dinners for the freezer, for example, can save you from resorting to fast food—which is almost always higher in fat and sodium, lower in fiber, and much more expensive than home-cooked meals. To jumpstart your better eating routine, consider spending a bit more on groceries to make snacks and meals simpler to prepare at home. It is easier to include fruits and vegetables in your diet when you use prewashed salad greens, prechopped vegetables for veggies and dip or stir-fry, precut fruit, salad bar items, and the like. (Frozen vegetables are also an easy alternative to fresh, and they contain more vitamins and less salt than canned.) Bringing lunch to work may give you healthier options than buying it. Life doesn't get any easier after you have a baby—good health habits now can only help you as you move on to the next phase of your life.

Here's some advice: Pack your lunch. Restaurant or cafeteria food can be full of sodium, which doesn't help with the swelling. (Mary Ellen M., pediatric nurse)

EATING OUT

One in five meals eaten in this country is prepared in a restaurant, and one in four Americans has a fast-food meal on any given day. Women who work long hours and those who entertain on the job may eat out several times a week. Although eating fast foods or rich high-sodium meals isn't ideal, sporadic indiscretions won't harm your baby. Just take an extra minute with the menu to find foods that are healthful—fruits, vegetables, and whole grains—and limit your intake of fats and sweets.

Sources of 300 milligrams of calcium.

Pregnant women need five of these servings a day

Calcium source	*How much will provide 300 milligrams?*	*Notes*
Milk	One cup	Whole milk has almost twice the calories of skim milk
Calcium-fortified soy or rice milk	One cup	Rice milk and soy milk that are not calcium-fortified have very little calcium
Ice cream	Two cups	Lots of calories here
Calcium-enriched ice cream	Half a cup	Fewer calories per gram of calcium than regular ice cream
Fruit yogurt	One cup	Most are sold in six-ounce containers, even though you will need a full eight ounces to make one cup. Check the label—some flavored yogurts are higher in calcium than others
Milkshake	12 oz.	A good source of calcium—and tasty—but watch those calories!
American cheese	Three slices	Try a grilled cheese with two cheese slices on calcium-fortified wheat bread
Cooked collard greens	Just over one cup	This is probably about three or four regular-sized servings
Cheese pizza	Two large slices	It's all in the cheese
Canned sardines or salmon	4 oz. tin	The tiny bones in the fish provide the calcium
Broccoli	Two cups	Broccoli is often listed as a good source of calcium, but this seems like a lot to eat!
Calcium-fortified juice	One cup	In general, juices are not as good for you as whole fruits are, but the calcium adds some benefit
Calcium-fortified cold cereal	A half cup cereal with a half cup of milk	Drink the milk when you finish the cereal
Sesame seeds	One ounce (about a third of a cup)	

Sources of 300 milligrams of calcium (Continued)

Pregnant women need five of these servings a day

Calcium source	*How much will provide 300 milligrams?*	*Notes*
Firm tofu set with calcium	A fifth of a block	Check the label to see that it is prepared with calcium and not with magnesium
Tums, OsCal, Viactiv, or any other calcium or calcium plus D supplement. (Avoid "natural" oyster shell-derived sources, which may contain lead)	One "Tums EX"	Tums is a great source of calcium and also a mild antacid. Some supplements have as much as 500 milligrams. If you aren't taking a prenatal vitamin, additional vitamin D helps build bone, particularly if you don't get a lot of sun

Publicly Pregnant

In the first trimester, pregnancy is usually more on your mind than in the thoughts of those around you. Soon, though, colleagues, friends, family, and even complete strangers will be aware that you are "with child." This may manifest itself by comments on how you are taking care of yourself and your baby-to-be. Although the advice may be well-meaning, you are the one taking care of this baby, and you need to make your own adult decisions.

I like to have a cup of coffee in the morning before I fly. When I was pregnant, I was often approached by what I called the "pregnancy police," women who were total strangers stopping to warn me that drinking coffee caused low birthweight babies—but my babies were over nine pounds, so maybe drinking coffee was a good thing. They might have been bigger! (Susan G., commercial airline pilot)

Don't be surprised that your pregnancy engenders opinions from those around you. Close colleagues may worry about how your absence will affect their workloads. Your boss may question your priorities. Your best friend may be bursting with happiness for you—or a little fearful about where she will fit in your new

CALCIUM SOURCES FOR WOMEN WITH LACTOSE INTOLERANCE

Many people have difficulty digesting lactose, the sugar in milk, because they do not have lactase, the lactose-digesting enzyme. Lactose intolerance leads to gas, bloating, cramps, or diarrhea after drinking milk. Although anyone can be lactose intolerant, it is most common in people of Asian and African ancestry. To help yourself get enough calcium in your diet, you might try:

- Small portions of dairy products
- Lactaid milk, which contains the enzyme that breaks down lactose, or a Lactaid pill before drinking milk
- Cultured dairy products like yogurt or buttermilk, which don't contain much lactose
- Non-dairy calcium sources
- Calcium supplements (note that supplements containing magnesium as well as calcium may be less constipating)

life. Friends who have suffered from infertility or miscarriage may, consciously or not, feel ambivalent about your good news because of their own experiences. If you get odd reactions, remember that your pregnancy may be difficult for others for reasons that you will never fully understand. Mostly, though, people are drawn to pregnant women; they feel connected by this common experience.

> ***The best thing about working when I was pregnant was how everyone had a story to tell, even the guys I barely knew. For the most part, my being pregnant made people smile and tell me stories about their children. That part was really nice in a workplace that was otherwise pretty stiff. (Elizabeth S., online producer)***

Your Relationship

On the home front, your partner may be more aware of the baby-to-be after seeing the little one on ultrasound or feeling kicks. If this is your first child together, now is a good time to start talking about expectations—what your families were like growing up, what aspects of their parenting you want to emulate and what you want to improve on, your fears and excitement, and how you plan to divide the work and share the pleasures of raising a child. As you start this exciting joint venture, take special care to communicate well about your hopes, dreams, and fears; you need to work together to prepare your relationship for the new arrival.

It wasn't real to him until he felt kicking and saw the ultrasound. He couldn't understand why I was so tired—but personally we felt much closer. (Heather H., real estate attorney)

I was adored during my pregnancies. I felt at the "top of my game." (Helene L., teacher)

Mid-pregnancy, many women become more enthusiastic about sex, perhaps because they feel more physically comfortable; others prefer just to cuddle. But you're not the only one adjusting to the "new you"—your partner may experience changes in his sex drive as well. As you each try to figure out how you feel about your changing body—proud? neutral? turned off?—you may find that you and your partner have very different attitudes about sexual intimacy. To make matters worse, the partner who is more interested often interprets any drop in the other's libido as a personal rejection. The best way to work through these differences is to gently communicate what you want, listen carefully to your partner's point of view, and agree to be generous with each other. Now is the best time to work on your communication skills and to practice the art of compromise: giving birth, breastfeeding, and having young children at home can challenge anyone's desire and ability to enjoy their partner sexually.

Right now we are on the no sex plan due to some bleeding. This is by far the toughest part! (Christi M., medical student)

You have a very small window in which you actually feel like having sex, around months four and five. Take advantage of it. About the middle of the

fifth month your body really starts to change and it's just too weird. Rick and I both know you can't hurt the baby, but it is right THERE. It's not like it's in a crib in the next room. (Jen B., dance teacher)

Bill was very nervous about "crushing the baby." (Beth L., computer science researcher)

After the first trimester, sex was great. I loved not having to worry about birth control. (Deb L., writer)

Sex during pregnancy? It was the greatest. My interest was the highest and orgasms the strongest. (Patsy H., midwife)

TIME TOGETHER

The second trimester is a great time for a vacation, if feasible. Most women feel pretty well, and complications of pregnancy are unlikely to occur while you are far from home. Just be sure to check in with your doctor or midwife before you go, to get their advice and approval.

If you travel to a sunny locale, your practitioner may remind you to be careful not to get too much sun on your face. A condition called melasma, the "mask of pregnancy," is caused by overexposure to the sun and can leave you with dark splotches on your cheeks and forehead for months to come. Women of darker complexions are more susceptible than those who are very fair, but every pregnant mom is at risk. Oddly enough, sunblock, which prevents sunburn and other sun damage, won't necessarily prevent melasma. So bring your big brimmed hat, or stay in the shade.

If you can't take a vacation, try to set time aside for the two of you. At the very least, plan a "date night" once every week or so. Spending time with just each other is one way to maintain your relationship and keep the lines of communication open. After the baby arrives, you may want to keep the tradition going, so that you can continue to enjoy and help each other as your life gets chaotic and your partnership takes a back seat to your newest family member.

This is how my Friday nights go now—we go out with friends and I get my Friday night coke, we're home by ten, and I'm up until one because I'm not used to caffeine anymore. (Jen B., dance teacher)

16 Communication at Work

Working while pregnant can bring a whole new set of challenges, many having to do with communication. Telling your boss you are expecting, dealing with others' reactions to the pregnancy, redistributing work, and starting to plan for maternity leave are just some of the tasks at hand.

> ***I was really nervous about telling my boss because we are such a small company, with only six people. I didn't want her to think I wasn't going to be able to do my job anymore. (Amanda O., meeting planner)***

How to Announce Your Pregnancy at Work

I wrote earlier about factors to consider in deciding *when* to disclose your pregnancy at work. Although no set of recommendations will be perfect for all situations, consider the following guidelines for *how* to share your news:

- Try to tell your supervisors before they find out from someone else. Sometimes coworkers find out early—your symptoms are obvious, or you can't resist sharing your secret. If you tell colleagues first, you'll need to decide if you are willing to risk having your supervisor find out indirectly, or prefer to tell earlier than you might otherwise have planned.
- Make an appointment to talk with your boss. Some mothers-to-be find it helpful to time this meeting for right after a completed project or a good performance review.
- Know the culture of your workplace—will there be support or criticism? If you're unsure, try to find out (discreetly) how others in your situation have been treated during pregnancy.

- Be upbeat and positive, since this is your good news. But don't take a neutral or negative response personally—your boss's initial response may be based on how your absence will affect the workplace and not on what having a baby means to you. You have the right to procreate, no matter how irreplaceable you may seem. If no one had babies, where would they find workers for the future?
- Understand that pregnant employees are often seen as having prioritized their personal lives ahead of their work. Your team may need reassurance that you plan to continue to pull your load. Showing that you have thought about how your work will get done during pregnancy and while you are away will reassure your supervisor and coworkers that you take your responsibilities seriously, and aren't abandoning them.
- Pregnancy is expensive for employers. At the very least, they will need to cover your job while you are on maternity leave. Understanding your employer's concerns will help you be responsive and successful when you're negotiating to get what you need for yourself and your growing family. And asking what you can do to help with the transitions is a good way to show that you're a team player.
- You don't need to talk about maternity leave the day you announce you are pregnant, but familiarize yourself with laws and the policies at your workplace and have an idea of what you want in case it comes up.

What worked for me: I made an appointment to tell my boss I was pregnant, and then emailed everyone else. This way no one got left out or felt slighted. (Brenda W., lawyer)

I told my boss really early—I was about three months pregnant. I think this made it feel like I was pregnant and out of the office a very long time to him. In the future, I would tell only when I had to because I was showing (for me this was at about seven months). I think this would have helped and I wouldn't have been "written off" on key projects so much. (Jane J., advertising executive)

The law firm had one prior experience with someone getting pregnant and she quit shortly after returning to work, and then was quoted in a legal magazine about how bad they were to her—which brought bad

publicity for the firm; so I knew they would try to be supportive when I got pregnant. (Kendra F., civil litigator)

Changes at Work

Many women find that their identity in the workplace becomes tied to their pregnancy. They go from being one of the gang to being the pregnant one. It can be hard to be seen as a productive member of the team while you are pregnant, even if you are working as you always have.

The guys were used to treating me like a man, and now I was so obviously a woman. (Tracy G., police officer)

I was trying very hard to prove that the pregnancy would not interfere with my work, and/or would not diminish my capacities. Some women are powerhouses, but not all of us are and we could endanger ourselves and our fetuses by not acknowledging that we are not the same as before the pregnancy. (Lisa K., city administrator)

I was the first woman to be pregnant in my store. I think everybody is always excited to hear their friend is pregnant, but there weren't really any adjustments made to accommodate my pregnancy. They would try to help with larger boxes, but a lot of the time, it ended up being my responsibility anyway. I still performed all of my duties; I don't think anything changed. (Zoe B., inventory manager)

I worked through all four pregnancies. I don't remember facing too much concern or criticism. That's probably because I didn't dote on being pregnant. I never looked at being pregnant as something out of the ordinary. I always felt that pregnancy was just another part of day-to-day living. (Helene L., teacher)

TIPS FOR STAYING ON GOOD TERMS WITH YOUR COWORKERS

- Do your job. Pregnant women are often seen as prioritizing their personal lives over their work. If you don't want this reputation, do your job as well as you can.

- Look competent. Although pregnant women often report feeling slightly confused, research doesn't really bear this out. People believe what you say about yourself, so don't undermine your credibility by complaining about "pregnancy brain."
- Dress for success. Try to wear the same sorts of clothes you wore before you became pregnant, with modifications to accommodate the pregnancy. Make the effort to look professional.
- Try not to complain. Whining is never good, and may be especially detrimental to your professional reputation when it is associated with something that is seen as your choice—having a baby. (And if your listener has suffered from infertility or early miscarriage, your comments could be hurtful.)
- Go the extra mile. This is a time when being generous can pay big dividends later, when you need it most. If you have a reputation for being helpful, others will be more willing to lend a hand. If someone covers for you or helps you out, be appreciative.
- Plan ahead. Prepare for your leave by talking about your workload and how it might be handled while you are away. Be professional in training your replacement; your re-entry will be easier if your substitute has done a good job and feels positively toward you.
- Don't overextend. Try not to offer to work during your time at home—most women find it extraordinarily difficult, no matter how competent they are at work, to recover from childbirth and manage a new baby—even without additional demands. Most new mothers, too, find that during their leave they are not as interested in the happenings at work as they expected to be.

There is nothing worse than a constant complainer. View pregnancy as a time of wellness and not as sickness. Don't be the pregnant mom who cries wolf! Your coworkers will be more sympathetic if and when a true problem does arise during your pregnancy. (Pam H., nurse)

One challenge is that my job is very physical. As I get bigger I can't lift the dogs any more and I need more help from the vet techs. Also I can't restrain an animal. I end up having to ask for a lot of help, but people

don't seem to mind. I just bring donuts every once in a while. (Karen D., veterinarian)

The only time I remembered I was pregnant while flying airplanes was when I had to scoot the seat way back from the flight controls, more as each week went by. And whenever it was getting close to landing, the kid would start kicking. Hard. It was like clockwork (or maybe it was the change in pressure as we descended!). I guess I'd call it the prenatal version of "Are we there yet?" (Susan G., commercial airline pilot)

Maternity Leave

Figuring out what maternity benefits you are entitled to can be surprisingly confusing. Federal and state laws determine the minimal maternity leave requirements for large employers, but many jobs have benefits that are better, and some smaller employers offer much less support. Company, state, and federal benefits may overlap or run consecutively. Your human resources department is required to provide written policies without asking you why you want to see them, but even the benefits staff may not be aware of all the ramifications of state and federal rules.

If you are the first woman in your workplace to become pregnant, your employer may not have developed a maternity leave policy. In this situation, you may want to provide information on the federal Family and Medical Leave Act (FMLA), state laws, and policies of comparable employers, then negotiate your leave and your return. Many parents also consider their short-term disability, family leave, sick time, and vacation days when determining how much time they can afford to take off with their new baby.

For more on planning your maternity leave, and examples of different leave arrangements, see Chapter 23.

We were surprised to learn that our "great" PPO had a wellness cap of $100 per year per child, and that immunizations were considered well care (resulting in $1,500 of charges that first year). We didn't know in time for open enrollment deadlines or we could have used the flexible spending account. (Christie H., editor)

MAKING CHANGES TO YOUR HEALTH BENEFITS

If you plan to keep the same health insurer after you have the baby, you don't need to do anything right now. You will have a month after delivery to sign your new baby onto your (or the baby's father's) health plan, and then the expenses will be covered retroactively starting with the baby's day of birth.

If either of your employers provides a flexible healthcare spending account, be sure to calculate the added expenses of having a newborn so you know what to set aside in the year that you will give birth. Flexible spending accounts allow you to use pre-tax dollars for qualifying healthcare expenses that are not paid for by your health insurance. Co-pays, deductibles, over-the-counter medications, lactation consultant visits, and even a breast pump may be reimbursable. Remember, though, that these accounts are "use it or lose it": money that remains in the account at the end of the fiscal year will be forfeited.

Laws Related to Pregnancy and Work

To know your rights, you will need to understand the federal laws that will affect how your pregnancy and maternity leave will be handled by your employer.

THE PREGNANCY DISCRIMINATION ACT

The Pregnancy Discrimination Act (PDA) of 1978, an amendment to Title VII of the Civil Rights Act, requires companies with more than fifteen workers to treat pregnancy-related disability just like any other temporary disabling condition. Under the PDA, if your company provides disability pay, they must pay for *medically related* pregnancy leave. In addition, if you can do your job, your employer can't fire you because you are pregnant, or move you to another position without your consent. Medical leave for pregnancy is not the same as maternity leave taken to care for the baby.

Medical leave can be necessary for:

- Pregnancy disability, like missing work for severe nausea and vomiting or when you take off to recover after childbirth
- Occupational demands that would be unsafe in pregnancy (if your employer has no safer work for you)
- Pregnancy complications

The PDA does *not* apply to:

- Jobs at a company with fewer than fifteen employees
- Maternity leave to care for your newborn after the six-weeks postpartum recovery period

The PDA can be important for many different work situations. Some examples:

- If your work is unsafe—for instance in law enforcement, where you might sustain a blow to the abdomen while making an arrest—your employer must find light-duty work for you if you request it. If they cannot provide an alternative position, you may need to go out on disability. If an employer accommodates partially disabled workers who cannot perform certain job assignments (such as lifting heavy objects because of a strained back), similar arrangements have to be made for pregnant workers.
- If you work with radiation or other potentially toxic substances, and wish to stay in your position during pregnancy, your employer can't require you take leave or change jobs unless you physically can't do your work. Similarly, your employer cannot prohibit you from returning to work sooner than company standards dictate.
- Pregnancy-related medical time off is compensated at whatever pay you would receive during any other medical leave. Accrual of seniority, vacation time, and automatic pay increases must be the same as if you were on medical disability leave.
- An employer can't refuse to hire you because you are pregnant as long as you can perform the major functions of the job.
- Your employer can't require that you use up all vacation days before going onto disability unless that is required of all workers with temporary disabilities.

- Pregnancy benefits cannot differ for single versus married moms.
- Disability payments may be taxed or tax-free, depending on how the premiums were paid. Be prepared: if the premiums were paid with pre-tax dollars and taxes aren't withheld from your disability check, you will have to pay taxes on your disability income at tax time.

I interviewed for a job while I was pregnant. I didn't tell them at the first interview, but when they called to offer me the job I told them right away. They couldn't very well take back the offer then, and I didn't want to just show up pregnant. (Brenda W., lawyer)

THE FAMILY AND MEDICAL LEAVE ACT

The Family and Medical Leave Act (FMLA) of 1993 addresses slightly different issues. Under the FMLA, companies with more than fifty employees (who work within a seventy-five-mile radius) must provide up to twelve weeks a year of unpaid leave to take care of yourself, a newly born or adopted child, or an ill family member. Your job must be held for you, or an equivalent job offered on your return. When it is applied to pregnancy, FMLA generally covers twelve weeks: medical leave to care for yourself while you are recovering from birth and then family leave to care for your newborn. FMLA also provides partial-day leave for doctors' appointments, and intermittent leave for a temporary medical condition, such as preterm labor requiring a few weeks off from work. FMLA doesn't guarantee any pay; only protection of your job. Smaller companies often model their policies after FMLA even though they aren't bound by it.

FMLA covers about half of all workers. When does it *not* apply?

- Your company has fewer than fifty employees.
- You have worked in your job less than a year or worked fewer than 1,250 hours the previous year (an average of twenty-five hours a week).
- You already used up your leave under FMLA in the calendar year or your company's fiscal year.
- You work for a large company, but in a small, isolated office. For example, if a large national rental car company has a twenty-employee office one hundred miles from the next site, the workers in that office are exempt from FMLA requirements even though they work for a large employer.

- Layoffs occurred while you were on FMLA leave and your position would have been eliminated as part of a larger reorganization.

In addition, it is important to realize that under FMLA:

- If both parents work for the same employer, their combined annual family leave to care for a newborn or ill family member may be limited to twelve weeks.
- Certain highly paid employees (those receiving the top 10 percent of company pay within seventy-five miles of their location) may not be eligible to get their job back after leave if "such denial is necessary to prevent substantial and grievous economic injury to the operations of the employer."
- Rules on family leave may differ by a few weeks for teachers if their absence or return affects the beginning or end of a school term.
- Maternity policies for state and federal employees are usually similar to the FMLA, but may not be exactly the same.

The FMLA has several important implications for pregnant moms. Consider these possibilities:

- Because a total of twelve weeks a year is covered by FMLA, if you take medical or personal leave before you deliver, you will have less time available to you after the baby comes.
- Even on unpaid leave, your employer is required to maintain your health benefits just as if you were working. If you choose not to return to your job, however, your employer can require that you pay back the health premiums that were paid on your behalf during your time off.
- As many as 40 percent of employed women aren't covered by FMLA either because they haven't worked in that job long enough to qualify or because their employer is exempt.
- If you and your partner work for different companies and are both eligible for FMLA, you can each take that leave any time in the child's first year of life. This means that, if you wish, your partner can take three months of unpaid leave when you return to work, delaying the need to make other childcare arrangements.

- If your employer agrees, you may be able to take your unpaid three months of family leave spread out over more time, essentially working part-time for a few months at partial pay.
- If your leave straddles two years, either calendar years or fiscal years depending on your employer, you may be able to take full FMLA twice for the same baby, increasing your amount of time off.

HEALTH INSURANCE PORTABILITY AND ACCOUNTABILITY ACT

The Health Insurance Portability and Accountability Act (HIPAA) of 1996 has two provisions related to maternity care:

- Health insurance provided by your employer must cover pregnancy-related care in the same manner that it covers other conditions. For example, the insurance may not charge an additional deductible for prenatal care or exclude it from coverage.
- If you are pregnant when starting a new job, you may not be denied pregnancy-related coverage as a "prior condition" when you enroll in your new medical plan.

OCCUPATIONAL SAFETY AND HEALTH ACT

The Occupational Safety and Health Act requires companies to provide a workplace "free from known hazards that are likely to cause harm." This act applies to all personnel, pregnant or not. Employers must also provide workers with information about potentially harmful agents—usually in the form of papers called material safety data sheets (MSDS). If you think your employer may be breaking these rules, contact the Occupational Safety and Health Administration (OSHA) at www.osha.gov.

Above and Beyond the FMLA

State laws, union contracts, and employer policies are often more generous than the FMLA. California, for example, has a disability pool that employers can pay into. Whether they purchase California disability insurance or private insurance, the employee must receive 55 percent of her income (up to a certain maximum) for as many as fifty-two weeks, when she has to be away from work for medical reasons. This usually covers four weeks before delivery, if you can't do your job, and six weeks postpartum, while recovering from birth, but doesn't pay for leave to take care of a newborn, which isn't considered medically necessary. Unpaid FMLA still applies for time off to care for the baby. Other state laws extend family leave for more weeks or include companies with fewer workers. For a listing of state-by-state laws, see www.nationalpartnership.org.

Since my department was primarily male, the other officers didn't feel it was an important enough issue to bargain for maternity leave in our police union contract. That left me totally without pay. (Tracy G., police officer)

My workplace has a pretty good family leave policy. Unpaid, unfortunately, but you can take up to six months off no matter how long you had worked there (that is, you do not have to be covered by the FMLA). (Janet G., attorney)

You may be able to negotiate aspects of your leave. Before approaching your employer, take a look at the best-selling book *Getting to Yes* by Roger Fisher, William Ury, and Bruce Patton. A good next step would be to do your homework on what other employers offer. My favorite guide for this research is *Working Mother* magazine, which every year surveys personnel policies and awards their "100 Best Companies" designation. The highest-rated businesses provide six to twelve weeks of fully paid maternity leave followed by up to 14–144 unpaid weeks beyond FMLA requirements. Several also provide one to eight weeks of paid leave for new fathers, and paid time off plus financial support for adoption. Many companies say that their family-friendly policies improve recruitment and retention of the most highly qualified personnel, saving money in the long run. For more information, talk to friends about their companies' maternity benefits, and check out any October issue of *Working Mother.*

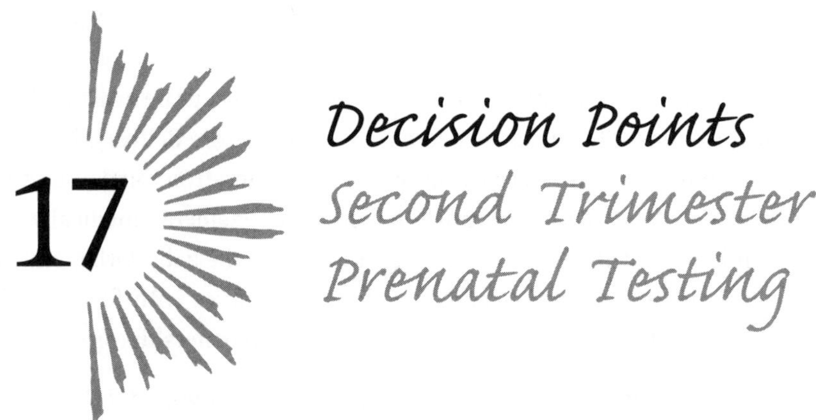

17 Decision Points: Second Trimester Prenatal Testing

During the second trimester, your pregnancy may feel steadier—you are truly on your way. Your close family members and friends probably know your good news at this point—and you may have ventured to tell others, too—so that many people are sharing your experience. Even the prenatal appointments start to feel familiar: you know by now that the nurse measures your weight and blood pressure, your urine gets dipped for protein and sugar, and your doctor or midwife checks how your uterus is growing. During your visits, you will probably also hear the baby's heartbeat. Unless you have symptoms like an abnormal vaginal discharge or risk factors for premature birth, you will probably not have internal examinations during the second trimester; they aren't necessary in a pregnancy that is progressing normally.

Ultrasound

Seeing a second trimester ultrasound is dramatic. Your little one has begun to look like a baby, and it's fun to imagine the joy to come, when you'll have a chance to snuggle together after birth. Often the pregnancy becomes more real to the parents after seeing the baby on the screen—dads may find it especially exciting, because they haven't been able to physically experience the baby until now. If you choose, and if the fetus cooperates, you might even find out if your baby-to-be is a girl or boy.

My son actually made the peace sign during our ultrasound—the tech just barely missed getting a picture of it, but we wrote it down for the baby book! (Sandy B., social worker)

Does everyone need an ultrasound? Although many doctors provide routine ultrasound scans, research studies haven't shown that having an ultrasound improves the likelihood of delivering a healthy baby. Sonography is important if you aren't certain about your last period, if the size of the uterus doesn't match up with how many weeks you should be, or if you are at risk for pregnancy complications. Insurance will usually allow one scan without argument, but if you had an early ultrasound, they may balk at a second one just to check on the anatomy. Families often want an ultrasound so they can feel reassured that the baby looks okay, but even a normal ultrasound doesn't guarantee that the baby is healthy: many problems can't be seen. Conversely, many "abnormal" findings are identified in babies who turn out to be fine.

> ***I had used fertility drugs to get pregnant, and then I measured seventeen weeks size at thirteen weeks so they said I needed a sonogram to see if it was twins. I waited in that room for ten minutes, which felt like an eternity, and all I could think of was I'll have to give one to my mother, because I can't deal with this. But it wasn't. (Laura K., attorney)***

HOW DOES ULTRASOUND WORK?

Standard ultrasound, also called 2D sonography, bounces sound waves off of structures to create an image of what is inside. A gel is used to improve the transmission of the sound waves. Ultrasound may be done transabdominally, which feels like rubbing a microphone over your gel-coated belly, or transvaginally, in which a condom-covered probe is placed into the vagina. Ultrasound doesn't hurt, although the full bladder sometimes needed for transabdominal imaging can be uncomfortable. Obstetrical ultrasound has never been shown to cause any problems for the baby.

WHAT CAN SECOND TRIMESTER ULTRASOUND SEE?

- The uterus and ovaries. Ultrasound can see the size and shape of these organs.
- The cervix. Transvaginal ultrasound can measure the length of the cervix. If you think of the uterus as being like a soda bottle, the cervix is the bottleneck. A long cervix is unlikely to open up prematurely.

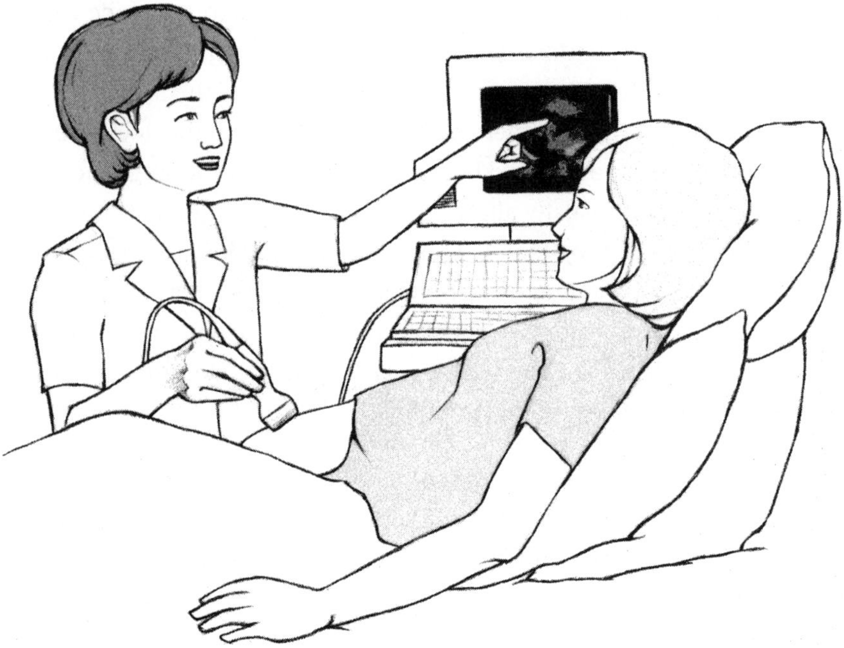

- The amniotic fluid, umbilical cord, and placenta. The placenta is located somewhere along the inner walls of the uterus. If it is close to the cervix, it may be described as low-lying, or if covering the cervix, placenta previa. Usually the placenta moves farther away from the cervix by the third trimester.
- The fetus. Ultrasound is often used to determine a more exact age for the fetus. Early in pregnancy, all embryos are the same size at the same age, so measurements correlate closely with how far along you are—during the first trimester, ultrasound dates the pregnancy accurately to within a week. By the third trimester, when babies grow to different sizes, though, age calculations are give or take three weeks. Your earliest ultrasound, combined with your last menstrual period (if known), provide the best estimate of your due date.

The baby's sex can also be determined by ultrasound. If the fetus is positioned in a favorable way, after about sixteen weeks ultrasound may show the genitals.

ULTRASOUND AND YOUR BABY'S SEX

Many parents equate having an ultrasound with finding out the sex of their baby. But although knowing whether your baby is a boy or girl may mean a lot to you, from a medical perspective, the sex isn't too important: instead, the baby's health is the biggest concern. This broader outlook may be worth keeping in mind, since if you really think about it, the sex is only one piece of information: you still won't know who the baby will look like, for example, or what the baby's personality will be. Sometimes, too, the sex can't be determined on ultrasound—the baby may be positioned in a way that hides the genitals from view. In this case, since finding out the sex doesn't qualify as a medical reason to have another scan, your insurance probably won't pay for it; unless another medical indication for ultrasound pops up, you may have to live with not knowing until you find out the old-fashioned way—at birth.

If you don't want to know the sex of your baby-to-be, be sure to tell the sonographer ahead of time. Conversely, if you want to know, ask. Still unsure? Some parents ask the ultrasound team to seal the news in an envelope so they can decide later if they want to know. Ultrasound technology is so good these days that the sonographer may be able to see the vulva if the fetus is a girl—so don't assume that your little one is a boy if the ultrasound team says they can determine the sex.

The anatomy of your fetus can be best seen after about eighteen weeks' gestation. A basic ultrasound scan, called a level one scan, will allow the sonographer to view the fundamental body structure. Level one scans, which are often done in the doctor's office and take about twenty minutes, can pick up some major problems, but can't assure that the fetal anatomy is entirely normal. If a problem is identified on a level one scan or by screening tests on your blood, you will be referred for what is called a level two scan, performed by a specialist with more advanced equipment.

SPECIAL TYPES OF ULTRASOUND SCANS

- Fetal echocardiogram. If heart problems are suspected, a fetal echocardiogram may be performed so the doctor can view the anatomy of the fetal heart in more detail. Fetal echocardiograms are usually recommended if the baby has a higher than usual chance of a heart problem—for instance, if someone in the family was born with a heart problem, or if the heart anatomy doesn't look normal during routine ultrasound imaging.
- 3D ultrasound. The 3D ultrasound, sometimes called 4D, allows a three-dimensional view of the baby. 3D scans visualize facial features with amazing detail. Entrepreneurial ultrasound units sometimes offer 3D scans for a fee, just for your enjoyment. While it may be tempting, most experts feel that scanning should be limited to medical necessity and not be done for entertainment. I always worry, too, that they will see something that may not look entirely normal, and won't know what it means (a common complication of new technologies). Currently, 3D scanning is used when routine ultrasound indicates a problem that could be visualized better in three dimensions.

At first I didn't want to know the baby's sex, but the longer the ultrasound took, I couldn't help myself. I finally asked when I couldn't take the doctor's silence any longer. "Is something wrong?" "No, no . . . well, I'll put it like this," the doctor said, "You have a baby Shaq (Shaquille O'Neal) in here." The doctor wasn't wrong. My baby was 8 lbs., 13 oz., and today, at twelve years old, he is 6' 3" and wears a size seventeen shoe. (Val P., administrative coordinator)

I hadn't decided for sure if I wanted to know the sex, and then the ultrasound doctor said "Look, it's a boy!" before I had a chance to tell her that I didn't want to know. (Maggie P., administrator)

I never wanted to know the sex of the baby, so I thought a lot about whether the baby was going to be a boy or a girl. I have never understood why anyone would want to know what the sex of a child is before it is born. It makes no sense to me. (Helene L., teacher)

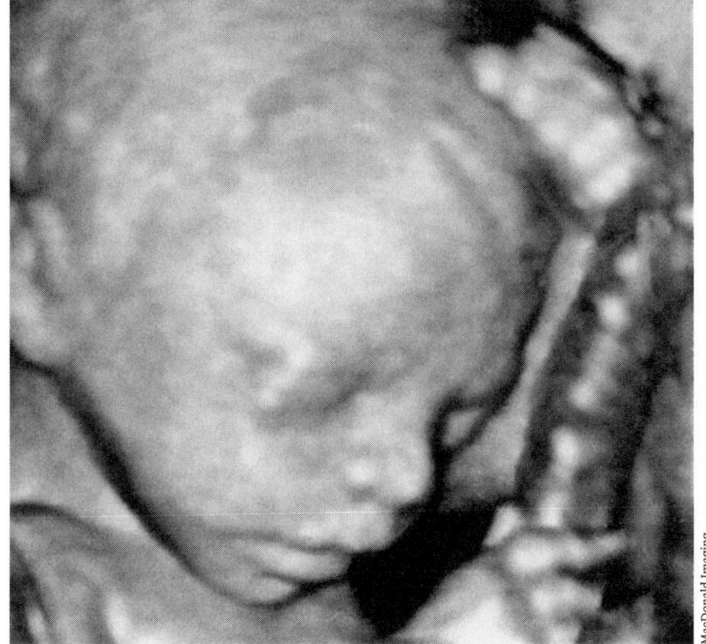
MacDonald Imaging

A 3D ultrasound profile at twenty-four weeks

> ***Some families want to know, while others choose to find out the old-fashioned way—at birth. I have a friend with four daughters who said the only time he had a son was in his mind, while his wife was pregnant. (Marge G., obstetrician)***

The number of tests available to assess a fetus has skyrocketed over the past decade. This may sound like great news; what parent wouldn't want reassurance that all is well? But when you ask a question (as you are doing when you have an ultrasound or other test to see if your baby is okay), you have to be prepared to deal with the answer. Just as with first trimester testing, it's really important that you understand what information can be obtained from each test and think ahead about how you would use that information. Some parents seek out tests for conditions that worry them; others decide that they don't want to have certain testing, especially if they wouldn't terminate an affected pregnancy.

SECOND TRIMESTER RISK MARKERS ON ULTRASOUND

Sonograms can't see the fetal chromosomes and won't identify a substantial percent of fetuses with genetic conditions like Down syndrome. Several ultrasound findings, though, are associated with genetic syndromes, and so are referred to as "markers." These findings, such as a bright area (echogenic focus) in the heart or small (choroid plexus) cysts in the brain, aren't really abnormal, but are identified more frequently in fetuses with genetic conditions. If a few markers are found, the chances of a genetic syndrome like Down's goes up, and further testing, including amniocentesis, might be warranted. Many families find these concepts very difficult. It is hard to believe that a marker isn't a problem in itself; it is just a statistical association. Consulting with a genetic counselor may help you to understand the issues, so you can make the right decisions for you and your family.

Multiple Marker Screening

Triple check, quad screen, alpha-fetoprotein (AFP), and second trimester maternal serum screening are all names used for a set of tests based on biochemical markers in the mother's blood. These tests, generally performed at around sixteen weeks, can be used for moms who didn't start prenatal care until after the first trimester and missed out on getting earlier screening, or as part of a combined or sequential testing protocol, in which the results of first and second trimester testing are used in concert. The quad screen may include alpha-fetoprotein (a protein that comes originally from the fetal blood but makes its way into the mom's bloodstream), and three placental hormones: hCG (the pregnancy test hormone), estriol, and inhibin A. The levels of these chemicals in the mother's blood, along with the mother's age, weight, and how far along she is in pregnancy, go into the computer, and out pops an assessment of your fetus's risk of having certain conditions, including Down syndrome and neural tube defects. If you already had a normal Down syndrome screening test in the first trimester, you may only need screening for neural tube defects in the second trimester, with ultrasound and/or AFP.

We had an elevated AFP with my third at age thirty-five. We hadn't discussed what we would do if something were abnormal. We went to the referral hospital for a genetics consult and they were surprised we had never talked about this before. I don't know what we would have done if the baby was abnormal. Tim would have wanted to keep it and I wouldn't have been able to. People should talk about these things before they get into the situation. I am grateful I never had to make that decision. (Deb L., writer)

Amniocentesis

In amniocentesis, a needle is used to draw a small amount of amniotic fluid from around the fetus while watching with ultrasound. The use of a needle may sound painful, but for most women, the procedure is only slightly more involved than getting blood drawn, and usually less painful than getting a shot. The amniotic fluid that is removed is sent to a lab for testing. One important fact to know about amniocentesis is that it occasionally causes a miscarriage—perhaps one for every two hundred to four hundred procedures, though more experienced practitioners may be able to offer better odds. The staff of the unit that does your amnio should be able to tell you their own statistics.

The amnio wasn't bad. I've had dental work that was far worse than that. Beforehand I was freaked out, having nightmares. My best friend said lie back, close your eyes, and don't look at what they're doing. (Jodi S., employee communications manager)

The fluid obtained from amniocentesis can be tested for fetal karyotype—the number and shape of the fetal chromosomes. Down syndrome, which is caused by an extra chromosome, can be detected with amniocentesis, as can many other genetic conditions. Preliminary amniocentesis results may be available in a few days, but the final results typically take several weeks. The fluid can be also tested for alpha-fetoprotein, a protein that leaks from the baby's system in certain anatomical conditions such as spina bifida.

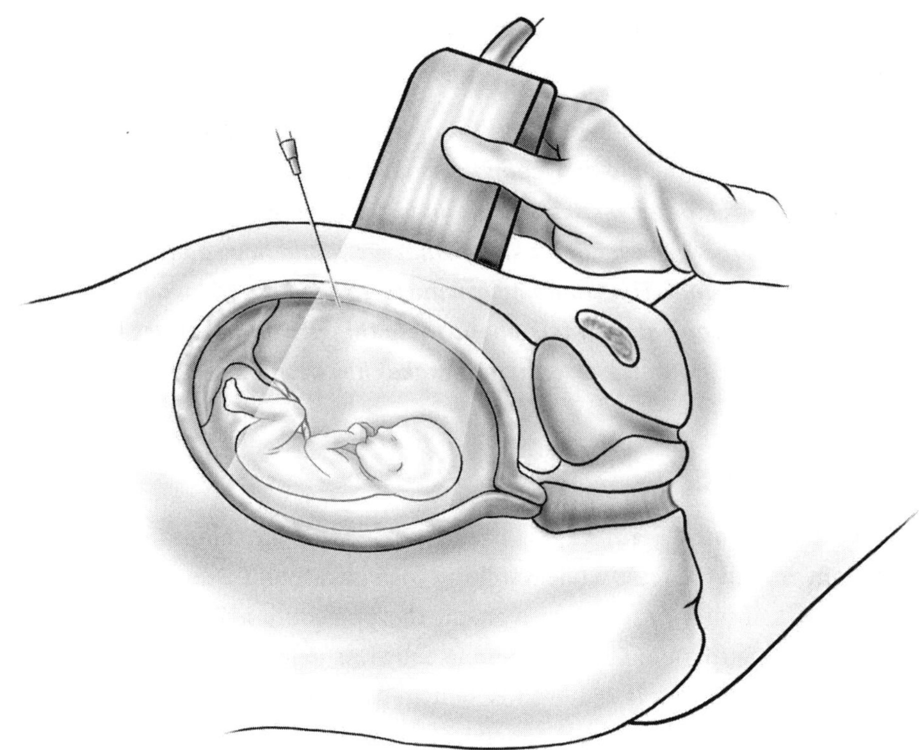

Amniocentesis

The waiting was the worst. You wait like two weeks to get the amnio results, and you have to face these questions and these possibilities that aren't really real yet. (Heidi R., law professor)

WHO SHOULD HAVE AMNIOCENTESIS?

Historically, amniocentesis was recommended to women whose Down syndrome risk was greater than the chance of the amnio causing a miscarriage—about a half of a percent. But that is a value judgment. One family might feel that a half-percent risk of miscarriage is unacceptable, particularly if they wouldn't terminate an affected pregnancy. Another family might prefer amnio even at a lower chance of Down syndrome, if they believe they couldn't handle a special needs child. Chorionic villus sampling, which can be done in the first trimester,

AGE AND DOWN SYNDROME INCIDENCE

*Mother's age at delivery**	*Likelihood of not having Down syndrome baby*	*Chance of Down syndrome at sixteen weeks*	*Chance of any major chromosomal finding*
20	99.9%	1 in 1,231	1 in 526
25	99.9%	1 in 887	1 in 476
30	99.8%	1 in 685	1 in 384
35	99.6%	1 in 250	1 in 132
40	99%	1 in 75	1 in 40
45+	96%	1 in 20	1 in 12

*Paternal age over forty-five increases the chance of some conditions, but not of Down syndrome. Tell your practitioner if your baby's father is over age forty-five.

Note: Many parents overestimate the age-related incidence of Down syndrome. The chance of finding a chromosome problem at a sixteen-week amnio is more than the chance at birth because chromosomally abnormal pregnancies are prone to late miscarriage—a miscarriage that occurs after sixteen weeks but before the fetus can live on its own.

may be preferred over amniocentesis, depending on its availability and how you feel about its slightly greater miscarriage risk.

I had an amnio with Alex at age thirty-six. I had already had two miscarriages. We wanted the information but we weren't sure what we would do if the chromosomes weren't normal. (Beth L., computer science researcher)

When Jonathan and I were deciding about an amnio, I was thirty-seven and had something like a 1 in 200 chance of having something wrong with the baby and a similar chance of having something go wrong with the amnio.

I thought that if Mother Nature gave us an abnormal baby, I could deal with it, but if I caused a problem for my innocent baby, I couldn't. He thought the opposite: that a miscarriage wouldn't ruin our lives, but an abnormal kid would. Same situation, two different spins. (Elisa R., ob-gyn)

My age played into all of my medical decisions. Like I got an amniocentesis. It was completely my decision. I'm a daughter of two physicians, I'm an attorney, so I'm probably better informed than the average duck. I came to the table with the idea that an amnio might be beneficial, and my doctor referred us to genetic counseling. From my perspective, it was a no-brainer. (Rebecca M., senior vice president, financial corporation)

Understanding the Risks and Benefits: True Informed Consent

If you don't want a test, you don't have to have it. After all, it is your body and your baby. And yet some tests will offer information that you might want or need. When deciding what to do next—about genetic screening, pregnancy care, labor interventions, or any other decision points in your medical care—understanding the pros and cons will help you make the right choice for you and your family. The questions here can guide your search for good advice. You might even try writing them on a card to carry with you to your medical appointments so you will remember what to ask.

The second trimester is a time of spectacular growth—for your fetus and for your identity as a parent-to-be. As dramatic ultrasound images bring your baby

---

What is the problem? How severe is it?

What are the risks and benefits of the suggested approach?

What are the alternatives to the suggested evaluation or treatment?

How much time do I have to make this decision?

What is the risk if I delay the decision or decline the intervention?

---

into focus, you may find yourself bonding with your little one in a way you never imagined. Prenatal testing, though it causes anxiety for many who choose to have it, eventually offers relief for most parents, as they discover that their fetus seems to be developing normally. No matter what you decide about testing, as you pass important milestones during your second trimester you may feel a new level of anticipation and joy: the baby is getting more real.

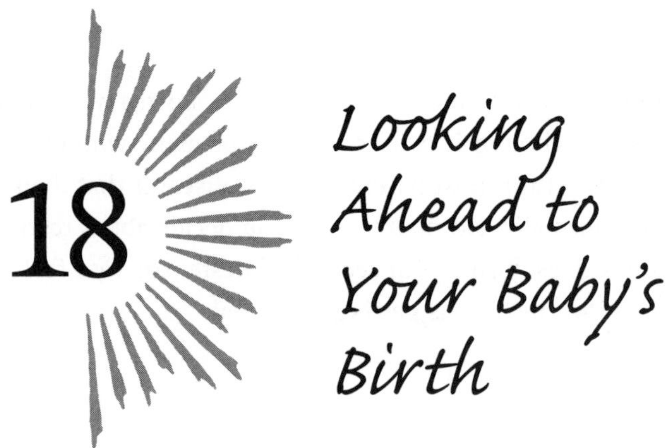

18 Looking Ahead to Your Baby's Birth

Late in the second trimester, many mothers-to-be enjoy daydreaming about holding their babies in their arms. They also often start mentally gearing up for their maternity leaves and their time at home being a mom. Labor and delivery, though, can be much less comfortable to imagine. If you're wondering what you and your partner can do now to prepare for your birth experience, you've come to the right chapter.

Childbirth Classes

Your first pregnancy takes you into unknown territory. You can learn about the experience from books and videos, but taking a class will compel you to set some time aside to get ready. In most prenatal classes you will learn about pregnancy and birth, and you can practice relaxation techniques while your partner practices coaching skills. You will also have an opportunity to bond with other parents in a similar stage of life. You may think of childbirth classes as preparation for natural, unmedicated birth, but nowadays many are quite mainstream, anticipating that most of the couples will deliver with an epidural. Families who desire unmedicated childbirth may actually be better served by seeking out classes that emphasize preparation for a more natural, less "medical" experience. Conversely, families who are planning on an epidural will be more comfortable if they avoid classes that are dogmatically anti-medical.

I went to a prenatal yoga class. All the people there are very earthy people who don't want medical interventions in labor. They teach you a lot of

positions to help with labor, and I guess I thought I would use things like that more. But with the Pitocin and the epidural, you don't really move around that much. This was a contrast to the "Great Expectations" class that I took at the hospital, where every woman there wanted an epidural, and I felt a lot more accepted. I felt really good being more prepared after the yoga classes, even though I didn't use much of it. (Amanda O., meeting planner)

Most of the people that told me their stories had never even considered a natural labor and had the idea that if you didn't have to experience the pain then why go through it? I took the opposite approach and said that I would at least try it without drugs and I could always ask for them if I really thought I needed them. (Danielle R., trust analyst)

STANDARD CHILDBIRTH CLASSES

In standard childbirth classes, which are usually based in hospitals, six or eight weekly two-hour sessions or a few longer weekend classes cover the events of pregnancy, labor, and birth. Instructors also teach Lamaze-style breathing and relaxation techniques for managing contractions. Unless you are lucky enough to have a very quick and easy labor, these classes generally will not provide adequate preparation for unmedicated birth. But if you are like most moms who take standard childbirth classes, you will not need extensive preparation for natural childbirth: although many mothers-to-be plan to keep an open mind, most who take hospital-based classes will have epidural anesthesia. Your practitioner or hospital will provide a schedule of sessions so you can choose a class that finishes up a few weeks before your due date.

LAMAZE

Lamaze breathing patterns were designed to distract a mother from the discomfort of contractions during labor. Lamaze classes that are oriented toward natural childbirth provide information about pregnancy and tools to cope with labor—such as different positions to labor in, breathing techniques, coaching, and birth options. Lamaze techniques have also been incorporated into many

NATURAL CHILDBIRTH VERSUS THE EPIDURAL

The decision to try for natural childbirth or plan on an epidural should depend on your personal beliefs and goals, as well as on how your labor is going. One way to think this through ahead of time is to consider how you have reacted in other situations. What is the greatest physical challenge that you have faced? A hard hike? Knee rehab? The Boston Marathon? If meeting challenges makes you feel good, natural childbirth may be for you. Women have given birth without drugs for thousands of years—you can do it too! And women who meet this challenge often find it to be the most empowering experience of their lives. If you generally avoid discomforts, though, and don't have a lot emotionally invested in "natural" birth as a rite of passage, you will probably be happier with an epidural. Epidural anesthesia makes childbirth more enjoyable for some women, because they don't have to work as much on coping and can focus on the miracle at hand. Even with an epidural, pushing out a baby can be a challenge. I don't believe natural childbirth is a moral decision; it is just a personal choice. Birth is fulfilling whether the baby is born in a cabin in the woods or by cesarean section in an operating room, as long as you have participated in the decisions and made choices that were right for you.

standard childbirth classes. For more information, see the Lamaze website at www.lamaze.org.

BRADLEY METHOD

The Bradley method, also called partner-coached childbirth, focuses on prenatal nutrition and fitness as well as relaxation techniques for drug-free labor and birth. Bradley classes typically start in the second trimester and meet more intensively than standard childbirth classes. Some Bradley instructors are hardline anti-medical, teaching the partner to "protect" the mother from the hospital team, whereas others encourage the families to work with their care providers to get the best experience. Talk to your instructor before signing up for class to be sure her style will suit your needs, and check out the Bradley website at www.bradleybirth.com if you want to learn more.

We had to go to the Bradley classes for twelve weeks; they're a lot more in-depth than the regular childbirth classes. (Kristen S., public relations)

HYPNOBIRTHING

You might think of hypnosis as the trance-like condition you see in the movies, but the self-hypnosis used in hypnobirthing is more of a deep meditative state. In the 1940s Dr. Grantly Dick-Read, in his book *Childbirth without Fear*, taught that much of the pain experienced during childbirth was caused by a cycle of fear and tension. The five-class hypnobirthing series follows traditional childbirth education topics; it also teaches the woman and her coach about the roles that anxiety and tension play in pain perception. Women using hypnobirthing respond to surges, the word that is used instead of contractions or pains, by putting themselves in a meditative state. Deep relaxation is believed to break the cycle of anxiety, tension, and pain. I am continually amazed at how relaxed and in control hypnobirthing moms seem to be; for details about this technique, see the hypnobirthing website at www.hypnobirthing.com.

BIRTHING FROM WITHIN

A British midwife created Birthing from Within after the personal, spiritual nature of her own birth surprised her. Birthing from Within classes are not about the physiology of birth, but rather an exploration of the inner meaning of birth through art, visualization, exploration of hopes and fears, and what they call "innovative pain coping practices." Classes typically meet for eight sessions, including two after the baby comes; see www.birthingfromwithin.com for more information.

Baby showers unfortunately usually turn out to be more like present-opening marathons, and aren't that emotionally rewarding. I read in a book called **Birthing from Within** ***about meaningful pregnant women rituals, but I never was able to figure out how to get one for me (and I even took a birthing class***

based on Birthing from Within, but they didn't do those rituals). (Cheryl L., lawyer)

BIRTH WORKS

This set of ten weekly classes teaches that every woman already possesses the knowledge of how to give birth and only needs to feel secure and confident in order to follow her own natural path. In addition to technical information about the birth process and common medical procedures, you will explore your beliefs and attitudes about birth, to give you more trust and faith in your body and in the natural process of childbirth. The website for Birth Works is www.birthworks.org.

Don't do the Lamaze breathing! I felt like it made me hyperventilate so I did some research and went with a natural childbirth technique where you focus more on deep breathing. I didn't actually attend any classes or get any training—I just read the books and practiced at home. It worked well for me! (Sandy B., social worker)

You watch the TV shows and you think you know about labor but you don't. The Bradley classes were good—even if I decided to get an epidural, I felt I would have learned along the way. (Danielle R., trust analyst)

We couldn't find a Lamaze class in our area, so we took standard childbirth classes, which had about two sessions on breathing and relaxation techniques. (Julie M., veterinarian)

Some of the folks that I dealt with while I was pregnant, like the people at maternity stores and Babies "R" Us, they talked to me like I was twelve years old. And some of the childbirth classes were clearly geared toward much younger women. They ought to change their approach when working with an older mom. (Rebecca M., senior vice president, financial corporation)

I think going to the childbirth classes sets up expectations about what the delivery will be like. Anyone will tell you who has been through it: it's not going to be like you expect. And anyone who has multiple children will tell you it's different every time. (Heidi R., law professor)

WEEKEND MARATHON CLASSES OR WEEKLY CLASSES?

Weekend all-day prenatal courses can be tempting, especially if you are busy: you can block out a day or two and get it all done. Unfortunately, this isn't the best way to learn. To really grow from new information, you need time to take it all in, and then the opportunity to ask questions and to practice new skills. (All-day classes can also be exhausting.) But if you can't commit to weekly sessions, compressed classes may be your best choice.

Prenatal Classes for Single Moms and Same-Sex Couples

Most prenatal classes assume that the mother is in a relationship with the father of the baby. Although the brochure might say that other support people are welcome to attend, you may feel uncomfortable if the teacher assumes that the father will have a major role. One option is to talk to the instructor ahead of time about the environment in the classroom, to see if the class will meet your needs. Alternatively, you can arrange a private class or a small group class of other nontraditional moms, or take out videos and books from the library. Many childbirth educators are happy to arrange a few individualized sessions. To locate a private childbirth educator, talk to the teacher of your local childbirth classes, ask your doctor or midwife, or contact the International Childbirth Education Association at www.icea.org.

As a single mother, I found the childbirth and parenthood classes offered by the local hospitals to be a complete disaster. They were totally focused on couples and appeared not to envisage the possibility of any single women giving birth without a husband or boyfriend. Less than useful comments included: "Guys, she can't do this on her own! When you come home at the end of the day, she will need you there to cook, to clean, to help her, she will not be able to do it without your help!" (Rebecca B., journalist)

A few women in childbirth class brought their mothers instead of the baby's father; my sister came with me, since the father had taken off. During

PREPARING YOUR BODY FOR BIRTH

No special preparation techniques are needed in the second trimester, but getting and staying in good shape can prove helpful. Labor and birth are very physical and may require strength and stamina. Aerobic conditioning, as well as lower body and some upper body exercise, will help you to move around in labor, push out your baby, and recover from birth. If you already work out, any combination of aerobic training and strength training will be beneficial. If you are out of shape, it is not too late to start walking or swimming to prepare for giving birth.

the breastfeeding class, I was the only one there by myself. I was a little embarrassed. (Myra K., courtroom assistant)

Labor Support

Now is a good time to start thinking about who will come with you when you have your baby. Will you be accompanied by your partner, other family members, close friends, a doula?

While I was pushing it was just me, the nurse, and my husband which was very nice. I went to my friend's birth and it seemed like there were fifty people in the room. (Galit A., tax attorney)

Brian's mom always talked about how wonderful birth is so I asked her to come to our baby's birth before we were even married! When I got pregnant I asked her and my mom. You don't get to see someone be born every day and I thought it would be nice to involve the grandparents. My mom, my mother-in-law, and my stepfather were all there with my husband and me. (Zenia M., nurse's aide)

The father of your baby, assuming he is involved and plans to be at the birth, should take childbirth classes with you. Remember, though, a few childbirth classes don't necessarily make a man an expert in labor or labor support. While some men are terrific coaches, fathers often worry about how they will handle childbirth. A man may feel that part of his role in life is to protect his woman from suffering—and labor can look a lot like suffering. He may not have the experience and perspective to know that in minutes you will be saying how proud you are that you did it, and how perfect the baby's little fingers are. He also may worry that he will faint or fail in some way. The dad has an important role witnessing the birth of his baby and he might be the person who knows you the best. But he may not be cut out to be your only labor support, particularly if you want natural childbirth. Penny Simkin's book *The Birth Partner* is a great resource for a dad (or anyone else) who wants to provide support for natural birth.

When I told my fiancé that I wanted natural childbirth he looked at me incredulously and said, "Why?" (Danielle R., trust analyst)

If you hope for an unmedicated experience, you may particularly want to consider additional support. Doulas (professional labor assistants) provide emotional and physical aid to mothers- and fathers-to-be. Doulas have expertise in comfort measures and often also teach childbirth classes. Their primary interest is helping you and your partner have a good birth experience. Doulas don't provide medical care or deliver babies, but research has shown that doula-supported labors are shorter, require less pain medication, and lead to fewer cesareans. We don't know exactly why doulas have better outcomes—maybe the continuous emotional support leads to lower levels of anxiety and stress hormones in the mother.

Often couples feel that labor is their time to go up against the world and do something difficult together; they feel that anyone else in the room might interfere with their relationship and with the role of the father as coach. But research on doulas shows that the fathers actually have the same or more contact with the mothers when a doula is present—probably because the doula encourages or models helpful behaviors. Satisfaction with the doula experience is very high for both mothers and fathers.

Doulas usually charge a flat rate—generally around four to five hundred dollars, so if your labor is short they get a good deal, and if your labor is long, they stick with you. Your doula will most likely talk with you before labor to learn about you and what type of experience you are seeking, then will drop everything to be with you when your labor begins. You can find a doula through your childbirth instructor, your OB, or Doulas of North America at www.dona.org.

If the cost is too much for you, or if you prefer a familiar face, consider asking a close woman friend or family member to come as extra support. One research study showed almost as much benefit (in terms of length of labor and need for medications) if a female family member or friend was there as from a trained doula.

If you are going to be delivered by a midwife, ask if it makes sense to have a doula in addition. Some midwives fulfill most of the doula's role in addition to taking care of you medically and delivering the baby.

Cord Blood Donation

Have you been contacted yet by a private cord blood storage company? If not, you may be soon: it turns out that the blood that remains in the umbilical cord after birth contains a type of stem cells that has the potential to develop into all the different components of blood. Normally, the cord blood is discarded with the placenta after delivery, wasting this potential resource. Cord blood collection by private companies, however, is somewhat controversial. Proponents explain that:

- Cord blood can be used like a bone marrow transplant, a potentially life-saving treatment for cancers and other diseases. Over time, more uses may be developed.
- If price is no object, there is no personal downside to cord blood storage.
- If you have a family member who is likely to benefit from a cord blood transplant, you may be eligible for a program that would pay for private cord blood collection. Ask your family member's physician.

Opponents of commercial cord blood collection, however, point out that

- Cord blood collection is expensive—on average, $1,500 up front and $100 per year for storage. Most new parents have many other uses for those dollars.
- Private cord blood companies market donation to families as "biological insurance" for their child. But a child's own cord blood would rarely be useful for that child. It couldn't be used to treat a genetic disease (since

it has exactly the same genes), and if the child developed leukemia, the doctors would worry that these were the same cells that turned into leukemia in the first place, and would probably prefer other treatment alternatives.

- The chance that a family would collect cord blood and then a close relative would happen to need it is miniscule. Very few samples of routinely collected cord blood have been put to use so far. Most of the samples that have been used have been from families who knew that another sibling was going to need it, and collected it for that purpose.
- If the company goes out of business, you could be out your payments as well as the sample of cord blood.

For these reasons, the American Academy of Pediatrics and many physicians do not recommend private cord blood banking except in cases where a family member currently needs a bone marrow transplant or is at high risk for needing one in the future.

PUBLIC CORD BLOOD BANKING

Another option for reserving umbilical cord blood, if your hospital offers it, is public cord blood donation. Similar to blood banking, cord blood is stored and kept available for anyone in need. The patient who needs it pays—a cost usually covered by insurance—and the donor is not charged. If the donating family ever requires a cord blood transplant, the sample will be given back at no charge. If the unit you donated is no longer available, another matched unit will be offered for free. In the United States, 150,000 units of donated cord blood would meet the needs of 80–90 percent of all patients, meaning that this valuable resource could help many more people if shared rather than hoarded by each family. For more information on public cord blood donation, go to www.nationalcordbloodprogram.org.

Picking a Doctor for Your Baby

Your baby receives medical care from you and your obstetrical team even before birth. But what about after the delivery? Who can provide the best medical care for your newborn, infant, and young child? The answers to that question will depend on your priorities. Some moms and dads want to become attached to a single doctor; others welcome the convenience of a large practice; still others weigh heavily factors like the affiliated hospital's reputation or the chance to see a doctor rather than a nurse practitioner at each visit. As you consider what kind of care provider you would like for your newborn, consider these facts:

- Pediatricians, family doctors, and nurse practitioners all can provide well-child care. Pediatricians are physicians who have completed medical school followed by three more years of residency in the outpatient and hospital treatment of children and adolescents. They usually provide for the medical needs of children from birth through age eighteen or twenty-one. Family doctors are physicians who have completed medical school followed by three years of residency training in the outpatient and hospital treatment of adults and children. They can provide medical care for your entire family from birth through old age. Nurse practitioners (NPs) are registered nurses, often with master's degrees, who have completed a two-year program of additional training either in pediatric care or family medical care and have passed national certifying examinations. NPs who provide well-child care usually see patients in the office in collaboration with a physician.
- Your insurance (or the father's) will automatically cover the baby from birth, as long as you notify your employer's human resource department within thirty days.
- You will most likely want to choose a practice that is covered by your insurance plan. Often the insurance company books and websites are not up-to-date; to be safe, try calling your preferred doctor's office and asking if they will take your insurance.
- A location near home will probably offer the best convenience. You won't want to cart a sick child all over town, unless that's your only acceptable option.
- Most doctors and nurse practitioners work in groups; you may see the same person each time or go to any member of the group, depending on how the practice works. Some groups have you see a consistent provider for well-child appointments, and whoever is on call for sick visits.
- If the group is affiliated with the hospital where you plan to give birth,

ask if they make rounds to see their babies. If they don't "round" at your hospital, the hospital pediatricians can care for the baby until you go home.

Choosing a professional to give medical care for your baby can seem like a daunting task, but it doesn't have to be. Ask your friends about their children's doctors, or ask your OB for a recommendation. My patients often bring me their insurance lists with the convenient office locations circled. Then I can scan through and refer them to someone I like and trust. Once you have a name, consider setting up a visit to be sure the practice is a good match for your family. Most pediatric practices will provide a prenatal appointment either for the cost of an office visit or free of charge. They will make up a chart for the baby with your family histories, and you can decide if the practice is right for you.

I was in the pediatrician's office for a prenatal consult filling out forms that asked for mother and father's names. I filled in my parents, until my husband pointed out to me that we were the parents! (Kathy H., software developer)

THE PRENATAL PEDIATRIC INTERVIEW

Who will see us when the baby is well?

Do you have weekend or evening office hours?

Can I call the office if I have a question? Who would I talk to?

What if my child is ill when the office is closed?

What hospitals are you affiliated with?

If you have strong feelings or questions on some aspect of parenting, like whether to have the baby sleep in the bed with you, breast versus bottle feeding, or circumcision, bringing those issues up for discussion at this visit serves two purposes: you become more informed, and it helps you to judge if this practitioner's style fits with your beliefs and preferences. Think ahead about what you want to ask.

Questions:

Did I feel comfortable asking questions? Were the answers useful and convincing to me?

Part 5

Double-Digit Growth (Week 27 until Birth)

At the beginning of the third trimester, your baby is growing quickly, and your body is getting ready for birth. Your prenatal visits become more frequent, and your practitioner will start to pay special attention to your blood pressure, the size of your little one, and any signs of imminent labor. Around this time, many working women will start fine-tuning their plans for the birth and care of their babies. How long should you continue on the job? What if your labor starts at work? This third trimester section will help you prepare both for the birth and for bringing the baby home, with information on work in late pregnancy, making a birth plan, breastfeeding versus bottle-feeding, obtaining baby supplies, and arranging maternity leave. Pregnancies that go beyond their due dates, and methods commonly used to induce labor, will also be discussed.

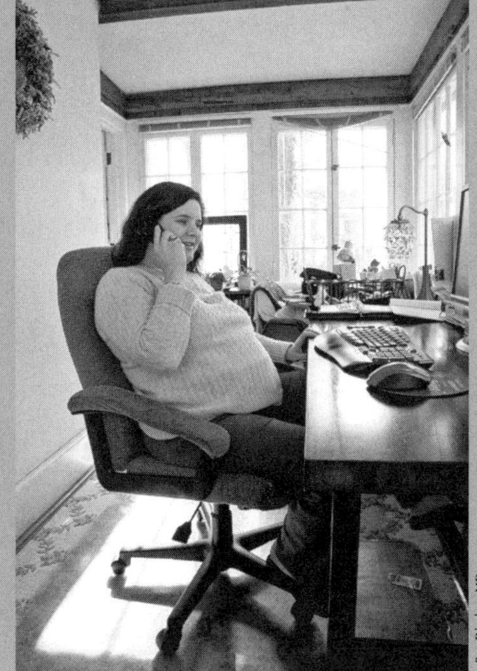

LeRoy Dierker, MD

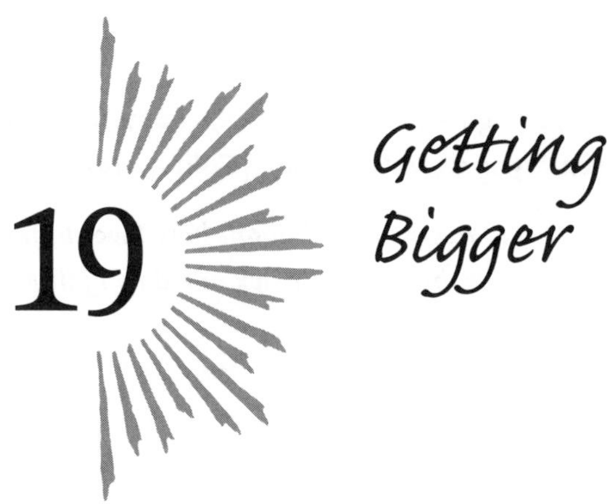

19 Getting Bigger

Congratulations—you've made it to the home stretch! Your baby is getting big, and so are you. You are now officially, conspicuously pregnant. I am always amazed at the range of feelings women have about their bodies at this point.

> ***It was difficult for me to imagine getting any bigger, and yet I kept getting bigger. (Elizabeth S., online producer)***

> ***Doing the weather in front of a green screen, my belly covered the western half of the U.S. My boss even joked about making maps to accommodate my belly. (Eileen M., weather reporter)***

> ***I was proud of how good I looked and felt. Each pregnancy I exercised and worked out and was very active until the day I delivered. (Helene L., teacher)***

> ***It was fun to have this big belly as an obvious sign of being female in such a male profession—I liked shattering the expectations. (Susan G., commercial airline pilot)***

> ***I felt very out of control during pregnancy, like someone else was calling the shots. I'm used to being in control. I got huge, I couldn't bend over, my breasts were leaking, and I was too uncomfortable to sleep well. I felt frustrated and angry a lot. I still fixed my hair and lipstick and exercised but I didn't feel like myself. (Sherri M., sales rep)***

> ***When I was six months along, a man at the ice cream store asked me if I was due that week. That was disheartening. (Zoe B., inventory manager)***

I am heavy and I was used to feeling I had to cover up my body, but now I was pregnant and I loved wearing maternity clothes. (Galit A., tax attorney)

My pregnancy was wonderful. I had been worried about how I would feel, since I had heard such terrible stories, but I wasn't sick one day. I felt great. (Kate R., financial analyst)

Body Changes

During the third trimester, your abdomen will grow as the baby gets bigger, and your breasts may continue to enlarge. If you need new bras after the seventh month, it makes sense to purchase a nursing bra if you plan to breastfeed, but don't get too many since you may continue to outgrow them. Some women whose breasts don't need much support find that tank tops with built-in bras accommodate their changing size. Leaking from the nipples is normal, but it is also normal not to produce any milk until after the baby is born.

My boobs grew and grew. It got to be a joke—every time I got a new bra I grew out of it. This lasted until I stopped breastfeeding. I think I went up four sizes. (Naomi B., attorney)

Body pigmentation tends to intensify in pregnancy. Your nipples may become darker, and you may notice the linea nigra, a dark line down the middle of your belly. This will revert to normal a few months after birth. About half of all women will develop some stretch marks or striae on their abdomen, breasts, or thighs. These will become fainter and more silvery over time.

You belly button may flatten out—or it may even protrude. A Band-Aid can help keep it from rubbing on your clothing or sticking out of tight tops. It will go back to normal after the baby is born.

My innie is now an outie, which is strange. (Jen B., dance teacher)

Your skin may be clear, or you may deal with breakouts. Your hair will probably be thicker than usual, and your nails stronger.

I looked great—my hair was great and my skin was clear, and I had a different kind of energy. (Galit A., tax attorney)

Third Trimester Days

Early in the third trimester most women feel terrific—energized and excited. As the months pass and you get bigger, you may start to drag. Try to protect yourself from getting run down. It's better to begin labor (and motherhood) feeling fresh and energetic than to start off worn out. Most women find that comfort becomes a high priority toward the end.

I just listened to my body; if I was tired or run down I would take some time to rest. My thought was that we've gone though the equivalent of three years of tuition (for IVF) to get this; it isn't worth jeopardizing it to get an extra ten minutes of work done. (Juanita G., research scientist)

Because of the twins, I was worried about preterm labor. I always carried a water bottle with me. When I was sitting down (not that often), I made sure to put my feet up on a stool under my desk. (Jane S., state governor)

Shoes were a huge problem because I became so swollen—I was wearing tennis sneakers at the end—something I would normally never do. (Jane J., advertising executive)

In my second pregnancy I was always tired, and it was hard to care for my two-year-old. Sometimes I would just let him play in the bath for an hour so he would be contained but still doing something fun. That way I could feel like a good mom without it being too taxing. (Julie M., veterinarian)

Third Trimester Nights

Sleeping may become difficult; either the baby wakes you, or your bladder does. Nighttime heartburn may require swigs from that liquid antacid you keep by the bedside. Getting comfortable may seem impossible—most women report that it takes a lot of pillows and arranging to settle in. Anticipation of labor, excitement about the baby, and worries about the changes in your life may also keep your mind churning. New research has shown that labors are shorter in women who get enough sleep in the weeks before childbirth, though, so try to allow for at least eight hours in bed each night.

TIPS FOR SLEEPING WELL

- Exercise early in the day.
- Have a bedtime ritual that helps you to settle down. Don't just hop into bed after racing around all day. A warm bath often does the trick.
- Avoid caffeine after noon. This includes coffee, caffeinated teas, large quantities of chocolate, and caffeinated sodas.
- When sleeping on your side, use pillows to prop up your belly and keep your arms and legs comfortably supported.
- If you and your bedmate have different temperature needs, use separate blankets.
- If your mind is racing, practice your breathing and relaxation techniques for labor.
- Remember that rest is almost as good as sleep; don't drive yourself crazy trying to fall asleep. If you can't sleep, get out of bed and do something quiet in dim lighting until you feel tired again.
- Some women take sleeping medication such as Ambien or Benadryl. Be sure to talk to your doctor or midwife before taking any medications, including over-the-counter sleep aids.

After a certain point, once you wake up, there is no falling back asleep. Period. You get to lie in bed and think about impending parenthood and all of the details that go along with it. So it doesn't matter if you wake up at six, five, or two-thirty. Last night I was awake from two-thirty until six. (Jen B., dance teacher)

I imagine what my child will like to do, what his or her interests will be, what they'll want to be when they grow up, what we'll do together, the games we'll play . . . whether I'll have any help, whether we'll be poor, whether I will send my child to school or homeschool him or her . . . whether we'll have friends . . . (Kate P., livestock farmer)

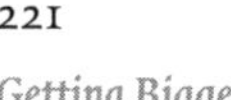

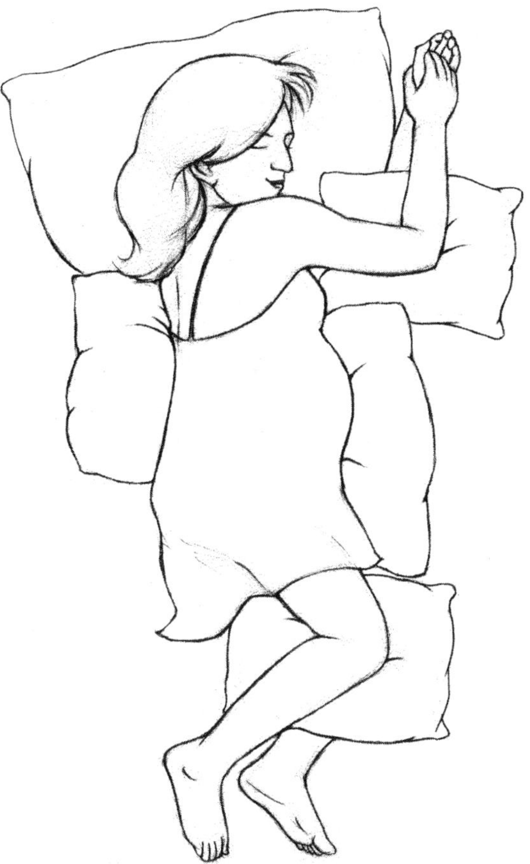

You might try using strategically positioned pillows to help you get comfortable during the night. Try lying on your side with a pillow under your tummy and one between your knees.

I was very uncomfortable late in pregnancy. Pillows were my friends. I used a body pillow in the bed, throw pillows behind me on the couch, a pillow behind me for driving. (Jennifer A., secretary)

Three days past my due date, sleeping was not something that came easily. I did my best perched atop the Great Wall of China—my husband's nickname for the pillow pile I had built during the last two months of the pregnancy. (Rebecca M., senior vice president, financial corporation)

During the night, many mothers-to-be have trouble with leg cramps. Medical science doesn't know why pregnant women get these painful spasms. Unfortunately there isn't anything proven to prevent them, although some people believe a teaspoon a day of yellow mustard helps keep them away (you can put it on toast). As soon as you feel a cramp starting, stretch the calf muscle by pulling your toes up toward your knee. Gentle massage may also provide relief. Some women find that a bolster or pillows at the foot of the bed reminds them not to stretch out their feet, since toe-pointing may set off the cramp. Leaving your blankets untucked may also help keep your toes from pointing.

I still cringe when I accidentally point my toes in bed—and it's been seventeen years since I've had a baby! (Maggie P., administrator)

A woman told me this story: she got a leg cramp in her ninth month, and screamed out. Her husband was up out of bed with the bag they packed for labor, dressed, and by the door before she was able to explain to him it wasn't that kind of cramp. (Marge G., obstetrician)

Practice Contractions

We'll talk about signs of labor later, but for now it's worth reviewing some of the normal sensations of late pregnancy, and how to differentiate them from labor. Practice contractions, also called Braxton-Hicks contractions, may feel like a tightening or balling up sensation in your belly or lower back, or like menstrual cramps. These usually last anywhere from a few seconds to a minute or so. A few contractions a day is totally normal; clusters may also be normal as long as they don't persist. You may notice a contraction any time your bladder is full or right after you empty it; when you get up from lying or sitting; during or after sex or exercise; if you get dehydrated; or when the baby gives you a big kick.

If it is still too early for the baby to be born safely, pay attention to contractions that come more than four to six times in an hour, and change your activities to try to make them stop. If they don't resolve after a few hours with rest and hydration, call your doctor or midwife.

Backaches

Backaches are quite common in pregnancy, even more so as you reach the last few months. These pains may occur in the upper or lower back. Pain in the buttock with or without radiation down the back of the leg may be sciatica. If the back pain is a tightening feeling, consider that it might be a contraction, and

BEFORE THIRTY-SIX WEEKS: COULD THIS BE PRETERM LABOR?

(Note that technically "preterm" refers to any birth before thirty-seven weeks, but since babies who have been inside the mom for thirty-five to thirty-six weeks do very well, we don't really worry about preterm labor unless it is before then. Your doctor or midwife can provide you with individualized guidelines.)

- Preterm labor contractions may be painless, so pay heed to any persistent balling up or tightening sensations in your abdomen or lower back—these are contractions.
- If you notice more than four to six contractions an hour, change your activities. If they don't go away within a few hours or if they are painful, phone your doctor or midwife, or go to the hospital.
- Breaking your water may produce a big gush, and be quite obvious, but sometimes it comes as a recurrent trickle. The fluid is watery, not gooey like the normal pregnancy discharge. If you think you might have broken your water, call your doctor or midwife to help you figure it out.
- *Any* bleeding before thirty-six weeks should be reported to your practitioner.
- An increase in pelvic pressure can be a sign that the baby will come early. Before your last month, persistent or recurrent vaginal pressure should be reported to your doctor or midwife.

follow the instructions for possible preterm labor. Back pain with a fever or very severe pain should be reported to your doctor or midwife right away to be sure you don't have a kidney infection or kidney stone. But if the pain is continuous, you probably have a garden-variety backache.

BACKACHE PREVENTION

- Start off pregnancy with strong abdominal muscles
- Use proper lifting techniques (see Chapter 9)

- Don't do things that make the pain worse. Take notice if wearing high heels, heavy lifting, exercising, or repetitive activities aggravate your pain
- Watch your posture at home and at work
- Use a six-inch cylindrical pillow for lumbar back support at your desk, when driving, and any time you are sitting
- Do back-strengthening and flexibility exercises (see later in this chapter)
- Get a weekly massage—you deserve it!
- Get help at work or home when you need it
- Try an elastic support for your abdomen, which may improve your posture and decrease stress on your back (for some examples, see www.babyhugger.com or call 1–888–770–0044)
- Consult with a physical therapist
- If you have severe sciatica, talk to your doctor or midwife. Sometimes a physical therapy referral or a short course of steroids (like prednisone) helps speed recovery.

I was having pelvic pain toward the end of pregnancy, and it was very difficult to walk from my parking lot to the office. I told my boss I might have to go out on disability if I couldn't park closer, and all of a sudden they were able to get me handicapped parking right in front. People don't make accommodations for you unless you ask. You have to push for what you need. (Brenda W., lawyer)

I had lower back pain in the third trimester. It was my low back and my sacroiliac joint. I went to a chiropractor who said my pelvis was tilted. She'd adjust me and I would feel better for a day or two. By the end I was going to her twice a week. (Julie M., veterinarian)

TREATMENT OF BACK PAIN

Back exercises for ten minutes a day can make a huge difference in your back pain. These exercises are good for flexibility and strength, too. The stretching exercises that you can do at your desk (illustrated earlier) are also helpful for back pain, particularly the shoulder pinch. If you're only going to do one exercise, the pelvic rock is often the most beneficial. Different exercises work for different people and at different times in the pregnancy. Try varied approaches to find what is best for you. Effective exercises can be used frequently throughout the day as needed.

The Last Few Weeks

Ready, set . . . during the final weeks of pregnancy, your body is busy preparing for birth. The experiences of these last weeks may seem unusual, but they are signs of progress. Your baby is on the way!

SHOW

"Show" or "bloody show" is an old-fashioned but still commonly used term for when the blob of mucus that was lodged in the cervix comes out. The mucus plug may pass days to weeks before labor, or you may never notice it. Often a little bit of blood comes out at the same time. A small amount of bleeding is also normal after you have an internal examination. Bleeding like a period, however, is not normal and should be reported to your doctor or midwife.

FALSE LABOR

Mild contractions may become more frequent, sometimes making it hard to tell if you are still practicing or if real labor has begun. Alternatively, some women don't notice any contractions until labor.

NESTING

Some mothers-to-be find themselves in a manic clean-up mode a day or two before labor begins. This is called nesting, but it doesn't happen to everyone; most mothers can't rely on nesting as a sign of imminent labor.

LIGHTENING

As the baby settles deeply (engages or drops) into your pelvis, you experience "lightening." You can eat more, and breathe more easily. The trade-off is that your bladder capacity diminishes, and you may feel like you are walking with a watermelon between your legs. The baby usually engages in the pelvis sometime

EXERCISES FOR YOUR BACK

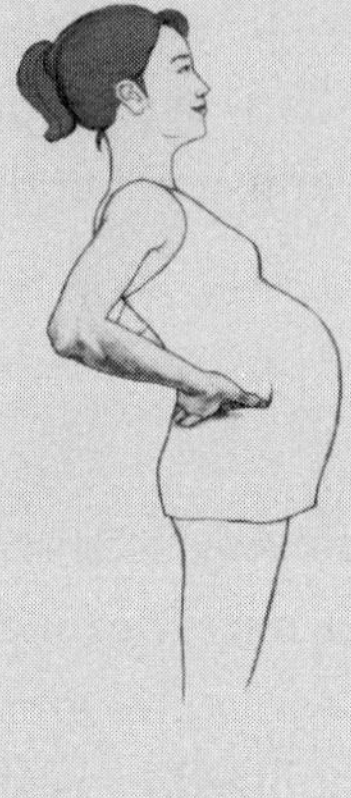

The standing back extension. Standing, place your hands at your lower back at the level of your waist. Using your hands as a fulcrum, bend your upper back backward and over your hands. Don't strain your tummy. Return to standing. Repeat five to ten times.

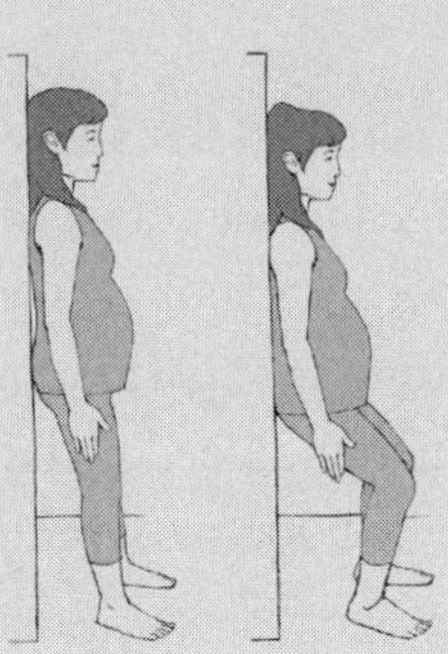

The standing pelvic tilt. Stand with your back against a wall, feet shoulder width apart, heels a few inches from the wall. Slide down the wall an inch or two and rotate your hips so that your lower back flattens against the wall. Hold for five seconds, then release and stand. Repeat ten times.

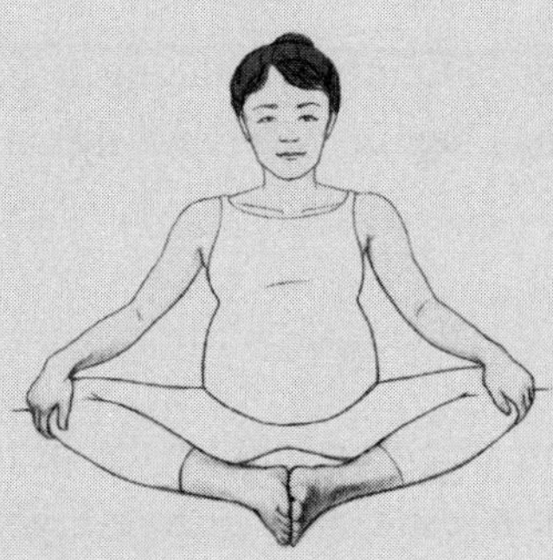

The tailor sitting stretch. Sit with the soles of your feet together. Apply gentle pressure to the insides of your knees with your hands. Be careful not to bounce your legs. Hold the stretch for thirty seconds, then release. Repeat ten times.

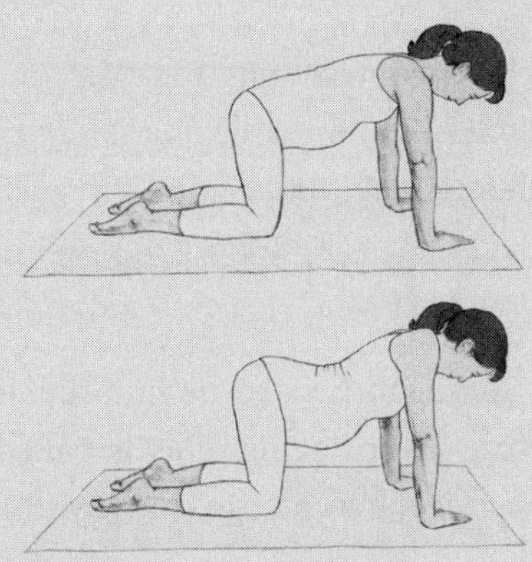

The pelvic rock. Get down on all fours, with your hands directly under your shoulders and your knees under your hips. Your arms should be vertical, not slanted. Rock your pelvis back to flatten out your back, then rock your pelvis forward and let your back sag. Repeat ten times. Don't allow your back to arch, particularly if you have sciatica.

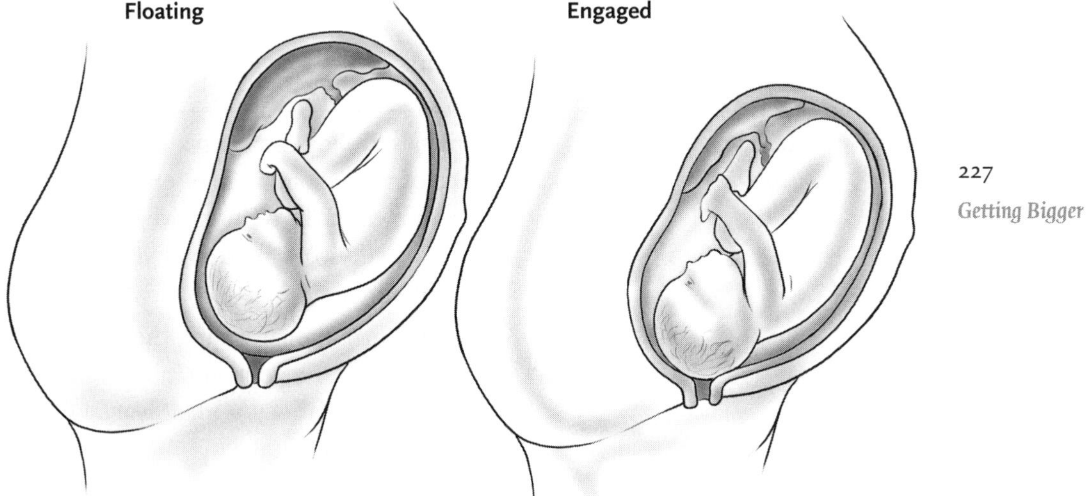

When the baby "drops," it descends from a floating position to become engaged in the pelvis.

between thirty-five weeks and when labor starts—earlier in first-time moms and later for those who have given birth before.

Your Soon-to-Be Baby

Your baby has reached the point where survival is possible, yet your body continues to provide for fetal needs better than any high-tech incubator can. The temperature and lighting are perfect, sounds are muffled, and oxygen and nutrients are plentiful. In fact, during each of the next several weeks in your womb, your baby will put on more than a quarter of a pound, gaining size, strength, and stamina. Although your body may be causing you some misery, think of all it is accomplishing. Inside you, right now, is a person you will love, and who will love you more than anyone has loved you before. It may be easier to endure the day-to-day discomforts if you remember to enjoy your body's miraculous and powerful achievement.

FETAL GROWTH

How is your baby growing? During the first two trimesters, most fetuses are pretty much the same size at the same age. But starting in the third trimester,

Fetal Milestones

Weeks	*Avg. Weight*	*Avg. Length*	*Milestones*
26	1 lb., 14 oz.	12″	The baby's eyelids can open and close; the chance of survival now is 80–90 percent (after many months of intensive care); about half of the survivors are free of serious long-term problems
28	2 lbs., 7 oz.	14″	With newborn intensive care, the chance of survival is over 90 percent, although the road may still be rocky, with at least a few months in the hospital
32	4 lbs.	16″	Babies born at thirty-two weeks usually do quite well, although they may have difficulties feeding or keeping their temperature steady. The odds of survival at thirty-two weeks are the same as at full-term
35	5 lbs.	17″	About half of the babies born at thirty-five weeks are ready to go home from the hospital in the usual two days
38	6 lbs., 6 oz.	19″	Beyond thirty-eight weeks there is no particular benefit to the baby from staying inside, but be patient—the baby may not send the signals that start labor for another few weeks
40	7 lbs., 3 oz.	20″	Babies continue to gain a quarter to half a pound a week up to and beyond the due date

Note: As the weeks pass, you can feel ever more confident that your baby will do well if born early.

babies start to grow at different rates. This means that the expected weights for fetuses in late pregnancy are just averages, and that the size of your newborn will be influenced by many factors, including:

- Your height and that of the father (big people have bigger babies)
- Your weight (overweight women have bigger babies)
- Your weight gain during pregnancy (excess calories can lead to bigger babies)
- The altitude where you live (babies are slightly smaller at higher altitudes)
- Whether you have uncontrolled gestational diabetes (the baby will use any extra sugar to grow)
- Whether you have high blood pressure (which may decrease blood flow and nutrients to the baby)
- Whether you are overdue (the baby has more time to grow)
- Your race (white babies are slightly bigger than babies of African or Asian ancestry)
- Whether you smoke cigarettes (babies whose mothers have a pack-a-day habit will, on average, be more than *half a pound smaller* at birth)
- The weight of your previous babies, if you have had any (typically, each pregnancy results in a slightly bigger newborn)
- Fetal sex (boys on average are five ounces bigger than girls at birth).

Even when all these factors are taken into account, though, weight isn't totally predictable. When researchers compared three commonly used means of estimating fetal weight—ultrasound measurements, the doctor's approximation by feel, and the mother's best guess—believe it or not, ultrasound was the *least* accurate. Even though ultrasound provides a number that sounds very exact, it's only an estimate made by applying a formula to measurements of the baby's head, tummy, and leg bone. A mother who had given birth before was most accurate at predicting the weight of the baby, comparing it to the experience of carrying her previous children. But even so, no one measurement was terribly accurate. So if your office pool is making wagers, check out the list of factors that affect weight, but don't bet the house!

The doctor predicted that the baby would weigh about nine pounds, but I thought bigger. She kept reminding me that my hips were big enough to

deliver vaginally. Not what you want to hear. When Ingrid came out at ten and a half pounds, it was a little shocking. (Peggy L., nurse-administrator)

I was worried the baby would be very big. Her father was ten pounds at birth. I thought maybe eight to nine pounds. Ultrasound predicted over eight pounds. The doctor thought around seven pounds. She was six pounds, six ounces at birth. (Danielle R., trust analyst)

After two babies, I sort of knew that I wouldn't grow a seven-pound baby. They were always in the sixes. I figured my third was about six pounds, the ultrasound said six, my doctor thought about six, and he was six pounds, ten ounces, so this is a case when everyone was right. (Jennifer A., secretary)

GUESSING THE SEX

Have people been speculating about the sex of your baby? Many folks believe they can predict the sex based on how you are carrying, or by other external signs. None of these legends has any validity—not even the rumor of faster heartbeats in boys (or was that girls?). By now you may have had the opportunity to learn the sex of your baby through ultrasound or other testing, but even if you know for sure, people often feel the need to make predictions.

In my first pregnancy I knew it was a boy as soon as my pregnancy test was positive. The second time around, I thought it was a girl but it wasn't as strong a feeling, and I thought maybe it was just because I wanted a girl. Then when I was five days overdue I was at the toy store and I found myself buying a pink bunny—I guess I was pretty sure it was a girl—and she was. (Julie M., veterinarian)

Everyone said because of the way I looked from the back they thought it was a boy. On ultrasound they said it was a girl but I wasn't sure if I should believe it. When she was born, I was so glad she was really a girl. (Sherri M., sales rep)

I've been sick a lot this time. I was never sick with Adam, so everyone said it's a girl, it must be a girl. Then I went for the ultrasound, and it's another boy. I think it's really just wives' tales. (Elizabeth S., online producer)

My friends and I were convinced I was having a girl. We did the string test, where I laid on the couch and someone tied my wedding ring to a string and spun the ring in a circle. The test predicted a girl, but I ended up with Jack! (Jen R., fashion merchandiser)

All of the old wives' tales were wrong with me. You know, the way you carry it, the slower heartbeat. (Amanda O., meeting planner)

I lived in Germany for one of my pregnancies. Whether in Europe or the USA, many folks felt that by the look/shape of the belly, they could tell if it is a boy or a girl. They usually have a fifty-fifty chance of being accurate! (Helene L., teacher)

FETAL ACTIVITIES

Whether your baby-to-be is a boy or girl, he or she is pretty much acting like a baby during these last few months. Third trimester fetuses swallow amniotic fluid and breathe it into their lungs, readying their bodies' systems for life outside. They suck their thumbs; they grasp if something touches their palms; they have sleep and wake cycles. If you feel occasional sets of evenly spaced rhythmic jumps, your baby probably has the hiccups. During the last month or so, the baby gets more crowded in the uterus; rolling or shifting motions replace kicks that used to be sharp and strong. But you should still feel the baby move multiple times a day. Fetal movement is a reassuring sign that the baby is doing well. I often wonder if babies that are wild during fetal life are the ones who are most active in childhood.

Johnny is always on the move. He didn't sleep when I was pregnant with him and he doesn't sleep now (at age three). (Kate R., financial analyst)

When my son got the hiccups I used to talk to my belly and tell him to drink some amniotic fluid to make them go away. (Marge G., obstetrician)

FETAL POSITIONING

Early in the third trimester your baby may be positioned breech (bottom first) or cephalic (headfirst). A rare baby will lie sideways, called transverse. Breech is common until about thirty-two weeks. By a month before the due date, though, most babies will have settled into the position they will be in during labor—usually headfirst. When the baby is headfirst you usually feel kicks up high, and smaller movements or just pressure at the bottom of your belly. Before the last month, don't worry if your baby isn't headfirst—most babies turn themselves around in time. Your doctor or midwife will determine the position of the baby as you get close to your due date.

Sometime during the last month, too, most babies drop lower, settling the top of their heads into the pelvis. In a first pregnancy, this "lightening" is a reassuring sign that the baby will probably fit through when the time comes. Your little one is moving into position, getting ready to join you out in the world.

During the final weeks of my first pregnancy, my son was in the breech position. My OB asked me if I spoke or sang to my son and I said "of course!" She told me that he was listening and that I should put music between my legs and have my husband talk to him there. Sure enough he "flipped" and was in "birthing position" during the last week or so. (Edie U., school psychologist)

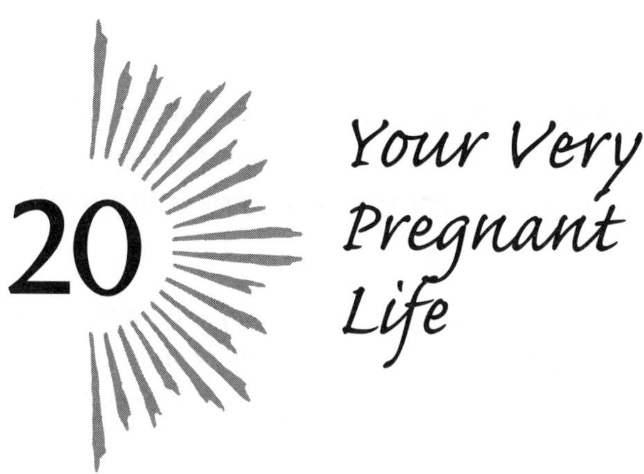

20 Your Very Pregnant Life

The newest member of your family will be here soon. No matter how uncomfortable you may be getting, or how uncertain you may feel, it is impossible not to be excited about the many changes to come. It's time to count down to the moment you will first hold your baby in your arms.

Alleviating Late Pregnancy Fatigue

The last trimester can be exhausting, but staying active will often help give you energy, whereas lying around may sap it. Try to continue to get some exercise each day. If you can work out, aerobics, weight training, prenatal yoga, and most other exercises are fine as long as the pregnancy is going well. Even if you have been sedentary, you can probably walk or do other light aerobic exercise. Swimming or any sort of water exercise is terrific if you have swelling; the pressure of the water on your body will push excess fluid from your tissues back into your veins, to be eliminated by your kidneys. You might spend extra time in the bathroom afterward, but your feet will thank you. Pelvic pressure may improve, too, after swimming. If you can't swim, even walking ten minutes a few times a day will be good for you, although it won't help the swelling and pressure. For all these activities, the usual pregnancy exercise rules still apply: don't get overheated or dehydrated, and don't push yourself beyond where you can talk. You might need to take a big breath at the end of each sentence, but you should be able to hold a conversation without stopping to gasp.

Toward the end of each of my three term pregnancies I climbed a 4,000-foot mountain in New Hampshire, just to prove I could do it. (Deb L., writer)

I ran throughout both pregnancies. With my first, I ran up to the last thirty minutes before I went into labor. I was going to a friend's house for dinner, and I decided to run there, and I started feeling my first contractions. (Kathy C., family therapist)

I exercised at least four times per week throughout my pregnancy, including the day I went into the hospital. I gained about thirty pounds, and didn't have any difficulty losing the weight afterwards. (Kafi P., teacher)

Exercise will help elevate your mood, enhance your self-esteem, control your weight, and keep your energy level high. It also will strengthen you for labor. You may have heard about specific exercises that are sometimes recommended to prepare for birth. These include:

- Kegels. Kegel exercises strengthen the muscles around the opening of the vagina. A correctly done Kegel will stop the flow of urine. (Kegeling on the toilet is recommended only as a test; it isn't good for your body to repeatedly interrupt the stream.) Kegels are very helpful if you are leaking urine—strengthening those muscles really works. But unless you are experiencing incontinence, the benefits of Kegels before birth are controversial: one school of thought says that strengthening the pelvic floor helps with labor and pushing; the other that Kegels make the birth canal tighter and more difficult to get the baby through. Practitioners generally agree, though, that Kegel exercises are very useful after the birth, helping you to regain pelvic muscle tone and bladder control.
- Perineal massage. This exercise involves daily stretching of the opening of the vagina in hopes that the baby will fit through more easily, avoiding the need for stitches. Instructions usually involve placing either your two thumbs or your partner's index fingers about two inches inside the vagina, and then pressing gently but firmly down and out for ten minutes a day to widen the opening, starting at around thirty-two weeks. You have to concentrate on relaxing the muscles as you stretch; a lubricant like KY jelly, baby oil, or mineral oil may make it more comfortable. You should feel mild burning but not severe pain, and if you are doing the exercise correctly, any discomfort should improve after the first week or two. The theory behind perineal massage? Vaginal tears are less common in second

or later babies because a first baby has stretched out the area during delivery—perineal massage tries to achieve the same effect before the first baby arrives. Unfortunately, research hasn't shown a dramatic effect of perineal massage; but it doesn't cause harm, and for some moms it might prevent the need for stitches.

- Balloon dilation of the vagina. I've read about a balloon device called the "Epi-No" which is inserted into the vagina daily for fifteen to twenty minutes, inflated a bit more each day for the last few weeks before birth in order to simulate the baby's head coming through. I saw one research study suggesting that use of the Epi-No decreased the likelihood of episiotomy and lacerations and shortened the duration of pushing, but I can't tell how the study was done or how valid it is. I don't know anyone who has tried it. Given that the procedure takes fifteen minutes a day and the device costs almost two hundred dollars, it sounds time-consuming and expensive, but potentially beneficial.
- Squatting. If you work with children or have young children at home, you probably find yourself in a squat quite often. Squatting strengthens your upper thighs, improves flexibility, and opens up your pelvis. It can be a great position for pushing during labor. If squatting isn't part of your daily routine, consider practicing it for ten minutes a few times a week.

I had a forceps delivery without an episiotomy. I think I didn't need the episiotomy because I was a hippie mom and had done perineal stretching exercises. (Kathy C., family therapist)

If You Are Told to Restrict Your Activities

Sometimes practitioners will ask a woman to slow down or avoid certain activities during the third trimester because of the danger of preterm birth—perhaps because of premature cervical dilation, excessive contractions, or vaginal bleeding. Terms used for this recommendation include *bed rest*, *modified bed rest*, and *house arrest*—but unfortunately each of these terms means different things to different practitioners, so you will need to ask specifically what you may and may not do. For example, can you work from home? Can you go to the store? How about childbirth class? Are you allowed to make yourself lunch? Do you have to arrange childcare for your older kids? Is it safe to have sex? (And if you aren't supposed to have intercourse, can you have orgasms, or are they worried about those contractions causing other contractions?)

Bed rest can be terribly stressful for mothers—both because of concerns about the baby, and due to the boredom that can accompany being inactive. If keeping busy at work is the way you cope with stress, you may suddenly have to learn new stress-management techniques. If you require prolonged bed rest, check out the terrific suggestions at www.sidelines.org, a nonprofit support network and information station for families with complicated pregnancies.

> ***I was the put on bed rest at home for a month. It was not fun at all. I would only walk around if I had to do something. I started crocheting and doing other crafts that could be done while sitting or lying down. Relaxation and getting into enjoyable things was key. I would curl up on the sofa with a book or a thousand-piece puzzle with a table in front of me with my food and other necessities. (Crystal W., customer service rep)***

Sex

Assuming you aren't under activity restrictions, sex is safe until your water breaks, as long as it feels good to you. Any position that is comfortable is probably okay; most couples avoid the "missionary position" with the man on top, though, because of the pressure it puts on the uterus. Research has shown that orgasm and intercourse don't cause preterm labor, premature delivery, or other complications for healthy low-risk women and their babies, so decisions about sex should just be based on what feels right to you, within the parameters of advice provided by your doctor or midwife. If your partner has ever had herpes (and you have not), or if he is at risk for other sexually transmitted infections, be sure to talk to your doctor or midwife so you know what precautions to take. And if either of you has other partners, condoms should be used to prevent transmitting infections.

Sex drive late in pregnancy is variable. Some women feel great about their bodies and enjoy sex and sensuality. Others feel self-conscious or just uninterested. Your partner may feel turned on by the pregnancy, or not, or you both may feel inhibited because of the baby. Most couples have sex less frequently in the last few months.

We had sex until the last six or seven weeks. My fiancé got scared he'd break my water. I told him to stop being a chicken. I think women know their bodies but men are afraid. (Jennifer A., secretary)

If sex usually makes you feel close, its absence toward the end of pregnancy may be hard on your relationship. And after the baby comes, you may need to wait six weeks or more so that you can heal before having sex. These changes to your intimate lives, combined with all of the demands that a new baby brings, make this a good time to consider your partnership.

Communication

Pregnancy can draw a couple together, but it may also be difficult. It's easy to forget about each other as the focus shifts to the new baby's arrival. One strategy is to set aside a "date night" each month, for a nice dinner and time to focus on the changes ahead. While you're relaxing together, you might ask each other:

- What excites us most about the arrival of the baby?
- What are our greatest concerns about adding an infant to our family?
- What are our worst fears about labor and birth?
- How are we each feeling about the father-to-be's part in the delivery room? (Be sure you both agree on what his role should be, even as you acknowledge that the delivery may not go exactly as planned.)
- If we have religious differences, how do we feel about religious practices (such as baptism or circumcision) surrounding our baby's birth?
- Do we want to make anyone the godmother or godfather for the baby? Who will we choose and why? What will that person's role be?
- What are our (and our parents') expectations about how much time our families will spend with us soon after the baby is born? And if there are differences in these expectations, how will we try to resolve them?
- How much parental leave will we take? Will we schedule our leaves at the same time, to enjoy being together as a family, or in sequence to extend the interval before we'll need to pay for childcare? How much time home with the baby do we think we will want, and how much time away from work can we afford?

- If we both will return to work, what are our criteria for choosing the right childcare? Do we want care in our home or would we rather have our baby go to someone else's home or a daycare center? Can we afford our preferred option? Who will research particular caregivers or centers?
- How will we try to preserve our relationship as a couple in the midst of the demands of a new infant?
- What other concerns do we have that would best be resolved now?

Donovan wasn't enthusiastic about the childbirth classes—I made him go. I worried that he wasn't paying attention in class and wouldn't be able to help me. He said watching the doulas in the Bradley class videos made him feel like she would take over his role and he would be useless. We finally agreed to disagree about the doula but I never did anything about it. When it came time he was more prepared that I expected. He also relied on what he knows about me. (Danielle R., trust analyst)

Many women turn emotionally inward toward the end of pregnancy. You may feel less connected at work and more focused on getting ready for the baby. It is normal too, to feel apprehensive about labor, and about the changes coming to your life. It can be an emotionally vulnerable time. I am repeatedly amazed at how people tell traumatic birth stories to women who are having their first babies. I think it is a form of hazing, in the guise of "making sure you are prepared." I tell my patients to avoid people who are still processing their bad experiences, and to seek out stories from friends who feel good about their births.

People try to be helpful but I don't know why they feel compelled to tell you all their harrowing birth stories. No one tells you about her beautiful, peaceful experience. (Naomi B., attorney)

I honestly believe that people were trying to be helpful by sharing their experiences, but for someone on the fence about how they want their labor to be I think it might push them more toward having an epidural. Long before I told people that I was going to have a natural labor I decided that I would be the only one to change my mind and that I was not going to be swayed by other people's experiences. (Danielle R., trust analyst)

Because you may already feel apprehensive about labor, hearing dramatic birth stories may be annoying, or even upsetting. But it is important to put your worries in perspective. No matter how easy or difficult your labor turns out to be, it is but a brief moment of your life; soon enough your little one will be out and in your arms, pregnancy will be over, and you will move on to new challenges and joys together as a family.

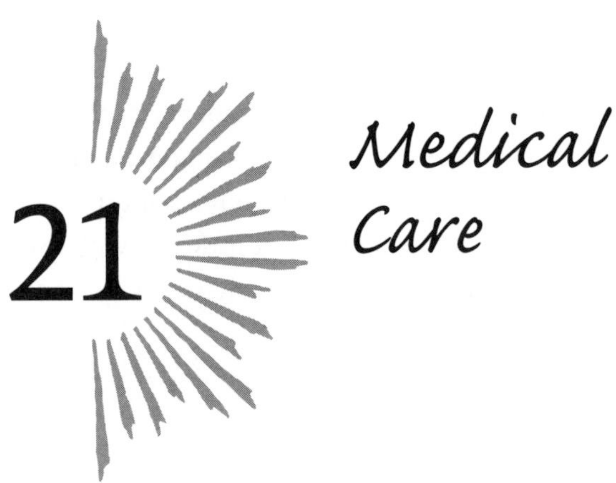

21 Medical Care

During your last trimester, you'll be at your OB's office so often that going there might seem like a second job. Starting at around thirty weeks, you'll be seen every two weeks, then weekly in the last month. (If your pregnancy becomes complicated, visits may be even more frequent.) There's a lot to do at each checkup: you'll be asked how you are feeling and how much the baby is moving; your weight and blood pressure will be checked; your urine will be tested for sugar and protein; your uterus will be measured; and you and your practitioner will listen to your baby's heartbeat.

The medical purpose of late pregnancy care is to screen for developing problems, such as preterm labor, gestational diabetes, and high blood pressure. These visits are also important emotionally for moms-to-be, as you plan for labor and delivery and imagine being the parent of a newborn. During each visit, be sure to ask questions and voice any concerns you may have.

> ***I really liked going to the doctor's appointments—hearing the heartbeat, scheduling the ultrasound, finding out how much weight I'd gained since the last visit (okay, maybe that wasn't so great, but it was a tangible way to measure something pretty amazing—the baby actually growing and developing!), talking about the due date, talking about taking the prenatal classes, etc. I guess the doctor's visits made it "official" that this was a pretty important thing going on! (Kristi V., professor)***

> ***I always had my OB appointments at 1 PM on Thursdays. Toward the end they were weekly and I really got into the habit. After the baby was born, one day I realized it was 1 PM on a Thursday and I wondered if my doctor missed me. (Elisa R., ob-gyn)***

Taking a Medical History

When your practitioner takes a medical history during the third trimester, she is trying to find out how you've been doing since the last appointment. You may be asked about any contractions, bleeding, leaking of fluid, and fetal movement, and how you are feeling overall.

Fetal movement is a sign of well-being. If the baby is moving less than normal, don't hesitate to call and tell your doctor or midwife: it is too important a concern to wait until your next appointment. Some practitioners recommend routine fetal movement tracking (called kick counts) in the third trimester; others use this technique only when there is a question about how the baby is doing. One technique I often recommend for my patients who need to count fetal movements is to choose a time of day when the baby tends to be active, and then time how long it takes to feel the baby move ten times. Usually you will be done in twenty minutes or so. If you aren't done in two hours, you must call in for advice.

Your prenatal appointment is a chance to report any unusual or unpleasant symptoms: both to differentiate serious problems from common annoyances, and to find out what you can do to feel better. If you are feeling poorly on the job, tell your doctor or midwife, who may be able to help you ask your employer to improve your working conditions. Some women will need to go out on disability to deal with discomforts or complications during this home stretch.

Checking Your Blood Pressure and Weight

At every visit, your doctor or nurse will take your blood pressure, and if it rises a lot compared to your norm, or reaches 140/90, they will look for other signs of pre-eclampsia, a pregnancy condition characterized by elevated blood pressure, protein in the urine, and swelling.

The scale may not seem like your friend, as you watch those numbers go where they may never have gone before. But watching your weight at each visit ensures that your overall weight gain is meeting the needs of the growing fetus. You'll also want to step on that scale to be sure you aren't experiencing the rapid weight gain associated with pre-eclampsia.

Date	Start Time	Movements	End Time	Elapsed Time

Copy this chart if you need or want to track fetal movements

Urine Testing

Why will your urine be tested at each visit? For the presence of protein and sugar. Although occasionally protein in the urine comes from vaginal secretions that have mixed in, or from a bladder infection, in general, protein doesn't belong in the urine and can be a sign of pre-eclampsia. Sugar in the urine, too, requires some follow-up testing. If sugar is detected in your urine, your medical team will test early for diabetes, rather than wait for the scheduled twenty-eight-week test. Once you have been screened and find out you aren't diabetic, it usually won't matter if some sugar gets into your urine.

The Physical Examination

By this point in your pregnancy, you will be familiar with much of what happens during a prenatal appointment. But your practitioner will be on the lookout for particular symptoms during this late stage. To help make sure your pregnancy continues to be a healthy one, she will probably:

- Check for swelling, also called edema. A little swelling in your feet is pretty normal in pregnancy, but severe edema, or any swelling of your face and hands, can be a sign of pre-eclampsia. If your blood pressure is normal, then you will know that the swelling is not a sign of a serious problem (although it may make you miserable). If your hands are puffy, remember to take off your rings (ice water and liquid soap work well) and leave them off until after the baby. You won't be happy if you have to have your rings cut off by a jeweler due to swollen fingers.
- Listen to the baby's heartbeat with a stethoscope (with the concave side, pressing firmly), an unamplified fetoscope, or a Doppler device. For convenience, most practitioners use the Doppler.
- Measure your abdomen. Your uterus grows about a centimeter (one half inch) a week. On average, the distance from your pubic bone to the top of the uterus (called fundal height—since the top of the uterus is called the fundus) measures the same in centimeters as weeks you are pregnant, give or take four centimeters. So for example, at thirty weeks the uterus typically measures between twenty-six and thirty-four centimeters. Fundal height provides a rough estimate of the size of the baby; fetal position, your shape, the amount of amniotic fluid, and other factors also affect this result. If the measurements are off track, or if you are heavy or carrying twins (so that belly measurements wouldn't accurately reflect the size of each baby), ultrasound might be used to follow fetal growth.

I am five foot nine and I guess I hid how big the baby was. My doctor estimated [my baby] to be eight to eight and a half pounds, but he was ten pounds, thirteen ounces. (Kendra F., civil litigator)

Screening for Gestational Diabetes

Although many women who develop gestational diabetes have risk factors, most have no symptoms, so generally all pregnant women are screened for diabetes at around twenty-six to twenty-eight weeks. You will probably be asked to drink a sweet solution called glucola and then have blood drawn exactly one

WHY DIABETES TESTING IS IMPORTANT

Pregnancy can interfere with a woman's sugar levels, making her temporarily diabetic. Gestational diabetes is pretty common—occurring in 2 to 14 percent of pregnancies. Untreated gestational diabetes can lead to excessively big babies with consequent difficult delivery, and (rarely) stillbirth. With good control of blood sugar levels and proper medical care, babies of gestational diabetic mothers usually do very well. The key is to find out at the right time whether gestational diabetes might be affecting your pregnancy. Since most mothers-to-be who develop gestational diabetes don't have trouble with their blood sugar until late in pregnancy, the test isn't routinely taken until the third trimester. But women at increased risk for diabetes (because of obesity or a family history of diabetes) may benefit from first trimester testing as well.

hour later. You won't need to fast overnight before this screening test, but you shouldn't have anything to eat or drink between drinking the glucola and having your blood drawn. If the results show that your sugar level is nice and low, you're off the hook. But if you "don't pass" your diabetes screening test, don't panic. Many women with high one-hour tests don't actually have diabetes—they just need further checking. Typically, the next step is a more definitive test: the glucose tolerance test, or GTT.

> ***I had diabetes for both of my pregnancies. I didn't find it that difficult to deal with, although it can be a bit unnerving when you first get diagnosed. It's a reality check, something to make you think about your lifestyle, eating habits, and weight. (Karen D., veterinarian)***

Testing for Anemia

A blood test to check for anemia (a low blood count) is usually done when you have blood drawn for the diabetes screen. Anemia may be caused by inadequate iron intake. If your blood shows that you have anemia, your doctor or midwife will let you know what to do next: you may need to change your diet, take an iron supplement, or have some more tests done.

Rhogam for Rh-Negative Mothers

Your blood type was checked at your first prenatal visit, and if you are among the 85 percent of people who are Rh positive (A+, B+, O+, or AB+), you won't need to do anything special before your delivery. (Even if your baby's father has a different blood type from you, no special prenatal treatment will be needed.) If you do happen to be Rh-negative, however, an easy treatment will keep your future pregnancies safe. Rh-negative blood (which could be O–, A–, B–, or AB–) means that the Rh factor is not present on your red blood cells. In the old days, before preventive treatment was invented, some Rh-negative mothers developed antibodies against their Rh-positive babies, leading to serious problems when the mother's immune system attacked the blood cells of their next Rh-positive fetus. Today, though, a woman who is Rh-negative can receive treatment with Rhogam (Rh immunoglobulin), which protects her from making antibodies against the baby's blood. Pregnancy problems from Rh incompatibility have become quite rare.

The Last Month

During your ninth month, your prenatal visits will change once again. You'll come for weekly appointments; your practitioner will determine the baby's position; you may begin internal (vaginal) examinations to check how your body is getting ready to give birth; and a few final tests will usually be done.

ABDOMINAL EXAMINATION

Toward the end of the third trimester, your practitioner will assess the baby's position by feeling your belly. Most babies lie in an up-and-down orientation, either head down or head up (breech). They usually curl up, with elbows and knees together in the "fetal position." If this is your first baby, you'll be glad to know that once first babies get into the head-down position they stay there; that

THE WHAT AND WHEN OF RHOGAM

Rhogam is an injection of antibodies that helps the Rh-negative mother to remove any stray fetal blood cells from her circulation before she has a chance to react to them. An Rh-negative woman should get a Rhogam shot any time that fetal blood may enter her circulation: during a miscarriage, when tubal (ectopic) pregnancy is diagnosed, at amniocentesis, after trauma to the abdomen (like in a car accident), or if she has vaginal bleeding. A routine dose is also given around twenty-eight weeks, to protect the mother from reacting to the small number of fetal cells that may enter her circulation during the remainder of pregnancy. After birth, a sample of the blood left in the umbilical cord is sent to check the newborn's blood type. If the baby turns out to be Rh-positive, the mom should have an additional injection of Rhogam within a day or two of delivery. If the baby turns out to be Rh-negative, it doesn't hurt that Rhogam was taken during pregnancy unnecessarily, but a postpartum dose won't be needed.

is, once your baby is found to be headfirst you don't have to worry much about him flipping to breech. Women who've had a lot of babies have a more relaxed abdominal wall, which doesn't hold the baby in position as tightly.

INTERNAL EXAMINATION

If your pregnancy has been uncomplicated, you probably won't have internal examinations until around thirty-five or thirty-six weeks. At that time the group B strep test will be done and your practitioner may check to see if your cervix is getting "ripe." A vaginal examination can also confirm the baby's position, since the baby's head is often low enough to be felt through an open cervix or through the vaginal wall.

As your body gets ready for labor, your cervix may start to dilate (open up) and efface (shorten), and the baby's head may drop low (engage) into your pelvis. But what does the vaginal examination tell you about when the baby will come?

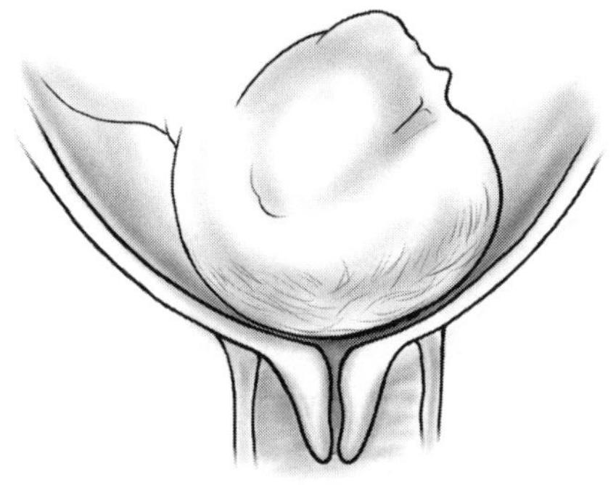
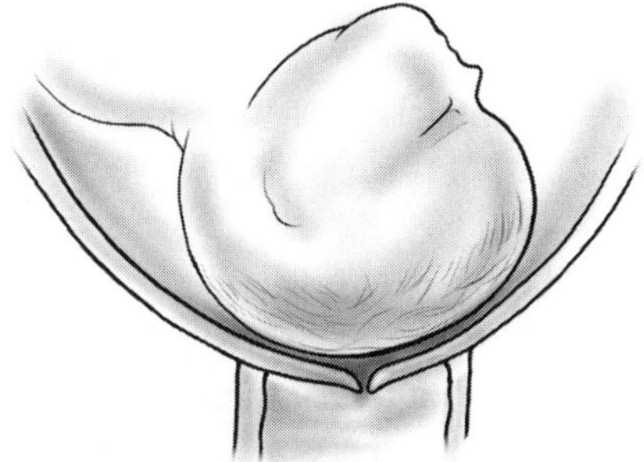

The cervix gets ready for labor

A sudden change in dilation between two weekly appointments often indicates that labor is imminent—but all guesses are just that, and the cervix can stay a few centimeters dilated for weeks, or go from long and closed one day to wide open for birth the next. Practitioners may be good at estimating the date of conception and the "due date," but predicting the actual day of delivery is clearly not a science.

GROUP B STREP TESTING

A culture for group B strep (GBS) bacteria typically is performed around thirty-five to thirty-seven weeks. A cotton swab is placed into the vagina (and usually the rectum too) and sent to the lab for culture.

TREATMENT FOR HERPES

If you have a history of genital herpes and get recurrent lesions, taking antiviral medication for the last month or so can help prevent an outbreak around the time of the baby's birth. Be sure to tell your doctor or midwife if you have ever been exposed to herpes or have had any genital blisters or sores.

AMNIOCENTESIS FOR FETAL LUNG MATURITY

Scientists believe that the signal that starts labor normally comes from the fetus, indicating that the baby is ready to be born. If you are going to be induced or have a scheduled cesarean earlier than a week before your due date, the American College of Obstetrics and Gynecology recommends that you have an amniocen-

THE GROUP B STREP STORY

We all know that bacteria live on the skin; similarly, bacteria are normally found in the vagina. For about 20 percent of women, group B strep, also called GBS or beta strep, is one of the bacteria present. This is not a vaginal infection and is nothing to worry about until labor. In the days before we screened for GBS, about one baby in five hundred would get very sick from group B strep picked up coming through the birth canal. So doctors devised a plan in which all mothers who harbor these bacteria would be treated with antibiotics during labor—and in this way they significantly reduced the incidence of serious neonatal group B strep infections. Since carriage of GBS can vary month to month (and pregnancy to pregnancy), we usually wait to check until the last month. If you carry GBS, you will be treated with antibiotics through an IV during labor. Keep in mind that the chance of your baby getting sick from GBS is pretty low even without treatment. Treating GBS is a public health measure—we treat a lot of mothers in order to prevent one sick baby, but it's worth it.

tesis before delivery to check that the baby's lungs are truly mature and ready to breathe air after birth.

The many medical visits during the third trimester help mark an important emotional transition for pregnant moms. Your baby may not be here yet, but clearly, with all the final checks and preparations, delivery is right around the corner. In the flurry of these visits, it can be easy to forget to bring up your own issues to your medical team, so make a list of your concerns, questions, discomforts, hopes, and fears. Now is also a great time to discuss with your practitioner, if you haven't already, what you are hoping for in your birth experience: voicing your ideas about labor and delivery early on will let you gauge the reaction and find out how feasible it will be to fulfill your wishes.

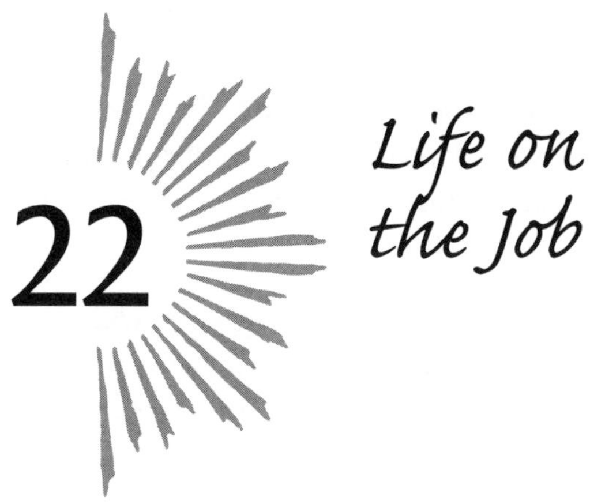

22 Life on the Job

Pregnancy is a transformative experience: it changes your body, your self-image, and your family relationships. How it affects your interactions with colleagues and friends at work and the way you do your job depends on several factors. What has your work life been like this trimester?

Changes at Work

Some women find that not much changes on the job during pregnancy, especially if they work in a traditionally female career. Others feel that they are treated either gingerly or dismissively. Studies of attitudes toward pregnant women show that they are often perceived as prioritizing their personal lives over work, and may be viewed as achieving less, even when their productivity stays the same. If you find your contribution undervalued in this way, the first step toward responding constructively is to recognize the problem.

An older male professor stopped me in the hall when I was about seven months pregnant and said, in a worried way, "How ARE you?" and I said "Fine, why?" And he said, "I just keep forgetting to ask how you are, because you don't SEEM pregnant." In other words, he'd never seen a pregnant professor before (there weren't many of us yet in my department), not to mention a woman who didn't make a fuss about the experience, and it threw him. (Lori G., professor)

The common comment becomes, "Oh, well, you're going to be gone." (Crystal W., customer service rep)

I interviewed for a job when I was in the third trimester. They were looking for a replacement because many employees were out on maternity leave. When he saw me his jaw dropped because I was pregnant as well, but they ended up offering me the job. (Sherri M., sales rep)

Sometimes pregnancy influences not only your relationships with your close colleagues, but also others' perceptions about how you can—or should—do your job. Customers, clients, patients, students, and other job contacts may respond differently to you when you are pregnant.

TV makes a woman who's six months pregnant look like she's two weeks overdue. This prompted many, many emails from worried viewers that maybe I "should stay home until the baby comes." (Eileen M., weather reporter)

When I got visibly pregnant, I was occasionally carted around to hearings and trials in federal court that were in front of judges known to show sympathy to pregnant women. (Janet G., attorney)

My boss called me the Mayor of Richmond Town Square Mall since everyone knew me and stopped in to see how I was doing during the pregnancy. (Annette M., store manager)

You may notice that people who would never touch you when you aren't pregnant reach out and touch your abdomen as you get bigger, just as strangers feel free to talk to and touch children. If this bothers you, try using body language to keep people's hands off.

Best advice that I received: if you don't want people patting your stomach (which isn't very professional, after all), carry a clipboard or legal pad in front of you to block their access. (Jane S., state governor)

Will you need to make changes at work? If your pregnancy is going well, you may feel able to plow ahead without any special accommodations, proud of your strength and serenity. But late pregnancy symptoms or complications can throw a wrench into your work life. Lengthy commutes, long hours, being on your feet, travel, and job pressure may become difficult to manage, especially if you don't have the easiest pregnancy.

I worked very hard to "prove myself" as a pregnant lawyer, to show that it wouldn't slow me down—at one point I did two trials back to back and was exhausted. (Janet G., attorney)

I felt pressure to stay dedicated to work and work every minute and was surprised by how late pregnancy slowed me down. In hindsight, I worked less and the world didn't stop spinning! (Kendra F., civil litigator)

Wear comfortable clothes and shoes. This is not the time to be fashionable. We all want to look good, but it's still all about comfort. (Mary Ellen M., pediatric nurse)

I was working full-time and commuting an hour, four days a week. I would leave the house at 7 and get home at 8 PM. I always wonder if the physical demands of my job led to my early delivery—I broke my water and delivered at thirty-five weeks. (Karen D., veterinarian)

I was being assigned to fly to Texas or California for an hour-long presentation without regard for how exhausted I was. My boss herself was a mother of four, from the era of toughing it out and proving that you could do it all. (Cheryl L., lawyer)

Travel

Business travel is a regular part of many careers. But as you get further along in your pregnancy, the demands of travel and being far from home should make you think twice about long trips. You should know that:

- Travel can be exhausting. Plan your schedule with more breaks than usual, and try to set up the trip so that you can cancel with short notice if you develop pregnancy complications or aren't feeling well.
- The risk of blood clots in the legs or lungs increases during pregnancy. On the road or in a plane, walk around every two to three hours to prevent blood from pooling in your legs. If you experience one swollen painful leg, sudden shortness of breath, or painful breathing, get medical help right away.
- If you develop problems while on a business trip, you can usually call

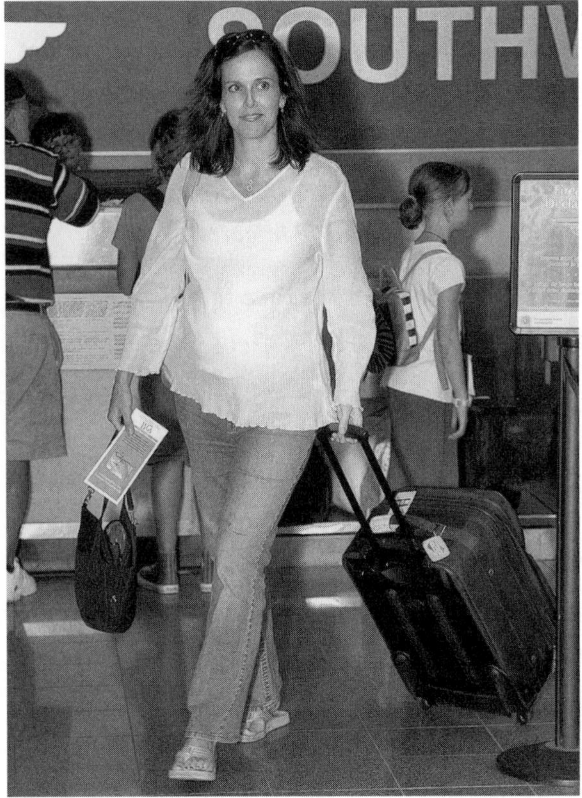

LeRoy Dierker, MD

your doctor or midwife for advice, but complications like preterm labor can't wait until you get home. Plan where you will go if problems arise; remember that some hospitals don't provide maternity services.

- Keep in mind that in the unlikely event that you deliver prematurely far from home, your baby could be in the hospital there for weeks.
- If you travel to a less developed area, you may not be able to get up-to-date, hygienic medical care.

If you must travel, take these steps to help make the trip safer for you and your baby:

- Tell your doctor or midwife of your plans, so before you go they can check you over for any developing complications, and provide you with individualized travel recommendations.

HOW LATE IN PREGNANCY CAN YOU TRAVEL?

Experts' recommendations on travel during pregnancy differ, and how late you should travel really depends on where you are going and how your pregnancy is progressing. Until about thirty-six weeks, a healthy woman with an uncomplicated pregnancy has only a small risk of developing a pregnancy complication while away from home. A woman with a higher risk pregnancy, a prior preterm birth, or whose cervix is opening up already, however, should not travel. Journeys to remote areas are probably not great at any time in pregnancy, and are most risky during the first trimester, when miscarriage might require treatment, and in the third trimester, when preterm labor and other complications are not uncommon. Airline policies vary, so check ahead. Most will allow you to fly throughout pregnancy with a note from your physician or midwife.

- Bring a copy of your prenatal chart with you. This way, if you need emergency care, the medical team will know your due date, lab test results, blood type, and so on.

During an event I managed in San Jose, I was eight months pregnant. My employer and event staff were very supportive throughout the week, and allowed me to sit down for most of the day, and to take breaks for meals as needed. They also worked longer hours to allow me to go to bed at a decent hour and get at least eight hours of sleep per night. For anyone who is in the meeting planning business, this rarely happens. (Amanda O., meeting planner)

In my eighth month of pregnancy I had to travel to an advanced statistics seminar in D.C. By the end of the seminar, my brain was exhausted. I got on the D.C. Metro, fell asleep, went past my stop to the end of the line; I was woken up by attendant to get off. I got on the return leg, went several stops, transferred at the right stop, got on the right train, and fell

asleep again. When I woke up this time, I was so flustered I ran off the train, leaving my briefcase behind. I gave up, decided to find it the next day, waddled to my hotel, and went to sleep. (Lisa K., city administrator)

Functioning on the Job

Many women perceive that they are intellectually less sharp or even slightly confused during the later weeks of pregnancy. While some of us call that "pregnancy brain" or "placenta brain," studies haven't shown true cognitive deficits in pregnant women. Pregnancy can be distracting, though, and tiring. Remember the 80/20 rule: 20 percent of your effort achieves 80 percent of your results. Efficiency on the job will help you continue to achieve, even if you can't work at your usual intense pace.

I was huge and not sleeping well and felt sluggish all the time. I am not sure if anyone noticed, but I could tell I wasn't thinking through difficult problems as easily. (Naomi B., attorney)

Alex would be so active during a meeting, I'd find myself distracted by his moving all around and I'd be trying to figure out if it was an elbow or a knee; I would totally tune out. (Beth L., computer science researcher)

My least productive time came early in the pregnancy when I was sick. At that time I would feel so bad I would say I was leaving early for an appointment and go home and sleep at 4 PM. But later in the pregnancy I became more productive because I was looking ahead and preparing for the time when I wouldn't be at work. (Peggy L., nurse-administrator)

Take it easy and don't push yourself too hard. Don't be afraid to say when you are tired, and take off from work if it just gets to be too much. Sometimes enough is enough. (Jennifer A., secretary)

Your Day-to-Day Well-Being

Comfort is a worthy goal as your pregnancy proceeds. Try to plan your work and your life so that you can manage, and you aren't stressed out or exhausted. You deserve to feel good during pregnancy, and your baby needs a mom who will be ready, mentally and physically, for the challenges and joys of caring for a newborn.

When choosing clothes for the last weeks of pregnancy, seek out simple outfits that are stretchy and comfortable; you can always brighten them with accessories. Do whatever works for you, and remember that many pregnant moms borrow maternity clothes, or find reasonably priced outfits at consignment shops. If you must wear a uniform for work, a larger-sized man's or woman's uniform may fit and feel better than the maternity versions.

Shoes can be a special challenge, particularly if your feet become swollen. Some women resort to wearing sneakers all day. If that isn't acceptable on your job, at least consider them for your commute; you can change when you get to work.

Limiting liquids or skipping meals makes pregnant women feel horrible. Drink fluids throughout your workday. If you don't eat regularly, you may find that your blood sugar drops and you feel poorly at inopportune moments. Always carry a snack, and plan your day so that you can eat every few hours. If you really don't have time for meals, bring healthful munchies (like nuts and raisins or a nutrition bar) or an energy drink, like Boost, that you can finish in just a few minutes.

Make sure you drink a lot of water throughout the day. A lot of workplaces are very dry and it's better to be in the bathroom all day than to go home thirsty, drink a lot in the evening, and be up all night going to the bathroom. (Mary Ellen M., pediatric nurse)

I felt that more attention should have been paid to my nutritional needs. For example, a client scheduled a five-hour meeting but never brought in food. This was not good for my diabetes, the baby, or me. I wish more people had been looking out for me . . . sometimes I felt like I was the only one who was defending my needs, but I felt guilty or a nuisance to do so. (Jane J., advertising executive)

How does a woman follow a strict gestational diabetic regimen at work when she is running from meeting to meeting, preparing presentations, working on spreadsheets, pulling long hours (past 10 PM), etc.? Discipline! Going on a low-carb/no-sugar diet brought my weight gain to a screeching

HOW PREGNANCY COMPLICATIONS MAY AFFECT YOUR WORK

Complications like gestational diabetes, gestational hypertension, and preterm labor don't usually begin until the third trimester, but any of these problems can influence your ability to do your job. A diagnosis of diabetes will require that you pay a lot more attention to diet and exercise, and you may need to check your blood sugar and take insulin injections during the workday. High blood pressure and preterm labor may require that you rest at home or in the hospital. You also may need to take time off from work for additional doctor visits for monitoring you and your baby.

halt. I'm happy I followed a very strict food regimen. I had a big baby . . . nine pounds two ounces . . . but healthy as can be. (Mary O., vice president, financial services corporation)

My supervisors were annoyed that I had to take so much time off toward the end. I tried to prepare them that I had gestational diabetes and my blood pressure was up, but I don't think they knew what that meant. Maybe I should have told them more, but really it was my private medical business. They were like, "My grandfather has high blood pressure and he doesn't see the doctor twice a week. What's the big deal?" (Danielle R., trust analyst)

Dealing with Third Trimester Symptoms on the Job

Whether or not your colleagues are perfectly understanding, it is important to take good care of your body during late pregnancy.

SWELLING

If your feet are swollen, try keeping them elevated whenever possible. Remember, too, that foods that are high in salt (for example, restaurant food) can cause water retention.

I put a box of files under my desk to put my feet up on. (Brenda W., lawyer)

I ate out a lot (on business) and didn't watch my salt intake; my last trip I arrived back in New York City with ankles the size of basketballs. My doctor rightfully told me to call a halt to the business-related travel. (Jean B., editor)

CARPAL TUNNEL SYNDROME

Carpal tunnel syndrome occurs when the wrist joint gets swollen and compresses the nerve as it runs through. The aching numbness of the thumb and first few fingers that characterizes carpal tunnel syndrome is usually worse at night and when typing or talking on the phone. Be sure your keyboard is at the proper height, with a gel pad to rest your wrists on. Consider using a headset for the phone. A hand brace might help, too, and can be obtained from your local drugstore, medical supply outlet, or physical therapist.

BACK PAIN AND SCIATICA

Pain in your back, including sciatica, can make sitting or walking difficult. Back exercises may help a lot (see Chapter 19 for suggestions, or ask your practitioner). If you sit at a desk, be sure that your chair is adjusted for comfort, use a six-inch lumbar roll for lower back support, and set a reminder to get up every thirty to forty-five minutes for a stretch. Professional, weekly back massages may also help you get through these last months. Talk to your doctor or midwife about a referral to a physical therapist if needed, and about any changes that you should make at work. If you are really struggling, you may need to go out on disability.

I don't think pregnancy really affected my work. I was definitely sore at night. I was used to working, but I did feel it in my back. (Annette M., store manager)

Toward the end of pregnancy I couldn't sit for the hour-long commute. I switched my hours to work 10–4 to avoid rush hour and worked some at home. (Heather H., real estate attorney)

I always felt better when I was working, but I left work at five months because it was too hard to operate on twenty cases a day or more. Plus I was wearing a respirator for protection from the anesthetic gases. It was hard on my back too, as my belly got bigger. It just got to be too much. I envied people who could work up until the end. I missed working and that identity. (Julie M., veterinarian)

GETTING BIG

There's not much you can do about growing—the baby, the fluid, the placenta, and the other changes in your body take up space. Just try not to gain excess weight, since the more you are carrying, the more uncomfortable you may be. Because of your size, it may not be possible to perform physically demanding work all the way until labor.

Overall I didn't have too many problems working while pregnant. Later in pregnancy it became really hard to bend over and carry things with my belly in the way, but that's about it. I worked until six days before he was born. (Stephanie B., FedEx courier)

I had a hard time driving because I couldn't get comfortable. (Danielle R., trust analyst)

At eight months I was coaching a chamber music group and they were having a hard time getting this piece right. Finally they did it fantastically and I get really into it so I screamed and fell on the floor and put my legs up in the air with excitement. Everyone was laughing at me—and then I couldn't get myself back up! (Annie F., classical violinist)

SHORTNESS OF BREATH AND DECREASED EXERCISE TOLERANCE

It's normal to feel out of shape late in pregnancy. Regular exercise can help you maintain your fitness level as much as possible, but expect to slow down as your pregnancy reaches its last stages.

Only one more week of teaching dance to four-year-olds. I can still do the older girls, but not preschool. Picture a moose in a leotard trying to skip

while waving ribbons and playing a tambourine. Not cute. (Jen B., dance teacher)

I worked until I was about seven to eight months pregnant with my first baby. It wasn't too bad because I worked a route with a lot of dock work; the guys that worked at the loading docks would see the pregnant woman and wouldn't even let me load my own truck. So I really had no reason not to work as long as possible. Later on, they added an extra twenty stops to my route, which became too much—I wasn't able to do all of that lifting, so I stopped. (Stephanie B., FedEx courier)

CONTRACTIONS

Many women have some contractions in the third trimester. These may feel like a balling up or tightening sensation, or like menstrual cramps. If it is too early to deliver and you have more than four contractions an hour, you need to change your activities and drink some fluids to see if you can get them to stop. This means that even if you are at work, you must listen to your body. If you have to go home sick, or spend half an hour with your feet up, do it. You are the only one who can take care of your baby right now; someone else will have to pick up the slack on the job. If you often get contractions at work, be sure to tell your doctor or midwife.

I started to have contractions at six months so my doctor asked me to sit on a stool periodically versus standing at the cash register all day. My employer had me bring a letter from the doctor. They felt as though I should not be sitting down; if I was, I was not doing my job. (Crystal W., customer service rep)

EXHAUSTION

Fatigue is normal toward the end of pregnancy. Expect to slow down during your last two months. You need to listen to your body and try not to exhaust yourself. If necessary, ask for help from your colleagues, or talk to your employer about reducing your responsibilities. Consult your doctor or midwife if you need help setting limits at work.

I had stools on either side of the classroom, so I would walk around the class, and sit down wherever I needed to. (Kafi P., teacher)

I was pregnant and pretty big and had two trials in a row. I got totally exhausted. The judge kept interrupting me and I felt like I was going to cry. The DA, who was a woman, noticed and asked for a break. I finally asked for a continuance. The judge was sympathetic; I just couldn't do it. (Jan R., state attorney)

Take breaks when you need them. Everyone understands that you may get tired more easily. You have to speak up. (Mary Ellen M., pediatric nurse)

Even though many women need to wind down their work lives during the last weeks of pregnancy, many other women feel terrific during this period and choose to work right up until labor begins.

I felt tired but so powerful growing this baby inside me and performing and teaching. I felt like I had superpowers. I liked the girls we taught to see the big pregnant woman teaching, going for it, to see pregnancy as "not a big deal." (Annie F., classical violinist)

I performed surgery earlier on the day I gave birth to Michaela. An older male anesthesiologist said later, "You girls today are entirely too casual about this stuff." (Elisa R., ob-gyn)

My baby moved a lot when I was at work. I felt like I had a little buddy with me all the time. (Kate R., financial analyst)

I planned my schedule to quit working the week before my due date because I was afraid of going into labor during an appointment. I stayed home for two weeks and did nothing. Bored, I went into the office to see a patient. At the end of the appointment she said she was relieved I had not gone into labor during the appointment. I never told her that I had! I went right from the office to the hospital. (Nancy C., dentist)

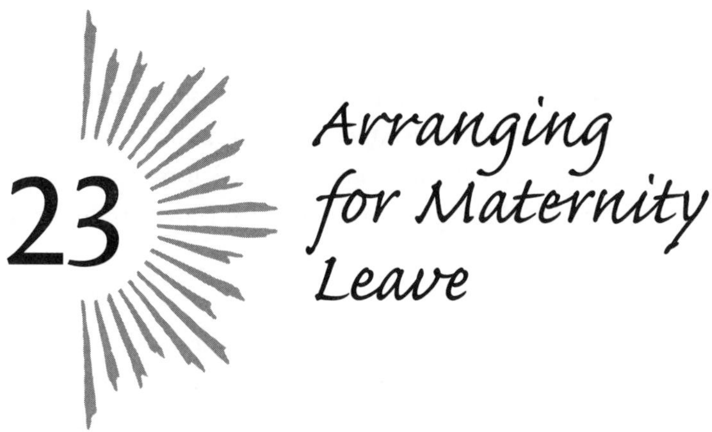

23 Arranging for Maternity Leave

Maternity leave shouldn't come as a surprise; after all, you and your employer have known for months that this baby will be born. Sometimes though, especially when moms work for a small company or their leave is path-breaking in some way, uncertainties will remain. Whatever your work environment, now is your chance to ease your employer's concerns, and importantly, show your continued commitment to your job. In particular, your efforts to plan and prepare for your time away can help ensure a smooth transition out and back again. Planning for leave includes assessing your options, negotiating your time away, organizing your work to be handed off, and arranging for your return to work.

A good maternity leave plan also anticipates the unexpected, because sometimes your baby is the one who determines when your last day will be. You should prepare yourself and your job for the possibility of an abrupt departure, in case you develop a pregnancy complication or go into labor sooner than expected. In fact, a substantial number of women need to take off from work at some point during their pregnancies.

Maternity Leave

How much time will you take off? Maternity leave serves two purposes: it allows you to recover from birth (disability) and it enables you to take care of your new baby (parenting). Even though you might feel fine within a week or two, six weeks is usually allowed for recovery, so for the first month and a half, your leave is both disability and parental. Beyond that, leave is for the care of the baby. This distinction becomes important because laws and company policies may treat these two purposes differently. Many new mothers don't take all of the leave that is allotted to them. For most, the lack of pay makes them jump back into work early; for others, the loss of stature and accomplishment at work is a factor; still others feel they aren't "baby people" and look forward to their return to the workplace. You will need to figure out how much leave is right for you.

THE FIRST SIX WEEKS

For most jobs, federal laws require that employers cover the six weeks of postpartum recovery just like they would handle any other disability leave. Depending on your contract you might use sick days, short-term disability pay, or, if you are out of sick time, leave without pay to make up the six-week period. Some contracts specify a maternity leave policy, but the first six weeks can't be less generous than disability leave would be for any other condition. And if you end up having a cesarean, you may be able to extend the "disability" time to eight weeks.

Although legally you take "disability" when you are pregnant, I did not like this terminology . . . it made me feel "sick" or incapable rather than just being in a normal state for a woman. (Jane J., advertising executive)

THROUGH TWELVE WEEKS

If you are covered under the Family and Medical Leave Act (FMLA), you are allowed twelve total weeks of parental leave, which includes any other paid leave. Generally FMLA allows you to get six more weeks after your first six "disability" weeks. You may be able to arrange with your employer to work part-time for several months or spread these six weeks of time off through the child's first year of life. The law doesn't require that you be paid during this time, though. And if you were employed less than full-time during the last twelve months, work for a small company, or haven't been at your job a year, you may not be covered by FMLA, and your employer will not be required to allow more time off than the six-week disability period. (Many smaller firms, though, have policies that mimic the FMLA.)

BEYOND THREE MONTHS

Some jobs and some states have policies that are more generous than required by federal law. Check with your company's human resources department to find out the policies at your workplace, and with www.nationalpartnership.org to learn about state-by-state requirements. You also may be able to individually negotiate leave beyond your employer's standard benefits.

I was fortunate to be allowed two years maternity leave for each child. I received about sixteen weeks paid time off for each child and then simply took my leave. (Edie U., school psychologist)

PLANNING TO STAY CONNECTED

When thinking ahead about how visible you want to be during your leave, be sure to talk to others about how they felt during their time away. While some new mothers want to stay in touch so they don't lose too much ground at work, most are surprised by how busy they are at home and how little interest they have in the job, at least for the first month or so. It may be a good idea to keep in touch with someone who can tell you what's happening and ask to be copied on important emails, but most experts recommend not promising to be involved with work during this time unless totally necessary. If you must be in contact, consider these guidelines:

- Designate one point person for communication. Anyone who needs you should work through this colleague.
- Use email if at all possible so you can write and respond when it is easiest for you.
- If you must talk on the phone, try to arrange that *you* call in at an approximate time during the day. This way you can choose a time when the baby (hopefully) won't need you.

I would have finished everything up, but some of my projects were dependent on other people doing their parts, so some things were still on my desk when I went on leave. They were upset, but I called them from the hospital and told them I would call Monday and go through each project and that appeased them. (Danielle R., trust analyst)

After my cesarean for the twins, I went onto a modified work schedule for a few weeks. I called in to my chief of staff each day. It was better if I called in, since babies can be unpredictable if you try to have work call you at a particular time. (Jane S., state governor)

PATERNITY LEAVE

The Family and Medical Leave Act (FMLA) isn't only for women. Depending on his employer, your baby's father may also be eligible for twelve weeks of leave to care for you and your new baby. Again, the law doesn't require pay, so you would need to check his employer's benefits. If he only has a week or two of paid leave, consider using it when you and the baby come home, rather than while you are in the hospital and have lots of help.

Factors to Consider When Planning Parental Leave

- How much time do you think you will want to be home with your new baby?
- What will you earn during your leave? Maternity leave may be partially paid time off, and partially unpaid. You may find that you can patch together sick time, disability pay, vacation days, and whatever your employer's parental leave compensation might be to optimize the number of paid days. Remember that disability pay may only be a fraction of your normal paycheck, and if taxes aren't taken out, you may owe money to the government next April.
- How will your leave affect any expected bonus pay, productivity incentives, accumulation of sick days, and vacation-day allocation?
- What other sources of income does your family have (partner's salary, other sources)?
- What can you afford to contribute from savings?
- What are your fixed monthly expenses?
- Can you cut some discretionary spending to make it easier to live on a smaller income?
- How will prolonged leave affect your stature and job security at work?
- How possible are part-time, phasing back in, telecommuting, job sharing, or other creative arrangements for when you resume work?
- What are your childcare options and how much will they cost?

I won't go back to work until after January, especially since the holidays are so hectic. I am using six to eight weeks of paid time off and two weeks of vacation, but I am taking a total of twelve weeks off so the rest will be unpaid. (Annette M., store manager)

I stayed home three months, because that's all the time I had. We don't really get maternity leave. I had just saved up sick time and vacation time. We get paid 65 percent. I think I had to use that for two or three weeks, because I had used up all of my paid time. I was still accruing time while I was off, so when I went back, I had a little time on the books. (Myra K., courtroom assistant)

The company I'm with now has a two-month maternity leave. I'll probably take a third month unpaid. (Elizabeth S., online producer)

My company has no policy of an extra two weeks for a C-section, so once my six weeks were up they cut my pay totally. I was off with no pay for a month, and back to work after the C-section when my baby was ten weeks old. (Heather M., telephone service technician)

Attitudes toward Parental Leave

Institutions and coworkers vary in their attitudes about maternity leave. If your workplace is family-friendly, you may feel supported and accepted as you plan out your departure and return. But in many jobs the philosophy is "work above all else," and your leave may be seen as disruptive, selfish, or even irresponsible. Your workplace may not have your family's needs in mind, but you still have to find a balance for all your obligations, including those to yourself and your children. Awareness of the culture of your workplace and where you can find support may ease a difficult situation. Chapter 16 has some additional information to help you figure out what you want and what you can afford.

When I was pregnant and working full-time as an internist, I was fortunate enough to work with men who were very gracious about my maternity leave coverage. They told me that when their working wives were home on maternity leave, someone else covered for them and so this was their

QUESTIONS TO ASK YOUR EMPLOYER ABOUT MATERNITY LEAVE

- How much leave am I entitled to?
- What will my salary be, if any, during leave? (Remember that medical leave to recover from delivery may be treated differently than time off to care for your newborn.)
- Do I have to use up saved vacation or sick days before my leave kicks in?
- What are my scheduling options when I return to work?

payback and they were happy to do it. I was VERY lucky. That is the way it should be. (Jenny K., internist)

Our office assistant just had a baby (cute and wonderful) but when she was pregnant, it was really tough to cover for her workload since there are only four of us. (Melissa G., mortgage broker)

Negotiating Leave

In some situations maternity leave is cut and dried—you know what you are allocated and you know that you will take the entire amount. Some women, though, manage to negotiate *more* than their job's standard leave. Your ability to negotiate will be determined by your value to the company and the culture of the organization.

When you sit down with your bosses to discuss your maternity leave, put yourself in their shoes and offer solutions rather than dumping the problem on them. Think about how your work will get done while you are away, and ask them what they need from you—you may identify compromises you can make that would help them without hurting you. Being flexible about issues that aren't too important to you can show that you're a team player. For example, if they are desperate for your involvement back at work as soon as possible, could you work one day a week after six weeks, or agree to call in every day or communicate by email to answer questions? Understanding their concerns can help you come up with a package that both sides can embrace. The more they are convinced you will return and become productive again, the more likely they are to negotiate. (For more on effective negotiating, read a book that changed my life, *Getting to Yes*, by Roger Fisher, William Ury, and Bruce Patton.)

Be sure you know the federal and state laws and the written policies of your job, so you are not taken advantage of during your negotiations. For more on laws, click on FMLA on the Department of Labor's website at www.dol.gov. For company policies and precedents, read your employee manual, talk with others at your company who have recently given birth, and obtain any written materials available through your human resources department. And if you want more than your job's policy allows (and you think you may be valuable enough to the organization that your boss would agree), try pushing for the extra benefits up front.

Another tip: when you're figuring out how to put together your maternity leave, try not to use all your vacation or sick time. Babies have a lot of routine doctor's appointments in the first year, and you never know when you or your baby will get sick. You might need some vacation, too!

I took twelve weeks FMLA with my first pregnancy, but with the second I wasn't working as much so I didn't qualify for FMLA. I had to request a personal leave of absence, which ended up being accepted for twelve weeks of leave. (Stephanie B., FedEx courier)

Many experts recommend following up your meeting about maternity leave with a written summary of what was agreed on, with dates. Remember that FMLA requires that you give your employer written notice at least thirty days before you begin your parental leave.

One piece of advice: don't make decisions about your job before you have the baby. I'd arranged to move to a lower-level job that could be done part-time, but my heart just wasn't in it. I went from my whole identity being in my work, to only wanting to be a wife and mother. I didn't realize how different I was going to feel after I had the baby. I'm just not that corporate person any more. (Kate R., financial analyst)

In my second pregnancy I was in a new job when I took maternity leave, so FMLA didn't cover. Based on my experience, I'd say if your employer promises to hold your job, get it in writing. (Jennifer A., secretary)

TELLING THE TRUTH ABOUT YOUR PLANS TO RETURN . . . OR NOT

Unless you are absolutely certain that you won't be going back to work, it's usually best to assume that you will. Try not to burn any bridges, even if you are unhappy about how your employer is handling your pregnancy or leave. If you have no intention to return, however, try not to lie outright, because that will undermine your credibility and may render you liable for health insurance payments made on your behalf during your leave. (It will also hurt mothers who come after you, who won't be believed when they say they intend to return.) And what if you plan to go back, but change your mind? We all know moms who intend to resume paid work but end up staying home full-time or shifting into a part-time career; after all, no one can know for sure how she will feel once she has held her baby in her arms. If you change your mind about going back to work, it is important to follow your instincts and do what's right for you and your family.

Many women worry about job security during their leave. If you are covered under the FMLA, you can't be terminated while you are out unless your job would have been eliminated anyway, which of course can be hard to judge. If you feel you have been treated unfairly, the Equal Employment Opportunity Commission (EEOC), whose national toll-free number is 1–800–669–4000, can get you in contact with your local EEOC branch.

The Work-Until-Labor or Take-Off-a-Few-Weeks Debate

Some employers will want you to work until whenever labor begins, while others prefer that you name a departure date that they can work around. Find out what they need, and think about what would be best for you, before deciding which plan best fits your situation.

Arguments for taking off a few weeks:

- You will have time to yourself
- You will have time to prepare for the baby
- You will feel rested before labor begins

Arguments for working until labor:

- You may feel bored and antsy waiting for the baby
- You may waste precious maternity leave, especially if you go overdue

In my first pregnancy I stopped working a week before my due date, and then I went a week late and was twiddling my thumbs for two weeks—and just WAITING. This pregnancy I am going to work up until labor. (Michele C., accountant)

The second time, I was so sure I was going to be early, like the first one, that I started my maternity leave early. When I still hadn't delivered by my due date, I decided to go back to work on a day-by-day basis. (Elisa R., ob-gyn)

I stopped working about one month before I was due, because I started getting really tired, and I wanted to make sure that I was well-rested for labor. (Kafi P., teacher)

They expected me to work up until labor. But I live forty minutes away and I wanted to take leave at thirty-eight to thirty-nine weeks so I wouldn't be so far if I went into labor. Plus I didn't want to be driving in labor, and it was winter and I was worried about the weather. They were very negative about me taking off before delivery. They seemed to think I was making excuses. (Danielle R., trust analyst)

They wanted me to take off starting at thirty-eight weeks so that they could plan for my absence. Then my baby came ten days late, which was tough—I wanted that time to be with him. Unfortunately you can't bank sleep, but when I look back on it I appreciate that time that I had to myself after working so hard in pregnancy and before my life changed after the baby came. (Kendra F., civil litigator)

One practical problem with taking off from work before labor: loss of leave at the other end. For many mothers-to-be, taking a few weeks off beforehand means they have that much less (paid or unpaid) time off after the baby. Some women set their schedule day-to-day for the last two weeks, just doing add-on work or last minute projects, so they can extricate themselves when they have to leave suddenly. Before you decide when to start your leave, be sure to check how your predelivery leave would affect your time at home after your little one arrives.

Getting Ready to Be Away

At least six to eight weeks before your due date, you will need to start preparing your work to be reassigned. Try these steps to ensure a successful handoff to your temporary replacement:

- Adjust your own mindset to the fact that you will be unavailable for many weeks.
- If your job is simple, a list of duties should be enough to help those covering for you do your work. If your job is more complex, consider creating a job handbook, listing all the tasks that need to be handed over in your absence. Include the names of those you report to and those who report to you on each project. Picture how they will do your work, and leave specific instructions in your notes. Don't forget the little tasks that have become second nature to you. For example, if you are the only one who uses a particular online tool, you might want to leave instructions on how to access it and do the basics.
- Talk with those taking over for you. Give them a tour of your projects and workspace. If possible, introduce them to clients or important contacts. If you need to train a replacement, start early.
- Clear your desk and your computer of personal information. Update your contact list. Leave only what will help your colleagues cover for you.
- If you password-protect files on your computer, write down any passwords that you may not remember when you return a few months down the road.
- Leave a trail. Organize projects and track your progress so that someone else can pick up where you left off.

- Try to work ahead so that your colleagues aren't thrown into a time crunch as they take on your job.
- Set up your email and phone-mail away message with contact information for questions or problems. Be sure a colleague will respond to any issues that are sent to your attention.

I "dropped" six weeks early and was dilated so they thought I might deliver early. This forced me to prepare for maternity leave. I worked frantically until I got things under control. Eventually I left all the new projects on a list for the next person to start. (Brenda W., lawyer)

Starting around seven months I made a spreadsheet with the status of each of my projects. I knew I might have to go from an appointment right to the hospital because the pregnancy was getting so complicated. (Danielle R., trust analyst)

Arranging for Your Return

Your colleagues will appreciate having you specify a return date before you leave. It also will help them to believe that you are really coming back. Remember that you can always resume work earlier than expected; they will welcome you, convinced that you are terrifically dedicated to the job. But once they are anticipating and planning for your date of return, extending your leave may be difficult, even if you are within the law. It is usually best, then, to arrange ahead of time for the maximum leave that you can get.

Being specific about a return date, as well as making a detailed, thoughtful arrangement for your own absence and likely return, are ways to show your colleagues and employer that even though you're going to be a mom, you still feel responsible toward your job. Although the transition into and out of parental leave may still be difficult for your and your coworkers, it can only help to try to anticipate and respond to an employer's needs during this time. Think of your investment in work now as potentially paying dividends in higher future earnings and more flexible scheduling down the road—benefits that you and your entire family may enjoy.

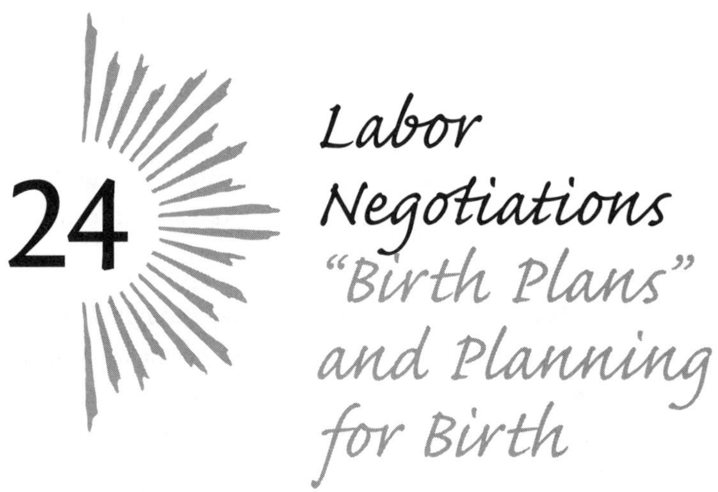

24 Labor Negotiations "Birth Plans" and Planning for Birth

What should you do now to get ready for childbirth? Although you can't plan for every eventuality, thinking ahead about who will support you during labor and how you will manage if the going gets tough can help you prepare for your baby's birthday. This chapter will help you create a list of preparations that can be done in advance: from packing your bags, to choosing your support team, to finding out where to park at the hospital.

Packing Your Bags

As your big day draws near, you will want to pack for your trip to the hospital. Luckily, you can expect the hospital to give you many of the things you'll need most: hospital gowns, towels, washcloths, soap, shampoo, sanitary pads, breast pads, and most newborn items. Because birth is messy, it makes sense to wear a hospital gown and save your own things for home or for later during your hospital stay. In fact, you may want to consider packing two bags: one for labor, and one "postpartum bag" to be brought after the baby arrives. And leave your valuables at home—you won't want to worry about them when you leave your room.

Taking a Childbirth Class

Although intense natural childbirth-oriented programs often begin in the second trimester, most childbirth classes are taken later in pregnancy, so that they will be completed a few weeks before your due date.

YOUR LABOR BAG PACKING LIST

- Insurance card
- Birth plan—if you have one
- Socks and slippers
- A robe
- Your toothbrush and other toiletries, contact lens solution, glasses, hairband
- Comfort items (based on your plans for how to manage labor): massage oil, lip balm, and the like
- Music (check if the hospital provides a CD player or if you need to bring one)
- Camera—still or video—with extra batteries
- Calling card (if you don't have a cell phone or won't be able to use it in the hospital)
- Phone list of friends and relatives
- Books, magazines, playing cards—things to do in case labor progresses slowly
- Snacks for dad, or change for the snack machines
- Medications you take that the hospital pharmacy may not stock

Many couples wonder if it is worth the effort and expense to take classes, especially if they are planning on an epidural. With a first baby, labor is such an unknown that some preparation is a good idea, just to be familiar with the range of possible events and experiences. Watching videos and reading are useful, but classes will compel you and your partner to spend some time thinking ahead, so you can get a sense of how you'll work together as a team. Education can also help both of you become more realistic about the challenges of labor and birth, so you can make choices (for example, about relaxation techniques and who will come with you) that will meet your needs.

I tell people that it definitely hurt and that I have never felt a pain like that before, but through the Bradley classes I was prepared to deal with the pain naturally. The class showed videos of actual labors and talked about the different stages of labor and how to recognize them and get past them. Having this knowledge allowed me to have an idea where I was on the

YOUR POSTPARTUM BAG

- A few pairs of clean underwear—maternity size
- Bras—nursing bras if you plan to breastfeed, or soft exercise-type bras
- A few pairs of socks
- Nightgowns, pajamas, or comfortable sweats if you won't want to wear hospital-issue attire

For the trip home:

- Soft, loose-fitting clothes for you (your mid-pregnancy sizes will be about right)
- A baby outfit (be sure it covers the baby's feet, or bring little socks)
- Baby hat
- Baby blankets
- Diaper bag with diapers, wipes, and a change of clothes for baby—you'll always want this with you when you take your baby out
- Car seat (installed ahead of time). Every state requires infant car seats. To learn the requirements in your state, check out www.infant-car-seats.com/seat-belt-laws.html.

journey to actually getting to see my baby and helped me to get through the next contraction. (Danielle R., trust analyst)

Even when it's not your first pregnancy, classes can be useful—particularly if you are trying for a VBAC (vaginal birth after cesarean), if you are seeking natural childbirth, or if it has been some time since your last pregnancy. In these situations, you may appreciate getting up to speed about the latest options.

If you haven't delivered at this hospital or birth center before, be sure to take advantage if they offer a free tour. Not only will you become better oriented to the place where you will give birth; you will meet some of the staff, have a chance to ask questions, and learn about their routines.

If you are terribly anxious about labor, you may find yourself not wanting to think about it at all—as if ignoring it will keep it from happening. Of course, preparation isn't absolutely necessary: the baby will come whether you have educated yourself about every nuance of labor or hardly thought about it. But if you really can't contemplate your baby's birth without panicking, you might consider seeking professional counseling, which can be very helpful in easing fears and phobias.

Choosing Your Support Team

Who will come with you when you have your baby? I have been a part of many lovely births with all sorts of arrangements of friends and family—from just the partner, to a mom and a friend, to what seemed like a boisterous family reunion. The people you bring with you will influence your experience. While your parents, siblings, and friends may want to be included, this is your time, and you need to decide who will (and who won't) be helpful. Do you want a quiet room, music playing, with just one or two loved ones to hold your hand? Do you mind cross-conversations while you are trying to relax? How private are you about your body? Will it give you and the father pleasure to share the baby's birth with your parents, or will inviting them to see your newborn afterward be enough? As part of your decision-making, find out your hospital's policies about the number of visitors and, if there is a limit, whether your visitors can take turns.

As you think about the people you would enjoy having with you, remember that labor isn't always pretty. One doctor I know tells her patients to only bring with them the sort of people they wouldn't mind seeing them throw up! And even if you invite only those friends and family you believe will be helpful to you, let them know that the invitation is conditional, because you can't know exactly how you will feel or how labor will go. Some mothers-to-be set up a code word with their nurse in case they want their extra visitors to be asked to leave.

In the room with me was my husband, my mother, my stepfather, and my mother-in-law. Everyone helped hold my legs up and whatever else I needed. (Zenia M., nurse's aide)

Many hospitals permit siblings over a certain age to be present at the birth if they have attended a preparation course and if an extra adult can see to their needs. Alternatively, children (and grandparents or other relatives) can be brought in immediately after the baby arrives.

Another factor to keep in mind is that the nurse will come and go during your early labor—she may have three patients or more; in addition, when her shift is over she will leave and a new nurse will be assigned. A midwife might stay with you throughout labor, or may function more like a doctor, coming in at key moments, and at the end to "catch the baby." So although the nurse, midwife, or doctors will provide support and help, it is your visitors who will stay at your side through thick and thin.

Another person who can help you during labor is a professional labor assistant, or doula. As explained in Chapter 11, a doula will provide emotional and practical support for you and your partner, and can advocate for you if you have birth preferences that are not standard for your location.

We hired a doula, and it was absolutely the right decision for us. It was so much easier and better to have someone who's always on your side and whose only job is to be there for you. (Cheryl L., lawyer)

When You Arrive in Labor

When you take your tour of the labor suite, ask about how you will be checked in and about their other routines: this is the time to find out what is standard procedure, and what you will need to request. For example, even though most birth plan worksheets on the Internet tell you to request that an enema and pubic shave not be done, most labor and delivery units haven't done these embarrassing treatments in decades. And speaking of birth plans—be sure you know how to get to the hospital, day or night, and where to park and enter once you arrive!

FETAL MONITORING

When you arrive at the hospital, nurses will check the baby, usually by placing you on the fetal monitor for twenty minutes or so. Many labor and delivery units keep the baby on continuous monitoring throughout labor. For some parents, this is reassuring; for others, it may feel unnecessarily medical or restrictive. Scientific research on low-risk pregnancies that compared continuous monitoring to listening at regular intervals, called intermittent auscultation, showed no difference in how the babies fared at birth—although more cesareans were done in the continuously monitored group. As long as labor is going well, then, listening to the baby at regular intervals is a safe alternative to continuous monitoring, but you may have to request it. Just be aware that some practitioners are most comfortable with continuous monitoring and really don't want a laboring mom off the monitor for long. In addition, if the nurses are really busy, intermittent auscultation might not be possible: they may not be able to come in at the necessary intervals to listen to the baby's heart. Concerns about how the baby is doing or how labor is going may also require the constant stream of information that a fetal monitor provides.

INTRAVENOUS LINES

Many practitioners feel safest if you have intravenous access, meaning an IV line or a small capped-off IV called a heparin (or saline) lock, so that medications or fluids can be given in case of emergency. The downside to an IV is that it is connected to a fluid bag on a wheeled IV pole, and can be awkward if you want to walk around or go in the shower, both helpful comfort measures for labor. A capped-off IV or "hep lock" doesn't usually restrict you, but it may feel like unnecessary medicalization. Remember, though, that the IV can also be useful. Antibiotics for group B strep must be given intravenously, epidural anesthesia always requires intravenous fluids, and in case of emergency, an IV line may be needed for treating you and your baby.

Your Labor Experience

Once you've been admitted to the hospital or birthing center, and your labor is in full swing, what will your experience be like, and what decisions will need to be made?

EATING AND DRINKING

Find out your practitioner's beliefs and your hospital's policies about eating during labor. During active labor digestion stops, and food can pile up in the stomach, to be seen again later (in a less appetizing form). In addition, in the rare chance of an emergency cesarean, a full stomach makes going to sleep for surgery more risky.

Even if you aren't allowed to eat, or don't feel like eating during active labor, you'll need fluids and calories to keep up your energy, especially if your labor is long. This can be done by munching ice or freeze pops, drinking clear liquids like apple juice or ginger ale, or receiving fluids through an IV line, depending on hospital policies, your medical circumstances, and personal preference.

MUSIC

Music can help you to relax and will personalize your labor room. Find out if CD players are provided or if you should bring your own. Choose a range of musical styles, so you can meet your needs for energizing or relaxing.

> ***I remember at one point the nurse asked if I wanted to change the CD (we'd been listening to Pachelbel for HOURS) and my husband knew by the look on my face that if they changed the CD my head was likely to start spinning! But then about an hour later, I wanted the CD changed and he knew exactly what one to put on—my son was born to a Mexican/Native American type blowpipe music—it was much more upbeat and had a good bass! (Sandy B., social worker)***

PHOTOGRAPHS AND VIDEO

Check your hospital's policies before you show up with a film crew. Some hospitals don't allow videotaping during a vaginal birth or cesarean, but most will be happy to have you film during labor and after the baby is born. If you are going to take lots of pictures, consider bringing someone with you for that purpose. You won't want your main support person to be fussing with a camera when you need attention.

STAYING STRONG THROUGH YOUR LABOR CONTRACTIONS

Labor is a different experience for every woman and in each pregnancy. Some labors are long and drawn out; others are quick and tumultuous. It usually gets pretty intense; with the help of your coaches you'll need to use your inner resources to keep yourself calm throughout the powerful physical and emotional happenings.

Your choices for managing the intensity of the contractions may be the most important part of your birth plan. Some hospitals don't have an anesthesiologist present at all times, so epidurals are only available with advance planning. In many hospitals, the default mode is to give an epidural when you enter active labor, generally around four to five centimeters' dilation. If that is what you want, it won't take much preparation ahead of time to make it happen. But if you have other ideas, planning can make a difference.

If you are worried about discomfort during early labor and don't like the idea of waiting that long for relief, you will need to educate yourself about nonmedical comfort measures and intravenous pain medications. Talk to your practitioner ahead of time about options. It is also your right to request an epidural before the protocol allows for it—after all, as long as you are really in labor, the worst that will happen if you get your epidural too early is that labor will slow down. As a result you may end up with more medical interventions, like Pitocin or a cesarean—which at that moment might not seem like such terrible possibilities.

If natural childbirth is your goal, be sure that those who come with you can help you toward that target. Your coach will need to know about nonmedical comfort measures and must be able to tolerate you looking uncomfortable, a difficult task for many husbands. If you or the baby's father has concerns about his ability to be your sole support, consider bringing a female friend or relative, or hiring a professional labor assistant (doula) to help you through.

For those who want the most natural experience, I do think it is valuable to specify to your coaches and the medical staff that you don't want to be offered pain medications. You know they exist, and you can always make a request if you change your mind. I saw a birth plan once that said, "Don't give me pain medicine even if I scream for it," but I don't think any caring medical professional would agree to that. You have to be allowed to change your mind, but we shouldn't undermine your resolve by continuously offering. This is one good use for a written birth plan: if you don't want medications or an epidural offered, be sure to inform the nurses and doctors who are taking care of you.

SPECIAL EQUIPMENT

Birthing beds and showers in the labor room are pretty standard, but other items may not be as available. Do you think you will want to use a birthing ball for labor? A squatting bar for pushing? A mirror to watch the birth? A bathtub for labor or delivery? Learn about variations, and ask about availability, so you will know your options when the time comes.

INDUCTION OR AUGMENTATION OF LABOR

Sometimes labor either hasn't started or is going too slowly, and induction or augmentation is recommended. Induction and stimulation of labor are very common, so learn about the different methods, both natural and medical, and under which circumstances induction or augmentation might be indicated. And keep in mind that stimulating a stalled-out labor with Pitocin may *decrease* the likelihood of cesarean.

The Big Moment: Your Baby Arrives

Ready or not, the time will come when your baby is ready to emerge. What will that experience be like for you and your support team? And what decisions might you need to make as events unfold?

WHO WILL DELIVER THE BABY?

Ask beforehand who will actually deliver your baby. Some practices have you meet all the OBs before you come in for labor, but some have too many doctors or midwives to make that a practical option. If a nurse-midwife or family doctor is caring for you, ask about their backup physicians, and how long it will take them to get there if a medical problem develops. If you plan to deliver at a birth center, learn about when and how you might be transferred to the hospital.

WHAT MEDICAL PERSONNEL WILL BE AT THE BIRTH?

You may be surprised at the number of staff members who may attend a hospital delivery—your OB, nurses for you and the baby, the anesthesia team if you have an epidural, a pediatrician or two if any problems are expected, as well as students and residents. At teaching hospitals, the residents are often the front line if any problems develop before your doctor arrives. Don't refuse to have them involved in your care: you won't want the resident to hesitate to come in if your baby's heartbeat is slow or some other concern arises. If you feel strongly

TWO ACCOMPLISHMENTS, ONE RECOVERY: GETTING YOUR TUBES TIED AFTER BIRTH

If this is your last baby, you may want to consider a permanent method of birth control. If you have a cesarean, tubal ligation adds little to the recovery, and may seem like a bonus. Tubal ligation can also be performed immediately after vaginal birth, though a small incision near your belly button, and if you had an epidural for delivery, your method of anesthesia will already be in place. This permanent decision should not be made on the spur of the moment—in fact, sometimes signing permission a month ahead is required—so if you think you want your tubes tied, be sure to ask about it during a prenatal visit.

about who will be in the room at the time of birth, discuss your concerns ahead of time with your doctor or midwife.

OPERATIVE VAGINAL DELIVERY

No parent hopes for a birth involving forceps or vacuum techniques, but sometimes their use is medically necessary. In fact, you will be wise to learn about operative vaginal deliveries in advance, because in some cases, these procedures are recommended but optional, which means you will have to make some decisions on the spot. Significantly, a cesarean birth may be the alternative, so you will want to learn a little about all the possibilities.

EPISIOTOMY

Episiotomy is an incision made to enlarge the vaginal opening before the baby is born. The pros and cons of episiotomy depend on the situation. Ask your doctor or midwife under what circumstances she is likely to do an episiotomy, so you can know what to expect. If you would prefer to avoid one, feel free to say so, but don't refuse to have one under any circumstances, since there are times when an episiotomy might be needed for you or for your baby.

WHEN THE BABY COMES OUT

Try to remember to open your eyes and look as your new baby emerges. As long as all is going well, do you want the baby handed immediately to you, or cleaned up and dried off first? Check on the policies of your birthing unit and practitioner if this matters to you. Do you want your partner or visitor to cut the umbilical cord, or do you want your practitioner to do it? Remember to ask early if you have preferences, since things move pretty fast right at delivery.

CORD BLOOD DONATION

If you are planning on saving or donating umbilical cord blood, arrangements usually need to be made ahead of time, and the doctor or midwife has to follow specific procedures after the cord is cut.

CESAREAN BIRTH

Many couples are shocked to be told that a C-section is needed, yet it shouldn't be that surprising; in the United States one in four babies is born by cesarean. Sometimes cesareans are planned; in other cases they become necessary during labor.

Because cesarean delivery isn't that rare, and because it can be a last-minute decision, it is best to think ahead about how you might experience a C-section. Even an urgent cesarean can usually be done under regional anesthesia (spinal or epidural) so that you can be awake and hear your baby's first cry. If you are awake for your cesarean, most hospitals will encourage your partner or another support person to stay with you in the operating room, but typically only one person is allowed. (Other friends or family members will have to wait to see the pictures, so find out your hospital's policies on taking photos and videos of cesarean births.) Your support person will sit next to you, up by your head, behind the surgical drapes. The surgery may be visible from there, but visitors who don't want to see what's happening can hunch down a little and look at you instead of into your incision. If you will be asleep for the surgery, visitors usually are not allowed because they aren't needed for your emotional support, and because they may find it unpleasant to see you under anesthesia.

Assuming that you are awake for the birth of the baby and all is well, feel free to request that your partner hold the baby as soon as possible. Sometimes the staff gets caught up in the routine newborn care, but often newborn procedures can wait, and your family can start bonding right there in the operating room.

You and Your Newborn

Anticipating the awesome moment when you first hold your newborn is an inspiring part of making a birth plan. What options will be available to you to make the post-delivery experience all that you dreamed it would be?

IMMEDIATE NEWBORN CARE

Newborns are wet, so they quickly become cold. Your baby will need to be dried off, and mucus may have to be suctioned from the nose and mouth. This can either be done in your arms (if you have a vaginal birth), or close by under a warmer, where oxygen and suction are available. After suctioning, the baby can stay with you if you want, being kept warm by your body and a blanket.

If there are any problems, even mild issues like mucus in the airways or meconium (the baby's first stool in the amniotic fluid), the nurses or pediatricians may take the baby to the warmer for assessment. If this happens, the staff may get caught up in the routine newborn care and forget to bring your baby back to you right away. Once your newborn has been stabilized, feel free to ask if what they are doing can wait, so your baby can be with you for the first moments of life. Routine newborn care, including antibiotic eye ointment, must be given by law, but can usually wait an hour or two.

ROOMING IN

One mother may want to have her new baby with her 24/7; another may want the baby to go to the nursery so she can get some rest. You don't need to decide in advance how much time your baby will spend with you in your room, but it's good to know there are options. If you have a private room (which may cost extra), your partner can probably stay with you and the baby, if you wish.

BREASTFEEDING

Do you plan to breastfeed or bottle-feed your baby? Do you mind if the hospital staff gives your baby a pacifier if she is fussy? Learn about these issues and the routines in the nursery, so that you can communicate your desires to the hospital staff.

CIRCUMCISION

Learn about the pros and cons of circumcision. Typically, medical circumcisions are performed while the baby is still in the hospital after birth. If you are planning on having a religious ritual circumcision, arrangements will need to be made with a practitioner in the community.

THE LENGTH OF YOUR STAY

Some mothers want to get home as fast as possible, while others feel best with the rest and support of round-the-clock nursing care within the hospital. New moms just learning to breastfeed can benefit from the education offered by the postpartum nurses and lactation consultants at the hospital, too. In 1999, the U.S. Congress passed a law that requires insurance plans to pay for forty-eight hours of hospital care after a vaginal birth and ninety-six hours after a cesarean, although most moms only stay three nights after a C-section. Leaving earlier than the days covered by insurance depends on your wishes and how you and the baby are doing. Typically, if you are discharged early, your insurance will pay for a visiting nurse to come to your home to check on you and the baby.

Your "Birth Plan"

As your delivery day approaches and becomes more real, you may find that you have strong feelings or ideals about certain aspects of your baby's birth. Do you want it to be as unmedical as possible? Do you imagine having a mirror to watch the baby be born? Are you picturing your husband's face as he views the baby for the first time and cuts the cord? Each parent's desires are different. Communicating these wishes to your doctor or midwife will help you to assess how realistic your wishes are for your individual situation. And because no birth goes exactly as planned, you might try to resolve now not to be too heartbroken about any parts of your experience that don't match your fantasy. While it is good to advocate for your preferences, try to educate yourself about all of the possibilities and most of all, be flexible when confronted with the unexpected.

We had a birthing plan. I had read a lot about medical intervention getting in the way of letting labor progress naturally. I was really committed to letting it happen on its own. I fought the interventions for awhile. I was in labor thirty hours and had pushed for three hours before I went to C-section. I think that my fighting the interventions probably made my labor longer than it needed to be. (Kendra F., civil litigator)

You might wonder why your doctor isn't as attentive to planning for your labor experience as you are. In medical training, we are taught that our primary job is to protect the health of the mother and baby; there is little focus on the birth experience. This medical approach works well for parents who share that biological view of birth, but it may not meet the needs of those who look at childbirth as a major life event and specially value the nonmedical aspects of the birth experience. Different hospitals and different practitioners are more or less flexible, depending on their philosophy, and on what you ask them to do. There are many ways to have a baby.

I brought up my labor preferences with my obstetrician. I spoke to her about her C-section rate, her stance on episiotomies, etc. She's had five children over the time that she was my gynecologist, so I expected her to be understanding, but she was very put off by my questions, which left a bad taste in my mouth. So I started looking into hiring a doula, a process that put me in touch with a wonderful midwife practice. I immediately clicked with them, and I transferred my care at six and a half months. (Linda S., creative director)

A birth plan is a written document that states your preferences. Advocates of birth plans will tell you that writing up what you are seeking will help ensure the experience you desire. The medical community's reception of birth plans is mixed: some obstetricians believe that birth plans interfere with their ability to care for their patients, while others welcome them as a communication tool. I have heard nurses and residents hypothesize that the more elaborate the birth

SETTING THE SCENE FOR A SATISFYING BIRTH EXPERIENCE

- Get a feel for the sort of experience you are seeking and choose an obstetrical or midwifery practice and birth location that fits with your beliefs.
- Educate yourself. Take childbirth classes, read, and think about what sort of person you are and what type of experience will probably suit you. Practice the relaxation techniques you plan to use. Learn about all aspects of labor and birth, even those you don't expect, like cesarean section.
- Talk to your partner and other coaches, so that you understand everyone's wishes, expectations, and fears.
- Find out about the routines at the location where you will give birth. Take a tour, and talk to other mothers who have delivered there.
- Talk to your practitioner about the sort of experience you are seeking. If your desires are off the beaten path, a written birth plan can help communicate your wishes to the many people who will be helping you on your baby's birthday. Only those aspects that are nonstandard or clearly optional need to be specified.
- Bring with you friends, family, or a professional labor assistant who can advocate for you and provide support.
- If an intervention is recommended that you are not sure about, ask questions.

plan, the greater the chance that the mom will end up with a cesarean; they feel that trying to control things too much increases the odds of getting the opposite of what you desire. I like to think of birth plans as a statement of preferences: if all goes well, these are our wishes.

It's understandable that obstetrical professionals would be unwilling to commit to a birth plan as a contract given the unpredictable medical aspects of labor care. What if we are concerned about the baby's heart rate? What if the mother hemorrhages and doesn't have an IV? What if the doctor feels an episiotomy is necessary to speed delivery when the baby is in trouble? The medical team isn't usually willing to sign off on a birth plan as if it were legally binding. But it can be very useful to communicate the kind of experience you are seeking, so those around you know what approach to try first.

WRITING A BIRTH PLAN

In general, birth plans should start with a statement of appreciation for the care you will receive, and an acknowledgment that things don't always go as planned. The medical team needs to feel that you are working with them, not against them. Keep the birth plan short, and focus on aspects that are important to you, and that are not routine at your chosen location.

Page 288 shows a birth plan that I received from one of my patients that was interesting because it was a statement of what the parents were seeking rather than a lot of rules for the team to follow. Templates for more specific birth plans can be found on many websites.

I'm not very big on childbirth; I didn't bond with the fetus. I was glad to have a midwife who understood that and whose only goal was to have a healthy baby and mother. (Lori G., professor)

DISAPPOINTMENT

Labor doesn't always go as planned, and most couples are not able to have every request in their birth plan fulfilled. Some labors are so fast there is no time for anesthesia. Others are long and rotten and in my opinion not made for an unmedicated experience. Sometimes pregnancy complications require strict bed rest during labor, or urgent delivery by cesarean. If you choose a team you trust and who communicate well with you, you will understand and feel well cared for overall, even if you don't have the birth of your dreams.

Despite the labors not being ideal, the end result is that I have two healthy, wonderful babies who don't remember their labors. (Linda S., creative director)

Remember, too, that the process of bringing a baby into the world takes but a day or two of your life; then it will be over and the important work of building your relationship with your little one will begin. Whether you obsessed about the birth or denied it for nine months, the baby will be here and life will move on.

BIRTH PLAN

Julie P. and Rob M.

Birth Team:
Dr. Marjorie Greenfield
Kim W., doula
And the MacDonald Hospital staff

This is our first baby and we are thrilled about welcoming him or her into our lives. We would love your support in experiencing the magic of birth.

Thank you for your support and for sharing your time with us.

Please help us encourage:

- laughter
- a sense of wonder
- trying various positions to assist labor
- a climate of safety
- working with Kim on pain relief
- bonding with baby

Please help us discourage

- artificial stimulation of labor
- pain medications
- fear
- intrusions on our privacy

In my generation (I'm fifty), there was a lot of emphasis on natural childbirth, and of taking back the experience of pregnancy and childbirth. The thought was that pregnancy and childbirth are what make you a woman. I think that's the wrong emphasis. Pregnancy makes a **baby** ***and your job is to take care of that baby. (Deb L., writer)***

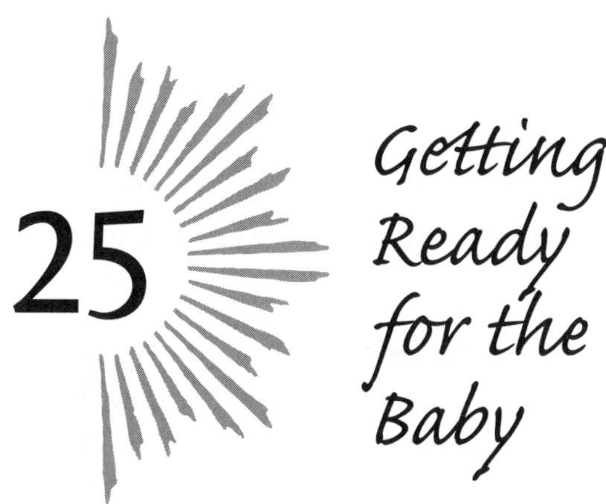

25 Getting Ready for the Baby

During a first pregnancy, especially, it's easy to feel as though childbirth is the most important job ahead: the experience is such an unknown that you may have difficulty picturing moving beyond the big day. But it's important to appreciate what is happening inside of you: the little person growing in your body will join your family soon. It's time to get ready for what comes after delivery—life at home with your new baby.

> ***I felt so productive when I was pregnant. Like, even when I wasn't doing anything, I was doing something really important. (Elisa R., ob-gyn)***

> ***Society does not do much to celebrate/honor pregnant women. I felt like I wanted a mom-welcoming ceremony that talked about what a wonderful and important role I would have. The one place that I went that was positive was prenatal yoga. Every class we would begin by bowing our heads to the "new life in our bellies" and think about it in a moment of silence as we started and ended the class. I am terrible at yoga and would have dropped out, except that I lived and died for those peaceful positive moments every week where I felt publicly thanked and praised. (Cheryl L., lawyer)***

What will your baby need at the hospital and for the first days and weeks at home? Many experienced moms have favorite answers to this question, but everyone will need to consider the basics: food, diapers, and essential baby gear. Read on for some tips for preparing your home and family for your little bundle.

Breast or Bottle?

Many working moms struggle with the decision of whether to breastfeed or bottle-feed their babies. There are many arguments to be made for going with the breast, including:

- Breast milk contains exactly what babies need. For the first six months of life, human milk is the *only* food they require. As they get older, the constitution of the milk changes to meet the requirements of their changing bodies. Even during a single feeding, the milk shifts from high protein (foremilk) to higher fat (hind milk)—like dinner and dessert!
- Breast milk contains antibodies that help fight off infections. The baby's own immune system is undeveloped for the first six months or so, and doesn't fully mature until a few years of age. When compared with babies who only received formula, breastfed babies are less likely to get several types of infections, and may be protected from certain autoimmune diseases.
- Breastfed babies score higher than formula-fed infants do on measures of intellectual development later in life (although of course we don't know if that is due to the breast milk itself or is because more educated mothers are likelier to nurse their babies).
- Breastfed babies' poop smells better than that of formula-fed babies.
- Breastfeeding is good for the mom: your uterus will shrink to its normal size more quickly, and the production of milk burns off extra calories. (The sagginess or stretch marks that some women develop in their breasts after having children are caused by pregnancy, not by nursing.) Breastfeeding also protects you (somewhat) from getting pregnant too soon, and helps to prevent cancer of the breast and ovary. You might think that breastfeeding will take calcium out of your body, but osteoporosis (brittle bones) is actually *less* common in elderly women who breastfed earlier in life.
- Working moms often feel good about supplying their babies with breast milk even when they can't be with them. It is something only you can provide.
- Breastfeeding saves money—on average you'll spend one quarter as

much on the extra food for you, compared with the costs of formula and bottles, leading to a savings of over a thousand dollars a year.

Breastfeeding quite possibly was the best part of the entire pregnancy and birth. After having the C-section, I can't think of any better way to bond with my baby. That little boy would place his tiny hands around my breast while nursing, like a little hug. It was the most precious part of becoming a mother! (Tracy G., police officer)

Breastfeeding is so much easier than preparing bottles. I would hate to get up at 5 AM to fix a bottle when I can just nurse my son and he falls back to sleep for a while longer. (Loren W., vice president of marketing)

Breastfeeding at night was one of the most wonderful times of the day because you are all cuddled up and it's just the two of you and it's very calming. After breastfeeding, it was actually easier to fall back to sleep than at other times. (Juanita G., research scientist)

But while many mothers love nursing, some find the idea overwhelming or distasteful. For other women, a medical problem may require medication that isn't compatible with breastfeeding, or may preclude breastfeeding in some other way. In these situations, alternatives are available. In areas of the world with a clean water supply, infant formulas are safe and nutritious, and are probably the best choice if breastfeeding isn't feasible.

Breastfeeding was not joyful for me. My boobs were always big and I felt self-conscious. They were even bigger while I was nursing. I didn't like wearing the special bra. I didn't like the giant shirts. I never relaxed; I just felt I was doing this to feed Sam. (Annie F., classical violinist)

BREASTFEEDING AND WORK

If you want to breastfeed but plan to go back to work, you have a variety of options: you can pump milk at work, run out to the baby during the day, have the baby brought to you to nurse, formula-feed during your work hours and breast-feed on nights and weekends, or switch to formula after you resume work. Just don't let your plans to return to work make you afraid to nurse: even six weeks of breast milk provides a lot of advantages for you and the baby, benefits that extend beyond the first few months. And if you enjoy it, you may find a way to continue at least part-time after your return to the workforce. Some lactation centers or childbirth education programs offer "back to work" breastfeeding classes. A lactation consultant also can give you individualized help as you plan for your return.

Pumping two to three times while at work kept my milk in and provided her with enough milk so that she never had to use the formula that was kept in the closet "just in case." (Brenda H., pediatric resident)

I loved nursing! When I returned to work after my first, I worked hard at maintaining a schedule of pumping and feeding, and tried to do that on weekends too. This drove me, my nanny, and my baby crazy. For child number two, I threw schedules out the window, and nursed whenever I could on weekends and nights. I allowed my nanny to supplement with formula if the freezer was empty. My supply was thin on Saturday mornings, but we nursed as much as he wanted, sometimes every two hours. I enjoyed being needed all weekend! On Mondays I was full at work, and occasionally leaked, but by midweek I was fine. (Jill H., gynecologist)

Consider the source when someone tells you that continuing to breastfeed after returning to work is "impossible" or "setting yourself up for failure." I was told both of those things and oddly one of those people never breastfed her children and the other was a stay-at-home mother. Despite going back to work, I nursed my son for two and a half years. (Kari S., librarian)

There is a lot of pressure on women to breastfeed. But in this day and age formulas are very good, and if you really hate nursing the baby will sense it, and that isn't good either. Do whatever makes you feel good about your body. Do whatever makes you feel good about being a mom. (Annie F., classical violinist)

BREASTFEEDING SUPPLIES

If you plan to breastfeed, you will probably appreciate having these items on hand when your baby arrives:

- Nursing bras and pads. Choose soft comfortable bras with flaps that can be opened with one hand. You will most likely wear your nursing bra (lined with disposable or washable pads) 24/7 for the first few weeks, until your supply and the baby's demand get in synch and your breasts stop leaking.
- Nursing gowns and tops. Gowns and tops designed for breastfeeding have hidden openings to allow you to nurse discreetly. Cropped tops also work well. Check out Motherwear at www.motherwear.com for helpful nursing clothes and nightgowns.
- Breast pump. Many women start with a good manual pump like the Medela Harmony or Avent Isis, and then figure out if they need something different. If you plan to pump at work, you may want an electric pump. Even if you aren't going back to work, some sort of pump (manual or electric) can be helpful if you need to be away from the baby during a feeding, or if you feel engorged and the baby doesn't want to eat. If you haven't nursed a baby before, it may be best to figure out what pump to get after you have established breastfeeding, so you can determine what type works best for you. A lactation consultant can also help advise you about pumps.

Many mothers-to-be take a breastfeeding class. Although breastfeeding sounds like it ought to be the most natural thing in the world, women who haven't been surrounded by breastfeeding since childhood typically have a lot to learn. For example, knowing how to help your baby get onto your breast in a comfortable, off-center "latch" can avoid sore nipples. And realistic expectations about how often newborns feed (a lot!), as well as knowing how to avoid the common pitfalls of breastfeeding, can help get you off to a good start. Finding a lactation support group, and attending a meeting before you deliver, may also prove helpful. Research has shown that women who take a breastfeeding class are more likely to make it work. So if breastfeeding is important to you, learn as much as you can before your baby arrives.

Women's concerns about their diet affecting their milk can prevent them from wanting to breastfeed. I know moms who wanted to quit breastfeeding just so they could drink coffee again. My pediatrician never suggested that I restrict my diet, and it made it easier for me to continue breastfeeding

for a full year. It's a mistake to think that your baby is cranky because of something you're eating—babies are just cranky sometimes! (Brenda W., lawyer)

While breastfeeding, I was just more aware of what I was eating. I didn't eat anything too spicy or too odd, and I mostly just increased my fluid intake. (Rebecca M., senior vice president, financial corporation)

Cloth or Disposable?

Most families these days use at least some disposable diapers, since they are much easier when you're out of the house. Cloth diapers are more environment-friendly, unless you are in an area of water shortage, and are good to have around for spit-ups, even if you aren't relying on them for diapering. If you do use cloth, a diaper service makes life easier, especially early on when the baby's stools are very soft, and when you may change a lot of messy diapers in a day. If you plan on disposables, keep in mind that for the first month or so a baby uses almost ten diapers a day—stockpile newborn diapers at home, so you don't have to keep running to the store. Most families try a variety of brands until they settle on one that offers the best balance of cost and convenience.

Circumcision

Now what about what's under that diaper? If you know you are having a girl, you're off the hook, but if a boy is on the way, you'll need to decide about circumcision. Circumcision, the surgical removal of the foreskin of the penis, is an ancient practice. Most American families who choose to circumcise have it done in the hospital a day or two after birth. Your family doctor, obstetrician, nurse-midwife, or pediatrician might perform the circumcision, depending on who delivered the baby and the custom in your region. Observant Jewish families circumcise their sons on the eighth day of life, at home in a ceremony called a bris.

Your decision about circumcision should come from your own values. Religious and cultural reasons usually trump all other arguments. Otherwise, I believe circumcision is mainly a cosmetic issue. Yet you shouldn't be afraid of the

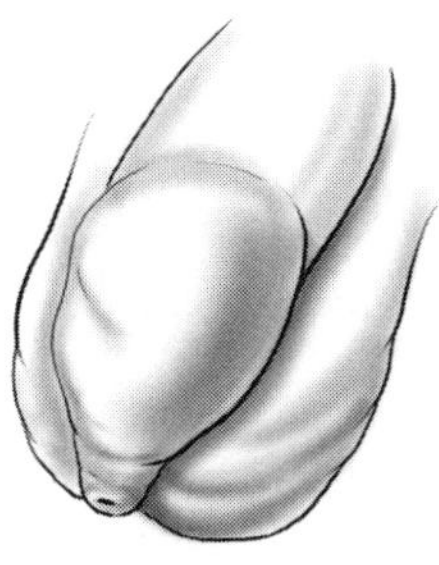
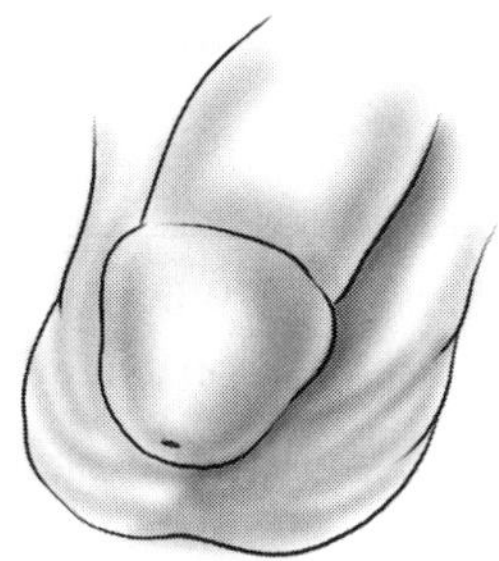

Circumcision: before and after

procedure. It takes less than five minutes in most cases, and surgical complications are very rare. Pain can be diminished with local anesthesia, and postoperative soreness can be offset with infant Tylenol. Often dads have strong feelings about circumcision, so be sure he is included in the decision-making. If you care about your son looking different in the locker room, ask your OB about the rate of circumcision in your area.

It may be helpful, too, to see where you fall in the common arguments for and against circumcision, but once you decide, don't drive yourself crazy with second guesses—in the long run, it will probably be fine either way.

THE AMERICAN ACADEMY OF PEDIATRICS' POSITION ON CIRCUMCISION

In a statement written in 1999 and reaffirmed in 2005, the American Academy of Pediatrics had this to say about circumcising newborn boys: "Existing scientific evidence demonstrates potential medical benefits of newborn male circumcision; however, these data are not sufficient to recommend routine neonatal circumcision. In circumstances in which there are potential benefits and risks, yet the procedure is not essential to the child's current well-being, parents should determine what is in the best interest of the child. To make an informed choice, parents of all male infants should be given accurate and unbiased information and be provided the opportunity to discuss this decision. If a decision for circumcision is made, procedural analgesia should be provided."

Common Arguments for and Against Circumcision

FOR	AGAINST
Will look like other family members (if other family members are circumcised)	Why do a cosmetic surgical procedure on a baby?
Will look like other males his age (if you live in a part of the country where circumcision is widely used)	Many factors determine if a boy will be teased—not just if he is circumcised
Most families in our area (Midwest, South) are circumcising newborn boys	Many families in our area (West Coast, Southwest, East Coast) are deciding not to circumcise
If circumcision ultimately is needed, it is better to have done it as a baby than later in life	Circumcision is medically unnecessary in the vast majority of boys (doctors who are inexperienced in the care of uncircumcised children may be more likely to say that circumcision is necessary later in life)
Fewer bladder infections	Males have very low rates of bladder infection—even uncircumcised boys get fewer infections than girls do
Less chance of penile cancer later in life	Penile cancer is very, very rare
Less chance of HIV infection	Not expecting this child to be at risk for HIV
Pain is minimized by local anesthesia, sucking a pacifier, or distraction with talk and touch	May be painful for some babies
Most men have plenty of pleasure with sex, circumcised or not	Some believe that circumcision diminishes sexual enjoyment
We come from a religious/cultural background that requires circumcision	No religious reasons to have a child circumcised
Circumcision is a fairly minor procedure that takes only three to five minutes	Rarely, serious surgical complications can occur

We're Jewish, so the circumcision decision wasn't really an issue. However, on the morning before the bris (ritual circumcision), my husband woke up and said, "Remind me—why are we doing this?" (Elizabeth S., online producer)

Picking a Name

If you think everyone has an opinion about circumcision and breastfeeding, just wait until you start talking about baby names. Selecting a name is very personal. It can be chosen to honor a relative, to specify characteristics that you are hoping to find in this child, or just because it sounds right. Your name influences how others view you. Many couples start off by each making a list of names that appeal to them, then looking to see if any entries are on both lists. Catalogs of baby names, in books or on the web, can help provide ideas. One fun source is www.babynamewizard.com/namevoyager, which shows time lines of the popularity of different names.

If you don't want input on your choice of name, don't announce it until after the baby is born.

There was a lot of pressure to use family names. Plus we had this rule about no names that could be shortened or cutened-up. That made things difficult. (Cheryl L., lawyer)

What to Bring to the Hospital for the Baby

After delivery, the hospital will provide your baby with disposable diapers, receiving blankets, infant T-shirts, hats, pacifiers, and formula/bottles (if you are bottle-feeding). You will need to supply clothes, blankets, and a car seat for the baby's trip home.

Newborns are safest in a rear-facing infant car seat set up in the back seat. This way if the car stops short, they will be pressed into the back of the car seat, which is relatively cushioned, rather than thrown forward. Choose a car seat that is easy to use and fits into your vehicle. Used car seats are safe, as long as they have never been in a serious accident, are in good condition, and come with instructions. Research has shown that many children's car seats are installed incorrectly, so if you have any questions, have your installation professionally checked before the baby comes. To locate a safety technician near you, call 866-SEATCHECK or visit www.seatcheck.org. For excellent information on car seat safety, check out the website of the American Academy of Pediatrics at www.AAP.org.

I wish the infant car seat that snaps into a stroller frame had been invented when I had Dan. He would fall blissfully asleep every time we took him in the car, but no matter how hard we tried to be quiet and gentle, he was wide awake (and not happy) by the time we moved him out of the car seat and into the carrier or stroller. (Marge G., obstetrician)

Baby Gear

Technically, newborns don't need that much at first: a place to sleep, diapers and wipes, clothes and blankets, and either bottles and formula or mom's breasts. You may find that hard to believe, though, if you have been to a baby shower lately. So many brilliant ideas for making life with baby easier and more enjoyable! Who thought of soft rubber faucet covers for the tub? The "Pee-pee Teepee" to put over a little boy's penis during a diaper change? A garbage can that vacuum-seals in odors? The "Miracle Blanket," with flaps to help swaddle the baby? And best yet, a warmer for tushy wipes?

All these fun and useful products mean that many babies end up with a lot of costly, extraneous stuff; yet much of what you truly need can be borrowed, and then passed along again later. If you are struggling to meet your baby's basic needs, be advised that some states or agencies provide assistance to families with new babies; even some working families may qualify. The hospital social worker should know your local resources.

Although every family has some products they feel that they couldn't live without (ours was the infant swing), once the baby comes, you may find that you need time and help rather than more stuff. If you are registering for a shower, or if anyone asks you what you need, consider some of these ideas:

- Postpartum doula or baby nurse
- Lactation consultation
- Gift certificates for take-out or (better yet) for restaurants that deliver

- Casseroles for the freezer
- Gift certificate for a good electric breast pump—I say gift certificate, because until you know exactly what you need, it may be hard to judge which one is going to work best for you.

I'm pregnant, I'm working full-time, and I have a toddler. When am I going to have time to stencil the elephants on the wall? The poor girl, we actually had her in a utility closet for a while. (Linda S., creative director)

Information and Support

I read lots of books on pregnancy during my first pregnancy, and just became immersed in it. I stared at my navel for nine months. My time would have been better spent reading about taking care of a baby. I wasn't prepared. (Deb L., writer)

I bought every book on babies and read them all while I was pregnant. But now I know I have to do a little of me and a little of the book. (Kate R., financial analyst)

Keep in mind that taking care of a newborn is surprisingly time-consuming. For the first few weeks at home, it is ideal if you can have another adult with you most of the time. When a baby is fussing and you can't tell why, you will feel less frustrated if you have someone there who can help you brainstorm about what to do or just how to cope. At a minimum, it's nice to have someone to answer the phone if you are trying to sleep, run out to get more diapers, or hold the baby so you can take a shower. If the baby's dad is taking paternity leave, he can participate fully in getting to know and care for the new baby. If not, try to line up other adults who can help out—family members, friends, or a professional postpartum doula or baby nurse.

Now, during late pregnancy, is also a good time to talk to your partner about the division of labor after the baby comes. Talk about your own families, about how work was divided between your parents, and about your expectations and hopes for each of your roles. Do you think you should be the primary parent, the one who is most intimately familiar with your child's world? Or do you plan to share the pleasures and responsibilities of parenting more equally?

Negotiate household jobs with your partner ahead of time—the home is not just the "woman's domain." Be clear about who will be responsible for cooking, shopping, and housework after you bring home the baby. Dads who take on substantial roles with the children—like bath time, diaper changes, or getting ready for bed—become competent and confident, which means that you both will be less likely to fall into the trap of the mom doing everything because she is better at it. (A lovely book for new parents that addresses this issue, and many others, is *Heading Home With Your Newborn* by Laura Jana and Jennifer Hsu.)

After I go back to work, my husband is going to take two months to stay home. I think that's going to help him to get a bond with the baby that he wouldn't have otherwise had. The reality is that there are a lot of dads who would like to have a part of that. (Cheryl L., lawyer)

Most of the couples in my circles are equal parents. Both parents change diapers, bathe the baby, put him to sleep. Some of the dads had fathers who worked all the time and didn't spend time with them—they don't want to be like that. (Annie F., classical violinist)

Just as with birth plans, your strategies for handling the immense responsibilities of parenting may need tweaking after the baby arrives. Maybe your partner, not you, will have that special knack for calming your crying newborn, or breastfeeding will be more time-consuming than you anticipated. But with good communication, flexibility, and a sense of shared commitment to your new little family member, you and your partner can work together to find the best possible balance between baby care, personal needs, workplace demands, and family responsibilities. It's not an easy juggling act, but the rewards of figuring it out together are immense—for you, your relationship, and your growing family.

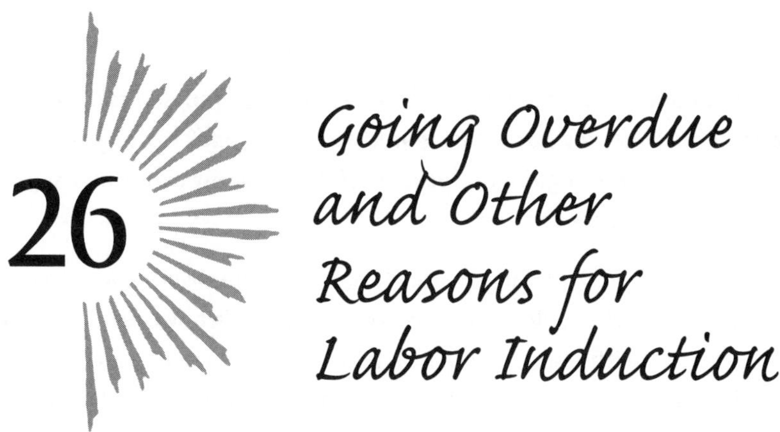

26 Going Overdue and Other Reasons for Labor Induction

Toward the end of your pregnancy, you may—quite understandably—begin to feel anxious. You are getting big and maybe physically uncomfortable; sleep can be difficult; and you probably can't wait to meet this little person who has been kicking and poking you for months. But sometimes the baby has other ideas, and nothing happens. In fact, about 7 percent of mothers-to-be will still be pregnant fourteen days beyond their due dates. Hopefully you listened to the recommendations earlier in the book and didn't get your heart set on a single due day—these assigned dates only suggest a likely midpoint in a four-week due "month." But even with the most realistic expectations, it can be hard to wait.

> ***I'm still pregnant. Damn all of those people that gave me the "so and so came three weeks early" stories. That's all I heard for months and now here I am twelve hours away from officially being due. Apparently my baby did not get the memo that first babies are supposed to be early. (Jen B., dance teacher)***

How Your Body Prepares for Birth

Before the cervix can open up, it must "ripen": specifically, it must become softer, shorter, and slightly open. Local hormones called prostaglandins play a role in this process. For some women, the cervix ripens during the weeks before the baby comes, and by the time they go into labor, the cervix is soft, effaced, and quite dilated. Others start off with a cervix that is long, firm, and closed, which makes for a longer labor.

I sit on the couch and yell at my belly—GET OUT! So far, no luck. I went to the doctor on Thursday hoping he would tell me to pack my bags (which they already are) but, again, no luck. He did tell me my cervix was slightly shorter. (Jen B., dance teacher)

No one knows exactly what initiates labor, why one woman's cervix ripens before labor and another's doesn't, why some labors start by breaking the water while others start with contractions, or why some babies gestate longer than others. It does seem, though, that the signal to start labor normally comes from the baby.

Haven't You Had That Baby Yet?

After thirty-eight weeks or so, in uncomplicated pregnancies, there is no benefit to the baby from prolonging the pregnancy. The problem is, natural labor doesn't always start the minute the baby and you are ready. You may worry that the baby is getting bigger and wonder whether induction would help you to have a better birth, with a smaller baby. After all, your baby is continuing to gain between a quarter and half a pound a week. Surprisingly, research has shown that inducing labor to prevent the baby from getting bigger isn't better than waiting for labor to start on its own (because induction itself, which can take several days with an unripe cervix, increases the chance of ending up with a cesarean). For most mothers and their babies, unless a medical reason for induction develops, patience is the best approach, at least through seven to fourteen days past the due date.

Rick has been great but he's at the point that anytime he calls me or talks to me the first thing he says is "Feel anything?" Of course I do: a seven-pound fetus that is only getting fatter by the day. (Jen B., dance teacher)

Myths and Facts about Jumpstarting Labor

Everyone has a story of a natural intervention that led to labor. From eating spicy food to having sex, urban legends abound. It is hard to judge what works, since women are generally trying these things when they are close to or past the due date, and labor may be imminent anyway. I have not seen research that proved any one of the common suggestions was effective, with the exception of taking castor oil, which causes diarrhea and uterine contractions that often progress to labor. The safety of castor oil induction hasn't been established, though, so I don't recommend trying it.

One week after my due date I was trying everything to go into labor, because if I went one more day I wasn't going to be able to have my planned home birth. I tried an enema, herbal treatments, sex, walking, driving bumpy roads. Finally a friend brought over some champagne, and Megan was born the next day. (Jan R., state attorney)

When I was overdue my mom was really funny. Everyone else around me was all sympathetic, and my mother was handing me her shopping bags to carry to bring labor on. When we went for walks, she would lead us up a hill. (Julie M., veterinarian)

I did try a night of jalapeño poppers and a chili dog last week but it didn't work. (Jen B., dance teacher)

I remember inducing labor a week post-due with a romantic dinner of rare steak and brie on crackers with a bottle of champagne, consumed in bed and followed by lovemaking. Naomi was born twelve hours later. (Deb L., writer)

My neighbor has eleven kids. When I told her I was overdue, she told me what works for her: leave dirty dishes in the sink and don't do the laundry—you'll have the baby. (Tammy L., accountant)

When I was four days late with Alex we had intercourse (very creatively). I used herbals, took long walks, and ate pizza—which I also vomited up upon arrival at the hospital the next morning. (Beth L., computer science researcher)

On the night that I was supposed to come in for induction, I decided to do a little walking to try to get things going. It worked, and I started contracting. (Shani M., student)

In the office, your practitioner may suggest sweeping the membranes (also called stripping the membranes) as a low-tech induction method. In this pro-

SOME NATURAL INDUCTION METHODS MAY NOT BE SAFE

Blue and black cohosh are herbs that have been used for "natural" labor induction. I believe that if a natural substance is capable of having biological effects, it is capable of causing negative effects; being natural doesn't mean something is safer than medical alternatives. Reports from midwives who use these herbal treatments indicate a possible risk of meconium-stained fluid and abnormally rapid fetal heart rates. I don't know of any studies that demonstrate the safety or effectiveness of blue cohosh and black cohosh, and some studies show risks, so I never recommend them. Most doctors and midwives consider these herbals unsafe.

Nipple stimulation causes the uterus to contract, but even a little tweak can lead to very long contractions that can stress out the baby. For this reason, I also wouldn't recommend nipple stimulation, except maybe under the watchful eye of your practitioner.

cedure, which may be a bit more uncomfortable than a vaginal exam, the examiner's finger is inserted inside the cervix, separating the bag of waters from its loose attachments to the lower uterine wall. Sweeping the membranes is believed to release natural prostaglandin hormones from the cervix, making the cervix more ripe and favorable for labor. Occasionally labor starts later that day, although it might have been going to start anyway.

Research on sweeping the membranes hasn't shown significant risk. In one study, a group of midwives swept the membranes of half their patients every week, starting at thirty-seven weeks gestation. They found no differences in the outcomes of the two groups, other than that women in the sweeping group were less likely to go past their due dates. Sweeping the membranes may be uncomfortable, but it's usually tolerable, and you can always say stop. You may notice more contractions and some vaginal spotting for a few hours afterward.

My doctor stripped my membranes when I was seven days overdue. I had contractions that evening, so we called my parents to come from four hours

away, but by the time they arrived the contractions had stopped. I went into labor three days later. (Julie M., veterinarian)

Deciding If and When to Induce Labor

As you pass your due date, your practitioner will probably recommend some steps to take to be sure the baby is doing well. (The placenta ages over time, and sometimes can't keep up with the needs of the growing fetus.) Fetal movement counts, fetal monitoring with nonstress testing, an ultrasound to check on the volume of amniotic fluid, or a biophysical profile may be recommended (see Appendix B). If fetal testing doesn't provide reassuring results, delivery is usually the best option.

I was two weeks late, I had to go in for a checkup, and they saw that my fluid was low, so I was scheduled for an induction that day. (Kafi P., teacher)

If the testing shows that the baby is doing well, avoiding induction is usually best, particularly if your cervix is "unripe" (unfavorable for induction). By seven to fourteen days past the due date, though, continuing to wait leads to a higher chance of cesarean than inducing labor does, because as the placenta ages the baby may not have the oxygen reserves to tolerate the normal stress of labor.

In general, then, induction of labor is indicated when the risks of continuing the pregnancy outweigh the risks of induction. Medical conditions like high blood pressure, diabetes, rupture of membranes without labor, and poor fetal growth can shift the risks and benefits of induction to favor delivering your baby before labor begins on its own.

I was ten days overdue, and my doctor wanted me to schedule a date for induction. I agreed but wasn't that excited to do it. You feel like once you start on that path of getting all sorts of medical interventions, you kind of continue to need more interventions. (Kendra F., civil litigator)

Labor Induction Methods

If your practitioner feels that induction is medically necessary, there are several techniques to use. The goal of each is to trigger your body's own labor process.

BREAKING THE WATERS

Natural rupture of the membranes often leads to labor, so sometimes a practitioner will manually rupture the membranes to encourage labor to begin. This option, also referred to as amniotomy, works best in a mom with a very ripe cervix who has already been contracting a lot, or who has had rapid labor in the past; that is, it is a good choice if labor is likely to be quick. If labor doesn't start within a few hours, an additional method of induction is usually added.

CERVICAL RIPENING AGENTS (PROSTAGLANDINS)

Prostaglandins are hormones involved in the natural process of cervical ripening; a few prostaglandin preparations are available for labor induction. Prostaglandin E2 gel (Dinoprost) and a sterile shoelace-like tape called Cervidil are both approved by the FDA for labor induction. Another product, misoprostol (Cytotec), is approved for treatment of stomach ulcers, but since it also contains a prostaglandin, it is often given "off label" for labor induction. All of these products can be given intravaginally and have local effects that may lead to softening, dilation, and effacement of the cervix, with or without contractions. Sometimes they work very well; other times they seem to have no effect at all. Often, multiple doses are needed before much of an effect is seen. Rarely, prostaglandins cause prolonged or strong contractions that can lead to slowing of the fetal heart rate (which can be scary). When this happens, preparations are usually started for cesarean, but removal of the tape (if Cervidil was used) or giving a medicine to block contractions usually solves the problem promptly. In the best-case scenarios, the cervix dilates and effaces painlessly over a dose or two, or, even better, the prostaglandin treatment initiates labor.

MECHANICAL DILATION (FOLEY BALLOON)

Once the cervix dilates to three or four centimeters, contractions are usually much more effective at opening the cervix further. Some practitioners use mechanical methods of dilating the cervix, instead of prostaglandins, to get to this point. The Foley catheter, a tube with an inflatable balloon on the end, was invented for draining urine from the bladder. When used for labor induction, the soft rubber tube is threaded up into the uterus just inside the cervix, and then the balloon on the end is inflated with water. As the uterus tries to expel the catheter, the balloon is slowly pushed through the cervix, leading to dilation. After a few hours, with or without low-dose Pitocin, the balloon falls out, letting the team know that the cervix has dilated enough to let the three- to four-centimeter balloon pass through. Usually Pitocin is begun or increased at that point.

PITOCIN INDUCTION

Oxytocin, a hormone naturally made in the mother's pituitary gland, stimulates uterine contractions. You may have heard of Pitocin, the brand name for the synthetic version of this hormone. To induce labor, Pitocin is given intravenously, in controlled amounts. The dose is increased every half hour or so until a good contraction pattern is established. Some mothers-to-be need only small doses of Pitocin to have strong contractions, while others hardly respond to it.

Continuous fetal monitoring is required during Pitocin treatment, so the mom is tethered to the monitor and can't walk far (unless a wireless monitor is available), or go in the shower or tub. If you are hoping for natural childbirth, talk to your practitioner ahead of time about any restrictions in your activities, and which comfort measures will be possible if you require labor induction.

The Experience of Labor Induction

Labor induction can go very smoothly, or be very frustrating. The more "ripe" the cervix is at the start, the more likely it is that induction will go well. When induction goes fast, you may wonder why you didn't do it earlier; but remember it might not have gone so nicely if your body hadn't been ready. Cervical ripening agents may require a day or two of repeated doses before either labor begins or the cervix becomes ready for rupture of membranes or Pitocin. During that time the mom may be kept in the hospital, where fetal monitoring requirements can interfere with some comfort measures. Sometimes labor just doesn't get going, and you and your care team have to decide between continuing to press on, returning home (and coming back another day), or proceeding to a cesarean birth. If you are scheduling an induction, be sure to talk to your practitioner about what to expect, so you will arrive at the hospital with a realistic outlook and be prepared for all the likely possibilities.

I had a scheduled induction. I went to the hospital for the appointment, and they were full. They sent me home, so I decided to go back to work that day. The day before I had been sent off to have a baby, and then there I am sitting at my desk. (Cheryl L., lawyer)

Your Emotions as the Due Date Comes and Goes

It's true that going past your due date may be aggravating, but labor induction can be frustrating too. Up to a point, patience is the best approach if you sail right on past that long-circled date on your calendar. Find some distractions, stay active, screen your calls, and if phone calls are getting to you, consider changing your outgoing voice mail message to "No, the baby isn't here yet—we promise to let you know!" Above all, try to keep some perspective: before you know it, your pregnancy will end and your baby will come; this delay of even a week or two really won't seem so long when you think about all the years you will have to love and enjoy your new baby.

Part 6

Exit Strategy (The Day of Birth)

The big day is almost here—but you still may have a lot of questions. How will you know when you are in labor? How can you improve your chances of having the birth experience you want, while not losing sight of the most important goal: a healthy mother and baby? Who should come with you for support during labor? Do you want an epidural, or will you use other comfort measures? In this section, an overview of normal labor (and some variations) will help you begin your decision-making journey. Along the way, I will explain common medical procedures and real moms will tell about their experiences. We will end our tour together with a miraculous new beginning: your baby's birth and first few hours of life in the world.

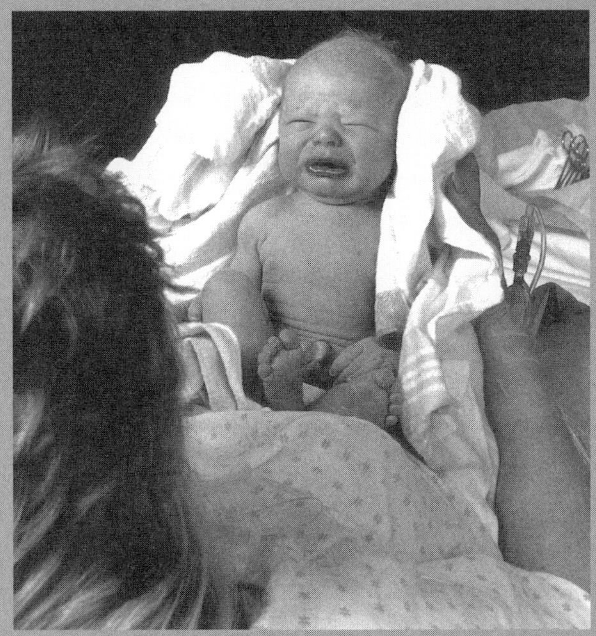

LeRoy Dierker, MD

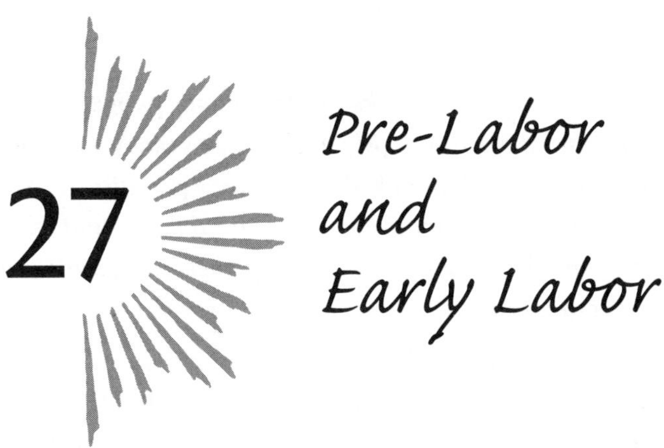

27 Pre-Labor and Early Labor

Some labors begin with a bang: the water breaks, or strong contractions start up without much warning. For most mothers-to-be, though, the onset of labor is hard to pinpoint. Maybe you will feel crampy for a day or two, like the start of a menstrual period. Or you will have a few painful contractions spread out over hours. Because these same symptoms can occur without consequence in late pregnancy, it may be frustratingly impossible to know—at least at first—if your labor is truly beginning.

Signs of Early Labor

Although each labor is somewhat unique, there are common signs that your baby will be arriving pretty soon:

WATER BREAKING

If your bag of water—the fluid-filled amniotic sac around the baby—breaks, labor is usually imminent. Sometimes the water breaking is obvious—a popping sensation followed by a warm gush. But sometimes a pregnant mom will feel only a subtle, intermittent trickling. The amniotic fluid is more watery and runny than the normal gooey discharge of pregnancy. If you see what you think may be amniotic fluid, call the number your doctor or midwife gave you for labor. The labor and delivery team will most likely check to see if you are leaking, and help you decide what to do next. Most women go into labor once their water has broken. If labor doesn't start on its own and the baby is full term, though, induction will be suggested: once the amniotic sac has been punctured, the baby is less protected from infection, and delivery is safer than continuing to be pregnant.

In the hour from the time my water broke until we finally pulled out of our garage, I changed clothes three times. (My husband was ready to kill me.) The amount of fluid that I expelled soaked through one pad after another. Nothing I read during my pregnancy prepared me for the fact that when my water broke, it would flow and flow and flow. (Rebecca M., senior vice president, financial corporation)

I was thirty-seven weeks and my husband was supposed to meet me at dog obedience class. I had been contracting all day, but didn't think I was in labor. Just as the class was starting, my water broke all over the stage. I was soaked. The people in class wanted to call an ambulance but then my husband came and I told him we had to go to the hospital. He had to line the car seats with plastic before he was willing to take me home to change and call the doctor. We made it to the hospital, and my son arrived eleven hours later. (Andrea S., nurse)

BLOODY SHOW

A small amount of blood mixed with mucus, called *bloody show*, is normal after an internal exam, or as your body gets ready for labor: the cervix may be loosening enough to expel the mucus plug that has been sealing off the uterine cavity from the outside world. (By contrast, bleeding like a menstrual period is not normal at any point during your pregnancy, and should be reported to your practitioner right away.)

CONTRACTIONS

In a healthy full-term pregnancy with an intact bag of waters, it's usually best to ignore the contractions of early labor . . . until you can't ignore them any more. You may want to go home from work (and locate your partner), but you don't need to rush to the hospital. We have all heard stories of women going to the hospital for labor, only to be frustrated when it turns out to be a false alarm. Sometimes this situation is unavoidable; if you have had a rapid labor in the past, you will not want to take any chances. But first babies usually give a lot of warning before they arrive.

My first contraction was not painful. I simply felt a tightening sensation within the lower half of my enormous belly. The contractions were approxi-

mately four minutes apart at that time. For the first hour or so, the contractions amounted to nothing more than a tightening sensation. (Rebecca M., senior vice president, financial corporation)

My labor was pretty fast. I called in and they said you sound like you can still breathe so come in a few hours. I started to get anxious about getting there in time, so I told my husband it was time to go. I thought he would go get his coat, but instead he went to the kitchen and started making sandwiches so he would have something to eat! (Kathy H., software developer)

Early Labor

My best advice: avoid the temptation to track every aspect of early labor. Don't time contractions that are mild—they may occur on and off for days before the real event begins. I can't tell you how many first-time parents exhaust themselves timing early labor contractions, showing up with pages and pages documenting every time the uterus tightened during the previous thirty hours. If you think you might be in labor, distract yourself. Go for a walk. Read a book. If possible, try to sleep. You won't sleep through real labor—and this may be the only sleep you will get until after the baby arrives.

For most moms-to-be, contractions aren't worth counting until you have to change your activities to get through them. At that point, they might be two to five minutes apart. If they stay that way for an hour, it is time to head on in. Of course, your situation may be unusual—your practitioner will give you individualized recommendations if you've had a prior cesarean or rapid labor, or if any other factors indicate that you should have a lower threshold for going in to the hospital.

For my second baby I woke up at 1 AM thinking this might be labor, but went back to sleep. Then at 5:45 I was pretty sure it was the real thing. The contractions were two minutes apart. I called the midwife and she said I sounded like it was still early labor and did I want to labor some at home. I said I needed to go in. I was admitted to my room at 7 o'clock and she was born at 8:12. (Julie M., veterinarian)

I thought I might be in labor, and when I called, the doctor told me to come down. We took a cab, and told the driver we were going to the hospital to

have our baby. He took one look at me and said, "No you're not." And he was right—it was a false alarm. (Emily H., executive director, nonprofit organization)

With my first, I was in surgery and started to feel contractions, mild at first, but persistent. I still had a couple of short cases to go. I didn't know what to do: if I cancelled the cases, or called one of my (male) colleagues to cover them, and then it turned out to be false labor, I would be subject to a unique kind of derision when I showed up at work the next day: "You're an obstetrician and don't even know when you're in labor?!" (Elisa R., ob-gyn)

The best way to avoid a false alarm is to look for signs that this is the real thing before heading to the hospital.

SIGNS OF REAL LABOR

- Your contractions are so strong that you have to change your activities to get through them.
- Someone looking at you would be able to tell something was happening even if you didn't want to be noticed, because you can't help but alter your breathing or facial expression during the contractions.
- Your contractions are coming at regular intervals—usually by the time they are strong, they are two to five minutes apart, from the start of one to the start of the next. Track them by writing down the time that each one begins.
- Each of your contractions lasts more than forty-five seconds.

I woke up in labor, and after awhile, I thought it was time to go to the hospital. But when I got there it was too early. So I walked around a while, but then I got tired, and decided to go home and sleep. (Karen S., nurse-midwife)

They said my labor was eighteen hours because they didn't start counting until my water broke, but I was contracting for four or five hours before then, which they didn't consider labor, but it felt like it. (Galit A., tax attorney)

Going into Labor at Work

If you plan to work right up until the end, or if labor starts a few weeks before you expect it, you might find yourself in labor at your workplace. Although you may have plenty of time to go home before you need to head in, have a plan for how you would get straight from work to your birth location if necessary (without having to drive yourself—it can be hard to concentrate while having a contraction!).

I started contractions with my second child at work on a Tuesday in the early afternoon and worked until five o'clock. I then told my supervisor that I wouldn't be in the next day and that I have to go to the hospital tonight! I thought she was going to pass out!! (Dana W., network technician)

One week early the baby's room wasn't ready and I was in complete denial. I was going to take leave from work one month beforehand but I never got around to it. I wasn't sure I was even in labor. I got to the hospital at 10:30 PM and she was born at 1 AM. (Laura K., attorney)

I was standing in surgery when my water broke. At first I thought it was sweat because the case wasn't going so well, but I'd never sweated down my legs before! (Elisa R., ob-gyn)

I wondered and worried for months where my water would break (in court?). Finally it happened as I went to see a friend's newly decorated home—and guess what! It doesn't stain! (Nancy G., lawyer)

Many women worry about breaking their water in a public setting, but in fact, only 10 percent of moms experience ruptured membranes before their labor begins. If you are concerned, you can keep with you a change of clothes, some large sanitary pads or newborn disposable diapers (they are perfect—absorbent and plastic-lined), and a plastic garbage bag (to sit on in the car). Typically, the amniotic fluid looks clear or yellowish. A dark green color can signify meconium, the baby's first stool, which may be passed into the fluid before birth.

I got up for my usual 4:30 AM trip to the bathroom. Half asleep, I realized the stream below me was strong and steady without showing any sign of

stopping. "Oh hell, now what?" And then it dawned on me that my water had broken. Finally. After weeks of wondering whether I would be one of those poor women whose water broke at an inopportune time—in my boss's office, on an elevator, or in the express checkout lane at the grocery where I would back up traffic—there it was in the still of the quiet night. No drama. No big deal. (Rebecca M., senior vice president, financial corporation)

Arriving at the Hospital

When you get to the hospital, your practitioner, a house doctor, or a nurse will most likely do an internal examination to see how dilated your cervix is. If you think you may have broken your water, they may test the fluid to see for sure. These steps will help determine if you are truly in labor and should be admitted to the hospital.

Labor is technically defined as regular contractions that lead to opening of the cervix, the neck of the womb. Early labor is the part of the birth process that is most variable. It can be intense or mild. It can be very short or very long. Sometimes what feels like early labor doesn't even technically qualify as labor, because the cervix isn't changing yet. This means that even if you are having regular contractions, the medical team may not call it labor.

But even if you are only experiencing pre-labor symptoms, the medical team may still want to support and guide you. In particular, if you are becoming worn out from a long pre-labor, or "prodrome," they may offer sleep medication to help you relax and rest. This isn't a bad idea. Research on long prodromes shows that after medication-induced sleep, about half of the moms will be in true labor, and almost half will have stopped contracting and can go home—only a few will continue to be in that maddening in-between state. And unless labor suddenly progresses rapidly, your body will have time to break down the medicines so that they are out of the baby's system before birth.

Once you are clearly in labor, you will be admitted to the hospital or birth center. You may feel a little frightened, or really excited (or both). The big day has finally arrived!

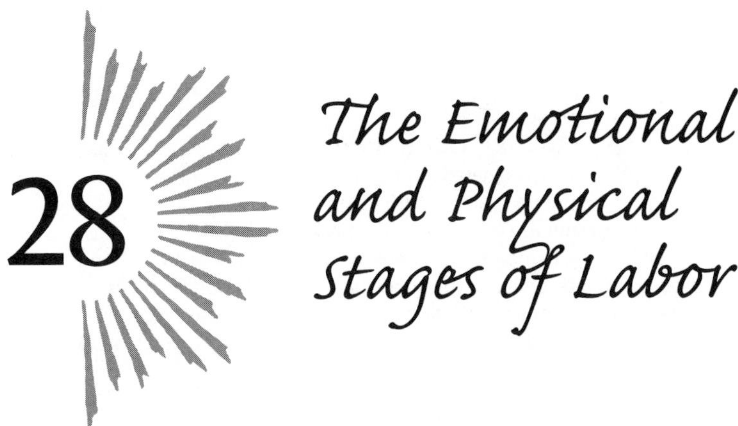

28 The Emotional and Physical Stages of Labor

It's not surprising that someone long ago decided to call the work of having a baby "labor"; this dramatic life event involves a lot of demanding effort. When everything goes as it should, strong contractions of the uterus help the cervix to open and the baby to descend into the pelvis—and the force of the contractions, along with the mother's pushing efforts, propel the baby through the birth canal and into the world.

Although every labor is different, each birth can be divided into recognizable stages. The first stage starts when contractions begin to be effective and ends when the cervix has completely opened; the second stage begins when you start pushing and ends when the baby is born; and the third stage involves delivery of the placenta (which we'll discuss later). To better understand the first stage of labor, we divide it into phases as well: the latent phase, the active phase, and transition. Where you are in this sequence typically determines how strong the contractions are and how rapidly you are progressing. It also (particularly if you don't have an epidural) plays a role in your emotional state.

My two sisters had very different perceptions of very similar labors. Sue thought her ten-hour labor was too long, but Karen was thrilled that her ten-hour labor was so short! (Elisa R., ob-gyn)

The progress of labor is gauged by dilation of the cervix, its effacement (shortening), and by the descent, or "station," of the baby. These measurements are made by vaginal examination. Wearing a surgical glove, the nurse, midwife, or doctor will place two fingers inside the vagina and feel the cervix, just like your doctor or midwife probably did during the last few weeks of pregnancy.

Contraction:
Coordinated tensing of the uterine muscle, which in turn causes the uterus to squeeze or ball up. This may at first feel like tightening, or menstrual cramps, typically becoming more like strong intestinal cramps or low back pain as labor advances. In early labor contractions may be irregular, lasting 30–60 seconds. Active labor contractions usually last from 45–90 seconds, with a break of at least a minute in between.

Dilation:
During labor the cervix dilates (opens up) to about ten centimeters.

Effacement:
The cervix starts off like a bottleneck, and slowly pulls up to become part of the lower uterus. This process of shortening is called effacement and is measured as a percent of a full-length (one and a half inch long) cervix. Full or 100% effacement is usually reached by the time active phase begins.

Station:
The descent of the baby is measured relative to the ischial spine, a protuberance of the pelvic bone inside the vagina. Centimeters above the spine are referred to with negative numbers, and below it, positive. By the time the baby descends to "plus four" the head will be visible, or crowning.

The lingo of labor progress. (The size of this circle is the same as the opening of a fully dilated cervix.)

Although these exams may be uncomfortable, many mothers-to-be welcome them during labor, because they bring news of progress.

The First Stage of Labor: Opening the Cervix

It's a go—you're on your way to having your baby! During the first stage, your contractions will start to really make a difference in thinning and dilating your cervix, and your body will get ready for the pushing to come.

THE LATENT PHASE

During the early part of labor, called the latent phase, it takes a lot of contractions to get the cervix to start to open. This part of labor can last hours or even

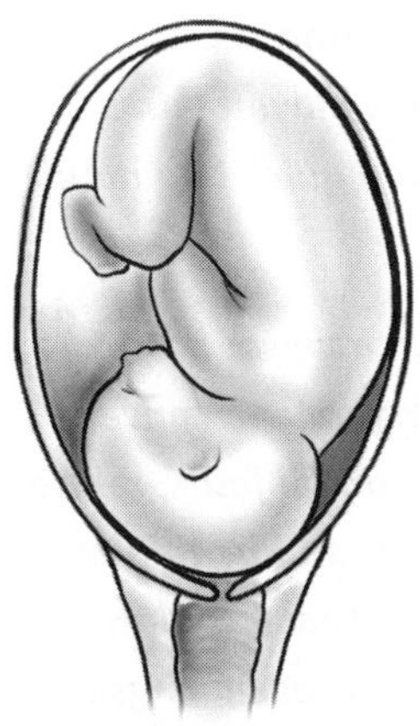
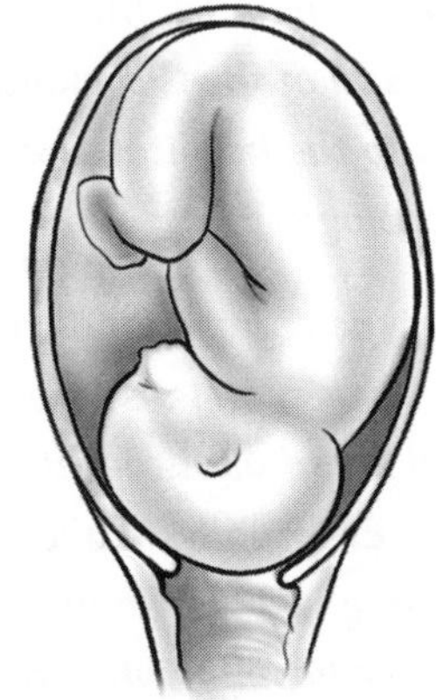
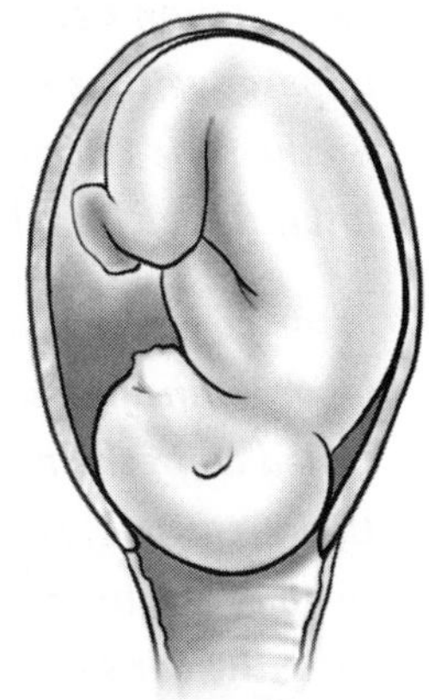

Cervical dilation. The cervix progresses to ten centimeters, or "complete dilation," during labor.

days. Yet although the contractions of early labor may be strong, most women get a good break in between, and feel pretty normal. Excitement, followed by boredom and fatigue (if it goes on a long time) are the most common emotions of early labor. In general, the length of latent phase doesn't have medical implications—a long latent phase, while frustrating and tiring, can precede a very normal active phase and birth.

> ***One of the surprises for me was the complete absence of any discomfort once a contraction passed. I had always focused on the fact that contractions would come at various intervals of time, but I had never really thought about the fact that when the contraction ended, I would feel absolutely fine. Being able to have two to four minutes of recovery time made the contractions all that much more manageable for me. (Rebecca M., senior vice president, financial corporation)***

> ***I just remember an overwhelming sense of relief when I went into labor. I had such an anxiety-ridden pregnancy, both from a medical and professional standpoint, that I was just overjoyed to feel those labor pains. (Melissa G., mortgage broker)***

> ***I felt in no rush to get to the hospital when I went into labor with my daughter. After twenty-four hours of dysfunctional labor with my son, being prepped for a C-section and then having a vaginal delivery in the operating***

room, I didn't expect anything too quick this time around. And it was imperative that I watch the end of the Cleveland Cavaliers playoff game. By the time I decided to get to the hospital, she was born a quick two hours later! (Loree R., school psychologist)

I started getting menstrual-type cramps, and when I took a warm bath, labor intensified so I knew it was real. I also stopped being able to converse. I tried all of the methods I'd heard about—getting down on all fours, relaxation breathing, swaying, etc. Eventually, I called the doctor and he told me to go to the hospital. At midnight, I was so uncomfortable that I couldn't sit in the car so I walked to the hospital while my husband drove alongside in the car. I had to stop and hold the trees during a labor cramp. (Peggy L., nurse-administrator)

FETAL POSITION DURING LABOR

How the baby's head is descending into your pelvis has an effect on whether you will feel your contractions in front or in your back, and how fast your labor will progress. Which way the baby is facing is described by where the back of the baby's head (the "occiput") is relative to the mom: facing sideways is called occiput transverse, or OT; facing up toward your pubic bone is occiput posterior, or OP; and facing back toward your spine, the most common position, is known as occiput anterior, or OA.

How do we know the baby's position? Your doctor or midwife may be able to determine which way the baby is facing by pressing on your belly or by feeling the bones of the baby's head during a vaginal examination. Sometimes the baby's position is just presumed, based on where you sense your contractions and how labor is proceeding. While we used to think that the position of the baby at the beginning of labor stayed constant until birth, research using ultrasound has shown that babies may turn several times as labor proceeds.

The shape of the mom's pelvis, gravity, and probably also random chance determine the baby's orientation. In the occiput anterior (most common) position, the baby presents its smallest head diameter into the birth canal, and tends to fit through most easily. A more difficult situation involving the baby's orientation can occur when the baby's back lies against the mother's back, pressing into the mother's lower spine during contractions. This scenario, called "back labor,"

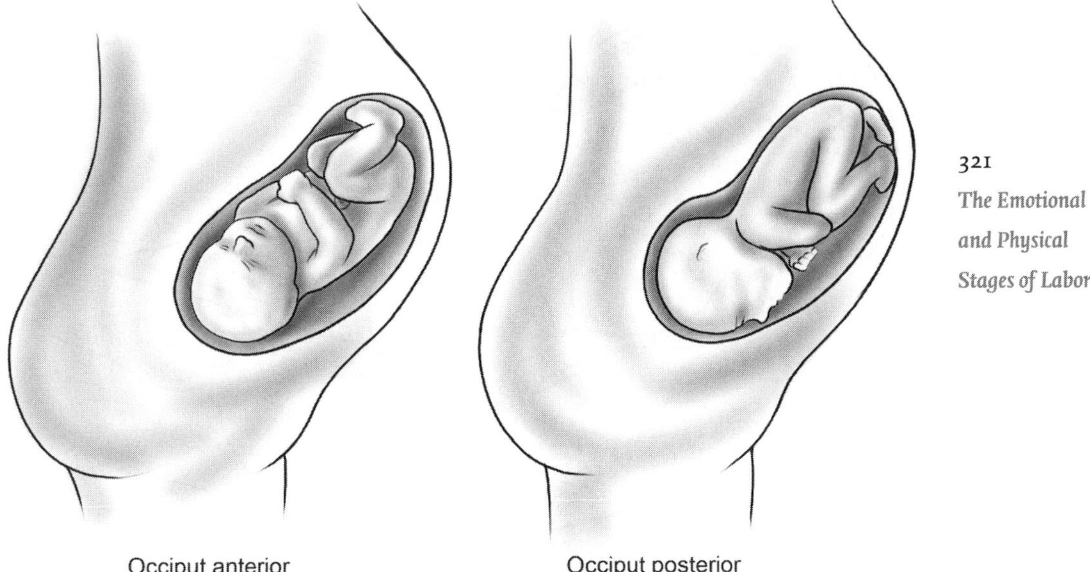

Positions of the baby's head during labor

may cause a slower and more painful labor. Maneuvering into a hands and knees position, or standing and lifting up your belly during your contractions, may help reposition the baby and stop the back pain. For more information on back labor, see the excellent book *Back Labor No More!!* by Janie McCoy King.

WHEN WILL MY WATER BREAK?

If you are one of the 90 percent of women whose water doesn't break before labor begins, your bag of waters will either break on its own at some point during labor, or the doctor will pop it, a procedure called "amniotomy," or assisted rupture of membranes. Amniotomy may be suggested to speed up labor, to allow internal monitoring of the baby, or to check for meconium (the baby's first bowel movement) in the fluid. Once the bag of waters is open, warm fluid will continue to leak out until birth.

It was nothing like I expected! I started having minor contractions about forty hours before giving birth. They finally got painful when my water started leaking about sixteen hours before birth (not gushing—just dribbling out). (Sandy B., social worker)

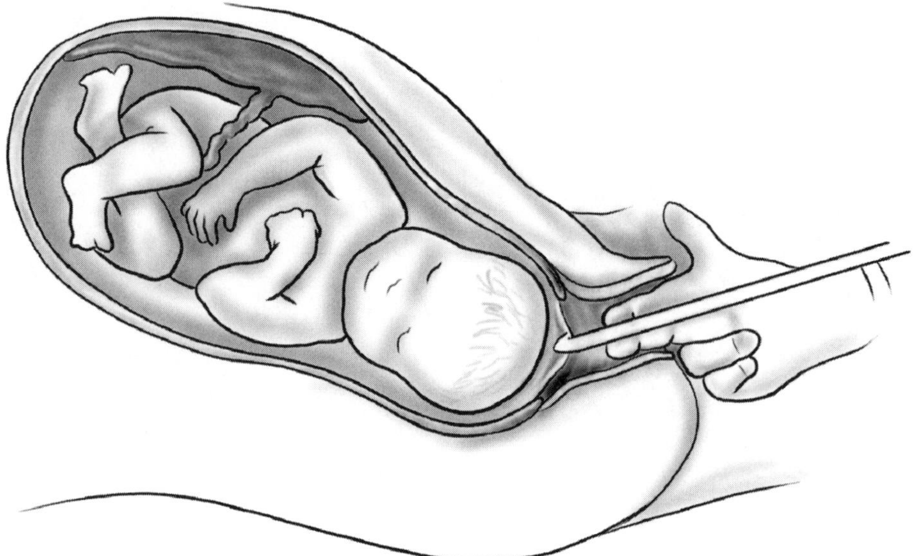

Assisted rupture of membranes. To break your water, an amnio hook, which may look like a long sterile crochet hook, is placed through the vagina and cervix, where it is used to snag the amniotic sac.

ACTIVE PHASE

Somewhere around three to five centimeters' dilation, the active phase of labor begins. During this phase, your contractions will feel more intense and will be more effective. They often last a full minute each, with maybe a minute or two break in between. Most women who are hoping for natural childbirth can manage through active phase using the techniques they have learned and practiced. Moms who plan on getting an epidural normally seek it out at this stage.

After running a dozen or more marathons, doing Ironman Hawaii, and completing other athletic challenges, I was shocked at how uncomfortable labor was. (Peggy L., nurse-administrator)

As I am lying in the labor room, Randy has the book out. He tells me I am in latent phase and it will be another six to twelve hours, then active phase begins, which will be six hours or so. I tell him no way. I call in the doctor and tell him I'm leaving. He asks where I am going because the head is

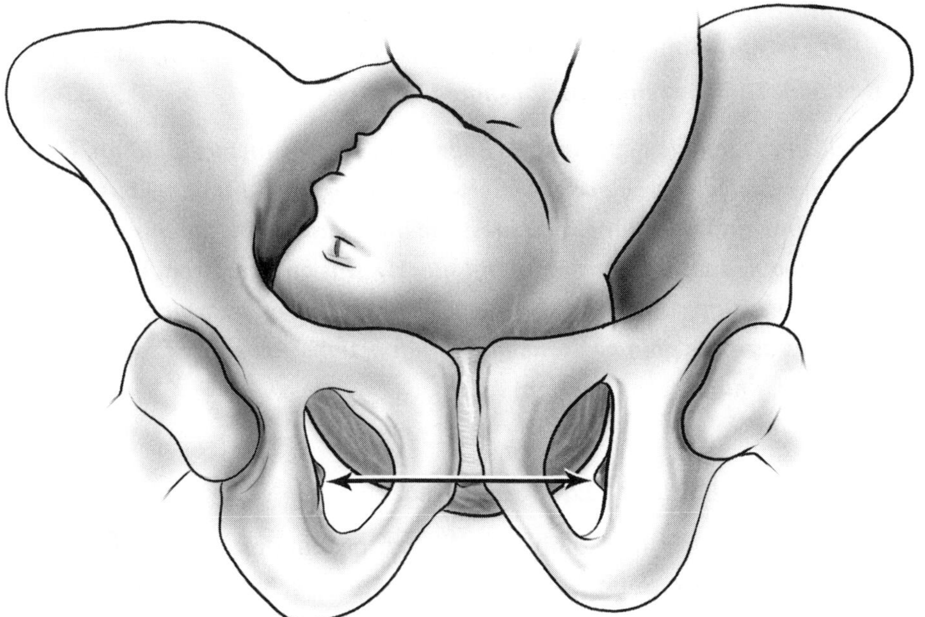

The fetal descent through the birth canal is measured in the distance above or below the "ischial spines," protuberances of the pelvic bones inside the vagina.

crowning! Jessica (my first) came after a total one-hour labor. (Nancy G., lawyer)

TRANSITION

Right before it's time to push, many women (particularly those without epidural anesthesia) go through an emotional stage called transition. During transition, mothers often feel panicky, like they can't do it. Many shiver or tremble involuntarily, and some even throw up. Often, women who ask for pain medicine during transition are expressing their distress, rather than truly changing their minds. This is when it's most important for your coach(es) to understand the normal process of labor, and to know what you want, because you may be saying you can't do it. It is a vulnerable time; if you are offered an epidural at this stage, you may take it even though you didn't want one; you won't believe that the finish line is close. Women seeking natural childbirth usually need lots of support and encouragement to get through transition.

I smacked my husband in the face with a washcloth. I was in active labor, and he tried to put a washcloth in my face, and I just took it off and threw it at him. That, he remembers! (Andrea S., nurse)

While in the middle of pacing the hallway at six centimeters' dilation, I had two unexpectedly strong contractions quickly together. I told my husband that I thought it was time to request the anesthesiologist. On our way back to the room, another contraction hit quickly, this one the strongest of all up to that point. As it gripped me, I could not think of breathing through it. It was as if the pain overrode all brain function. (Rebecca M., senior vice president, financial corporation)

The Second Stage of Labor: Pushing

Once your cervix has completely dilated, pushing may be a relief, giving you something active to do. You might feel an intense urge to bear down. An epidural can reduce this urge, so women with epidurals often need to be coached about when to push, but women without anesthesia can listen to their bodies.

I only pushed three times and it was my first baby. The urge was so strong and when I pushed it was a big relief so I knew I was pushing right. (Danielle R., trust analyst)

My doctor didn't realize the baby was so big but he turned out to be ten pounds, thirteen ounces. I pushed for three hours and then had to have a cesarean. My labor was long, but I was comfortable most of the time because I had an epidural. It was mostly a matter of waiting and being patient as my labor progress was very slow. (Kendra F., civil litigator)

When I was pushing I remember one of the nurses saying, "less face and more butt," and I had no idea what she was talking about. But eventually I figured it out. (Linda S., creative director) (Note from author: This means the pushing effort should be centered in your pelvis, not up in your chest and face.)

It's really nothing like it looks on TV. I was expecting lots of pain, but for me, it just went so smoothly. After I had the epidural, they told me to rest, and I

A NOT-SO-SPECIAL DELIVERY

The effort of pushing is very similar to moving your bowels, and (sorry to tell you) often some urine or stool is expelled during this phase. While it doesn't happen every time, you and your visitors should be aware that it may occur as a natural part of the birth process. Your nurse will wipe you off, to clean things up for birth. There's no need to feel embarrassed: doctors and nurses who are bothered by this don't choose obstetrics as a career!

did. Then they came back and woke me up when it was time to push, and I did. (Amanda O., meeting planner)

Then they said it was time to push. They asked whether I could feel my lower regions. I thought for moment. No, I can't really feel them, but if I admit that, will they take away this fabulous epidural? Yes, I said, I can feel things just fine. I watched the monitor closely for when to push, and pushed out my baby girl. (Heidi R., law professor)

Thanks to the epidural, the pushing phase was—to use my recurring adjective—entirely manageable. Yes, the delivery of the head was really uncomfortable, but I did not experience actual pain. The feeling I remember was pressure. Lots of pressure, but no pain. (Rebecca M., senior vice president, financial corporation)

First-time moms may push for five minutes or several hours—depending on the effectiveness of the pushing, how far up the birth canal the baby is at the start, and how easily the baby is fitting through. Epidural anesthesia may eliminate the sensations of the second stage, which may mean no pain, but also a lack of an urge to push, which can make pushing less effective. Without anesthesia, the descent of the baby typically leads to a strong pressure sensation, followed by a burning, pulling, or tearing feeling as the opening of the vagina stretches to accommodate the head.

SOME PUSHING POSITIONS

Sitting

Squatting using the squatting bar

On hands and knees

Lying on one side

Lying back

My friends with epidurals told me pushing wouldn't hurt, but it did and it was kind of scary, but also the whole thing was really fun. I had a strong urge to push and only pushed for forty minutes. (Galit A., tax attorney)

Changing positions while pushing can help the baby to fit through the pelvis. You can push sitting up in bed, lying back with your knees drawn toward your chest, on your hands and knees, sitting on the toilet, squatting on the floor or with a squatting bar in the bed, on your side with your legs drawn up, or any other way that feels right. Even with an epidural that requires you to stay in bed, numerous positions are usually feasible. Because your baby is both large and small in places, and because the birth canal is unevenly shaped, changing your position (in order to open up your pelvis differently, and allow gravity to work in varied directions) may help the baby to inch down its path. Reorienting every fifteen to twenty minutes not only will help keep you energized, but also will identify the positions that are most effective for you and your baby.

Some babies come quickly: by the time the cervix is fully open, just a few "umphs" are needed. More typically, pushing with a first baby feels like two steps forward, one step back: progress often seems slow. If the second stage takes a few hours, you may start to feel like the baby will never come. Although occasionally a baby won't fit through and a cesarean will be needed even at this late point, getting to full dilation is a positive sign that the baby will be born vaginally. You are really close to the finish line!

At about two hours of pushing, the OB came in and told me that if I hadn't made good progress by the time I'd been pushing for three hours that they would do a C-section. I did NOT know they had a time limit, so then I really, really started pushing (not that I felt I had been slacking up until that point, let me tell you!). At three hours, I had made good progress so they let me keep going another half an hour until my son came out at ten pounds, two ounces! (Sandy B., social worker)

29 Comfort Measures

Labors are so different from one another, and women's responses to labor so varied, that it is very hard for me to prepare you for the experience without knowing anything about your pregnancy, your coping style, or how your labor will go. Some women sail through labor like it is no big deal—one mother of six calls them labor "pangs" rather than pains—while others find labor to be the most difficult and painful physical trial of their lives.

> ***While I no longer remember the actual pain, I do know that those fifteen or so minutes after it got really painful, before the epidural took effect, presented the most difficult physical challenge I have ever encountered. (Rebecca M., senior vice president, financial corporation)***

> ***I had feared pregnancy for many years by listening to the horror stories of labor pains. But the physicians I worked with kept me at ease, and the best advice I can give anyone is to be knowledgeable about what your body is going through during the pregnancy and labor. My delivery was a breeze. (Val P., administrative coordinator)***

Preparing for Labor

Because every labor is unique, it makes good sense to educate yourself about the various possibilities, and plan to stay flexible. Rather than setting your heart (or your fears) on one vision of labor, create a "plan A, plan B, and plan C" for how you might deal with different events. Videos and educational television programs may help you envision different types of births, although some parents shy away from these as too frighteningly realistic. At the least, read about labor, take classes if possible, tour your birthing unit, and talk to your practitioner about routine procedures; if you plan on epidural anesthesia, find out under what sorts of conditions it might be encouraged or delayed. All this so you can have realistic expectations for the day that will stay with you forever—your baby's birthday.

Will I Be Able to Handle Labor?

There are two problems with pain. The first may seem redundant: pain hurts. Pain tolerance varies hugely between individuals, and between circumstances. Some mothers-to-be are willing to tolerate even severe pain for what they see as a good cause; others want immediate and complete relief. Think about where you fall in that spectrum. The second problem with pain is that it can be frightening, and fear leads to anxiety and a heightened perception of pain. Nonmedical comfort measures, like verbal encouragement, relaxation techniques, distraction, and understanding what is happening all help to diminish fear, reduce tension, and de-escalate pain. This is probably why research has shown that women who have doula support in labor are less likely to request an epidural.

I am really into natural medicine, except when it comes to pain control! I am a longtime marathon runner and triathlete, with very competitive times, and so when it came time to decide what to do, I thought I might want to be brave and go without pain medication. I tried everything—got down on all fours, panted like a dog, breathed deeply, took a warm bath, swayed with my husband, but nothing worked. Maybe I was less tolerant because I was used to controlling my pain when racing by just backing off a little (slowing down) when I started to feel uncomfortable. (Peggy L., nurse-administrator)

With my second, I stayed at home longer. We stayed in the bath, with my husband pouring hot water on my belly with each contraction. It was really helpful. This time, I achieved my goal of having a completely natural labor. When I reached the hospital, my water broke as I was getting up on the bed, and the baby came with less than an hour of pushing. It was such a rewarding experience. I felt very proud of myself for being able to do it without anesthesia or much intervention. (Shani M., student)

WHAT CAUSES LABOR PAIN?

Each aspect of labor may hurt in a different way. Contraction pain comes from the strength of the cramp itself, and from a decrease in oxygen to the uterine muscle as it contracts. Some women describe contractions as feeling like severe diarrhea cramps. Others primarily feel contractions in the lower back. The cervix also may hurt as it dilates—often this pain miraculously improves once the cervix is completely open. Some (but not all) women experience a surge of relief and joy as the time to push arrives; it is time to take an active role. Finally, the stretching of the birth canal as the baby descends can cause a burning, tearing, or severe pressure sensation. Once the birth is done, most mothers feel great relief: labor is over, and the new baby has arrived.

We all know from our own experiences with mild pain, like headaches or minor injuries, that we're more aware of pain when worried, and less aware when busy or distracted. This effect is not imaginary. Pain signals are modified by other inputs as they travel up nerves to the brain. That's why you may not notice your toothache until you are trying to fall asleep, why your headache may seem to resolve when you have something fun and diverting to do, and why some athletes aren't aware of their injuries until the game is over. It's why yogis can meditate so deeply that they don't react despite apparently painful stimuli, and why nonmedical comfort measures are effective for labor. For better or worse, external and internal factors actually modify the perception of pain.

How Difficult Will Labor Be?

It is impossible to predict how easy or difficult someone's labor will be, because each labor is different. Typically, active labor is intense enough that during contractions women without an epidural don't act or feel like they usually do. This means that you may not be able to advocate for yourself, ask questions, weigh options, make decisions, or think of things to do to make yourself feel better. You will be absorbed by the job of coping with your moment-by-moment experience and will be relying on your coaches to take on those other challenges.

Even moms-to-be who are planning to get an epidural should prepare to deal with early labor (when you may still be at home), and for the unexpected, in case the anesthesia team gets waylaid with emergencies or your progress is too swift for an epidural to be useful.

Nonmedical Comfort Measures

It may surprise you to learn how many different kinds of comfort measures are available, and how simple they can be. Here are some that my patients find most effective:

ENCOURAGEMENT

To my mind, reality-based encouragement is the cornerstone of coping with natural labor. The value of reassurance and positive thinking can't be overestimated. It truly helps, both emotionally and physically, to have someone with you to remind you that you can do anything for a minute, and that soon labor will be over and your baby will be in your arms. Choose your companions by who will support and nurture you. Many men are up to this role, but parents hoping for natural childbirth often appreciate additional support from a doula or another woman who understands the normal process of birth and knows how to "mother the mother" when the going gets tough.

Prior to the epidural, we used changing positions, having my husband massage me, and the birthing ball. These things really helped a lot. (Karen D., veterinarian)

I had a thirty-four-hour labor. Through the process, my doula was with me, which was very helpful. I would recommend it to everyone. She really helped me stay focused and work through the various positions. My midwife said we tried every position. She said we did everything possible to have a natural labor. (Kristen S., public relations)

For me, I was thinking about the personalities involved with my husband and myself, and that having a doula was the right thing for us. I think my

husband didn't think of it or didn't realize, because there's so much focus and attention on the pregnant mom, just how much a doula could help HIM. (Cheryl L., lawyer)

I was worried about my husband being my coach, but he was great. I didn't want a cheerleader, but he was just helpful, holding my leg for me since it was weak from the epidural. (Galit A., tax attorney)

RELAXATION

Anxiety amplifies pain and slows labor. Conversely, relaxation diminishes pain perception, and may improve the efficiency of your labor. What relaxes you? Massage, soft voices, hypnotic music, a calm environment, self-hypnosis, standing in the shower, a warm tub bath? Think ahead about what might help, get educated, and plan for what you may need—especially given that hospitals aren't always relaxing places. Be sure those who accompany you will advocate to keep your environment upbeat and serene.

During labor I had a really cold, nasty resident taking care of me before my doctor came. I told him that this was my first baby and I was frightened and he was making me feel worse. His behavior then changed for the better! I don't know where I found the courage to say that, but I felt proud of myself afterward. (Sonya G., secretary)

It took me three babies to really learn how to have a baby. The secret is . . . to let it happen. I know that sounds simple, but the more you hold on or try to get away from the pain, the more it hurts and the longer it takes. Let the baby push down and open your cervix. I didn't really get the hang of it until my last one. (Patsy H., midwife)

DISTRACTION AND FOCUS

The classic distraction technique is Lamaze breathing. Focal points to look at, warm or cool compresses, light massage, and position changes all can help. Changing position periodically also may assist the baby to move into a more favorable orientation, diminishing back pain and speeding labor. Deep massage or counterpressure on the lower back can help to ease back labor. Your coach,

LABOR AND BIRTH IN THE BATHTUB

Immediately after immersion in warm water, many women experience a deep relaxation and diminution of pain. For this reason, some hospitals and birth centers have tubs in the labor rooms; others have wheeled tubs you can bring in, or collapsible tubs that can be reconstructed and filled with a hose. If a tub isn't available, you may be able to rent one.

There are some drawbacks to using a tub during labor, however. It will be important to make sure the water temperature isn't hotter than body temperature, so you and the baby don't overheat. A special instrument will be needed to check the baby's heartbeat under the water. And warm bathing in early labor may stop the labor process, so immersion isn't usually recommended until five or six centimeters of dilation has been reached.

Tub use for delivery, rather than just for labor, is quite controversial. Only a limited number of practitioners are comfortable with a mother giving birth into a tub, in large part because of concerns about the baby's safety. If labor or birth in a warm tub appeals to you, talk to your practitioner early on in your pregnancy about the availability and safety of this option.

doula, nurse, midwife, or doctor may have more suggestions. Some women turn inward and are irritated by any contact, while others feel best with continuous massage or touch. Think ahead about what might work for you, and bring lots of ideas—comfort is often a matter of trial and error, and many different techniques may be used as your needs change.

My first labor was about ten hours. My husband was my coach, and basically spent the whole time helping me breathe through the contractions: in-2-3, out-2-3 for about eight hours. I have no recollection of the hours going by during labor—I think we invented our own hypnobirthing. It was a good experience. I didn't need an epidural. (Julie M., veterinarian)

I found that I could manage the pain for the most part by doing deep breathing and focusing on a picture I had brought. I listened to a Pachelbel

CD over and over as well. I was telling my husband that the contractions were about a nine in terms of pain (ten being highest) and the only way he could tell was by a slight grimace on my face. (Sandy B., social worker)

The doula really helped to keep me focused. With Bradley, that's what you do . . . keep focused. (Kristen S., public relations)

EDUCATION

Education is valuable both to understand the general course of labor and to learn about different comfort measures—but you can only do so much ahead of time. Much of your education will happen on the scene: you will identify which relaxation techniques are working the best; your coach will help you to understand what you are feeling and why; and your medical team will explain how your labor is progressing. Although doulas are usually employed to help with natural childbirth, even parents-to-be planning on an epidural may find it reassuring to have their own experienced birth advocate. A doula will also help to educate both parents—she can translate the medical team's feedback about how things are going, and help the mom discover which measures are most comforting.

I wanted that extra support for myself and my husband. I'd heard stories about deliveries and about women having doulas present. I just had no idea what to expect, so I wanted someone there for me who had seen childbirth before. (Elizabeth S., online producer)

We went to childbirth classes, and we kept thinking, "Thank goodness we don't have to remember all this." Having a doula took lots of pressure off my husband since he didn't have to be the only coach. (Cheryl L., lawyer)

At seven centimeters, I was just in horrible pain. I was in the shower, my husband was trying to direct the water on my back, and it just wouldn't get hot enough. I think this was a situation where a doula, or even an OB with whom I had built a solid relationship, would have been a lot of help, because someone could have told me that I was really just in transition, and that was why the pain was so great. A little encouragement that the end

GETTING THROUGH TRANSITION WITHOUT DRUGS

The transition phase of labor, right before it's time to push, is usually physically and emotionally trying for women without an epidural. Many moms-to-be who were committed to natural childbirth will ask for drugs around now. Simple reassurance that this panicky feeling is normal and a sign of labor's progress is often enough to get the mom through, but if the team doesn't understand why the mom is asking for drugs, they may run to get the anesthesiologist—just as mom starts to see the finish line. This is yet another way a doula who understands the normal events of labor can help—she can clue in your partner, and give you the support you need.

was near might have gone a long way. But who knows? In any case, I got an epidural. (Shani M., student)

Why Would Anyone Want Natural Childbirth?

Pain, triumph, and joy can coexist. If you're able to look at the experience of giving birth as a personal challenge, similar to climbing a mountain or running a marathon, natural childbirth will bring a feeling of empowerment, rather than powerlessness. Instead of viewing contractions as "bad pain," you may be able to see them as the forces required to bring your new baby into the world.

When I talked to other people they all asked, "Why would you not want drugs?" Even my mom said, "No harm in getting the epidural." I did natural 90 percent because I wanted to for myself, and 10 percent to prove to all these people that I could do it. (Danielle R., trust analyst)

Women who have unmedicated childbirth often speak of the confidence they gained from meeting the challenge, and the new respect they received from those who attended the birth. One new mom told me it made her feel like she could handle anything. What a wonderful way to start motherhood!

I feel like I proved my strength and when my baby cries I am stubborn: . . . I can figure you out. (Danielle R., trust analyst)

In addition to the sense of accomplishment women get from natural childbirth, there are some minor medical benefits. Babies of unmedicated moms are a little more alert, and may nurse more readily.

Natural childbirth made me feel powerful. If I can do that there's nothing I can't do. It was the hardest thing I have ever done. Donovan says I am a rock. I feel ready to attempt things I never would have before. (Danielle R., trust analyst)

I chose natural childbirth because I thought it would be cool to know what it felt like. It was a macho thing. Now that I've done it, the wisdom of experience tells me that it's the baby that's important. I'd like to do natural again, but I'd take an epidural if I needed one. (Kristi V., professor)

Why Some Laboring Moms Choose Pain Medication

Natural childbirth is not for everyone. Some women's labor experiences are extraordinarily drawn out and painful. Other women wish to save their emotional and physical energies for newborn care. And still others just don't see any point in avoiding the use of available medical advances. If after considering your options, you decide to pursue pain relief measures during labor, don't feel guilty for a moment—the only truly important outcome of labor is a healthy mom and newborn.

The Epidural

Epidural anesthesia has become a staple of American birth. About 60 percent of U.S. mothers give birth with an epidural—and in some hospitals as many as 80 to 90 percent of laboring women choose this option. An epidural numbs the nerves as they emerge from the spinal cord, taking away the pain of contractions and cervical dilation and sometimes relieving the pressure of the baby descending through the birth canal (although many women still feel strong pressure).

"I WANT TO FEEL IN CONTROL"

Many mothers-to-be have said to me that they are planning natural childbirth because they want to feel "in control" and don't want their legs to be numb or weak from an epidural. That's fine if it works for you, but for many women, natural childbirth doesn't feel very controlled. Panicky feelings are normal during the transition phase of labor. At least from the outside, mothers typically look more "in control" with an epidural than when dealing with the intensity of natural childbirth.

BENEFITS OF AN EPIDURAL

Moms who choose epidural anesthesia have several reasons for embracing this method of pain relief:

- Great respite from the pain of contractions. Many women find that having an epidural allows them to relax, enjoy labor, and feel excited about their baby's birth.
- Epidural anesthesia tends to lower the mother's blood pressure. For women who are predisposed to hypertension or who have the medical condition pre-eclampsia, this effect may be desirable, given that the pain of labor may increase the mom's blood pressure.
- If tension and anxiety are impeding the birth process, and especially if the mother is exhausted from a long, drawn-out labor, an epidural can actually speed labor along.
- Epidurals offer clear-headed pain relief. Moms can enjoy the experience of pushing out their babies and feel emotionally available for their newborn right after birth.
- If the mom is getting worn out, an epidural may allow her to sleep before she needs to gather her strength for pushing.
- Having an epidural in place may prevent the need for general anesthesia (and its increased medical risks and emotional stress) should a cesarean suddenly become necessary.

HOW IS AN EPIDURAL GIVEN?

During epidural anesthesia placement, you will sit with your feet dangling off the side of your bed, leaning forward, or will lie on your side, curled into a ball. Because this procedure is done in a sterile setting, family members are often asked to leave. Everyone present (except the mom-to-be) must don a surgical mask and cap. If you are sitting, someone—usually the nurse—will stand in front of you for physical and emotional support. The anesthetist will wash your back with an antiseptic, then numb an area over your mid-spine with a small needle. A larger needle will then be placed through the numb area, between two backbones, to the area outside the spinal cord. A thin tube called an epidural catheter is then fed through that needle. After the needle is removed, the soft thin tube is left in place, taped to your back and draped up over your shoulder. Pain medication, which drips on the nerves as they emerge from the spinal cord, can be given through this catheter. Some hospitals use a "patient-controlled" system in which you push a button when you need a boost of anesthetic. You can't overdose yourself; it locks out for ten or fifteen minutes after the bolus so you will see how it is working before you take another dose.

After I had the epidural put in, I was fine. I started pushing and everything was quick. It was all worth it. (Annette M., store manager)

I was amazed by how manageable labor was. I'd never do it without an epidural, but it was a great experience. If I weren't so old, I would do it again in a heartbeat. (Rebecca M., senior vice president, financial corporation)

When I got the epidural, I had no idea that this meant I was not allowed to get up. I felt like I was cheating because I felt nothing. Eight-pound, ten-ounce Brigid was born at twelve noon, and I didn't feel a thing, except extreme happiness. (Peggy L., nurse-administrator)

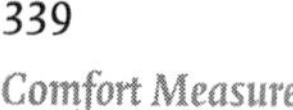

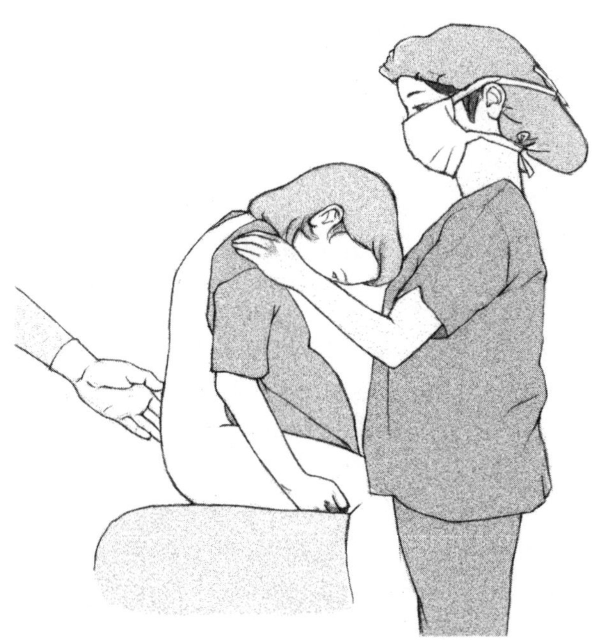

Getting an epidural

After the epidural took effect . . . I took a nap. Yes, a nap, while those contractions were pumping away. When I woke up, I asked if anyone wanted to play cards. Was I the same maniacal killer who was in labor earlier? When I looked up at the monitor, I could not believe my eyes. The contractions were twice as strong and coming right on top of one another, and I could barely feel a thing. Bliss. (Heidi R., law professor)

As an added benefit, the epidural enabled my husband to remain calm—and present—throughout the labor and delivery. To this day, he tells me that he could not have handled watching me experience the extended pain that I felt shortly before the epidural. (Rebecca M., senior vice president, financial corporation)

I now understand why so many babies are named after their anesthesiologists. (Melissa G., mortgage broker)

Whoever invented that epidural, they need to be canonized. I mean, we should know their name like we know Einstein's name. It was just the most magical thing. (Linda S., creative director)

As soon as the epidural took effect, both the memory and the reality of the pain evaporated. (Rebecca M., senior vice president, financial corporation)

DRAWBACKS TO EPIDURAL ANESTHESIA

Although epidurals are considered very safe and effective, you should also know that

- Some experts believe that an epidural, especially if given early in labor, increases the chances of needing a cesarean or of requiring a vacuum or forceps for birth. But the current evidence is contradictory; some studies indicate that epidurals received in early labor actually accelerate labor's progress.
- Epidural anesthesia makes the whole labor experience more medical: if you choose an epidural you will be given intravenous fluids through an IV line; your baby's heart rate and the contractions will need to be continuously tracked on the fetal monitor; and if the epidural interferes with your urge to push, you may require coaching to bear down effectively.
- Even with an epidural, labor may not be a walk in the park. Moms need to be realistic about how tough labor may be, and come emotionally and physically prepared to meet that challenge. Occasionally, too, the epidural isn't as effective as one would like. In this case, the anesthetists may be able to fix it, but sometimes they will need to start all over again and put in a new one (if delivery isn't imminent). With or without an epidural, pushing can still be strenuous and exhausting, particularly with a first baby.
- Most women stay in bed after the epidural is placed. Although many hospitals offer what they call "walking epidurals," using milder drugs so that your legs will remain strong enough to walk around, many moms still have numbness or weakness in their legs and are not steady on their feet. The medication also will require that your baby be continuously tracked on the fetal monitor, which is easiest to do when you are lying down.
- For unknown reasons, women with epidurals are more likely than others

to develop a fever during labor. Knowing that a fever might just be from the epidural can help the healthcare team to not overreact, but sometimes it's hard to tell if the fever is a sign of uterine infection, which can then lead to concerns about the baby becoming ill. If the healthcare team is worried, they may check the baby after birth for signs of infection, and may even give the newborn intravenous antibiotics for a few days to be safe. This treatment may require the baby to be in a separate nursery away from the mother—a deprivation for all involved.

- Sometimes after the epidural is placed, the mother's blood pressure falls, leading to a transient drop in the fetal heart rate. Usually the situation is not harmful and is easy to correct with intravenous fluids and changing position, but it can be frightening for the family, because the team may start to prepare for an emergency cesarean.
- Occasionally the epidural needle punctures the membrane around the spinal cord, allowing some spinal fluid to leak out which may lead to a spinal headache the next day. Effective treatment is available, so a severe headache after an epidural should be reported to the anesthesia staff.
- Mothers-to-be who want to have the most natural, noninterventionist labor experience may be disappointed if they end up with an epidural.
- Very rarely, a serious complication of epidural anesthesia may occur.

After I got my epidural, my baby's heart rate dropped; they gave me oxygen, and I had to get on my hands and knees. I didn't find out until afterward that my husband was terrified; he thought the baby was going to die. My doctor said it wasn't a big deal since they could deliver the baby by cesarean very quickly if necessary. (Maggie P., administrator)

When I became pregnant, I asked several anesthesiologists about whether I'd be able to have an epidural [given my recent back surgery]. They all responded that they could probably give me an epidural, but it might not work at all or there might be heavy side effects. I decided I would just avoid that and go for natural childbirth. (Jill H., gynecologist)

Laurel, my labor nurse, entered my room and spent several minutes getting to know my husband and me. We discussed my desire to have an epidural but to delay the administration so I could (a) keep my labor

advancing, and (b) remain mobile for as long as possible. (Rebecca M., senior vice president, financial corporation)

With an epidural they have to tell you when to push. I knew when to push, and I felt her come out. It made me feel incredibly connected with her. (Danielle R., trust analyst)

Last time I moved so fast I didn't have time to get an epidural. I felt so much better afterward, compared with my first two. I'm going to plan for natural childbirth this time, so I feel more prepared. It was just a better experience. (Catherine B., executive assistant)

HOW EARLY IN LABOR CAN I HAVE AN EPIDURAL?

In the past, epidural anesthesia was only made available when the mother entered active labor, usually after four centimeters' dilation. It was thought that having an epidural any earlier might increase the chances of needing other interventions, like Pitocin stimulation of labor or cesarean. Many doctors and hospitals still have policies for when an epidural can be offered—typically at four centimeters' cervical dilation.

The American College of Obstetrics and Gynecology, however, has taken a somewhat different stand on the subject:

> **There is no other circumstance where it is considered acceptable for an individual to experience untreated severe pain, amenable to safe intervention, while under a physician's care. In the absence of a medical contraindication, maternal request is sufficient medical indication for pain relief during labor.**

In response to this mandate, many labor units are offering earlier epidurals, or alternatives such as intravenous narcotic pain medication, during early labor. But even if you have the power to request pain medication during the early stages of labor, it might not be the right choice overall for your birth experience: an early epidural may increase the chance that you will need Pitocin stimulation of your labor. To become more informed, ask your practitioner not only about the policies at your hospital or birthing center, but also what strategies have worked well for other women.

I thought I might try natural because I wanted the experience, but after a few hours of contractions I felt like if this was going to go on many more hours I should get an epidural. (Galit A., tax attorney)

Other Treatments for Labor Pain

As popular as epidural anesthesia is, there are in fact several other options for managing pain during labor:

- Narcotic pain medicines. Nubain, Demerol, or morphine (taken as a shot or intravenously) or nasally inhaled medications like Stadol can take the edge off of contractions and allow the mom to rest. These are most useful in early labor, while the mother's body has time to remove the drug from the baby's system before birth. If a baby is born with high amounts of narcotic on board, he may have trouble breathing on his own, and may require ventilation or injections of the narcotic antidote, Narcan. Some mothers report feeling "foggy headed" or nauseated from narcotic pain medicines.
- Local anesthetics. Local anesthesia, similar to what the dentist uses, can be injected to numb the area between the vagina and the rectum, especially before an episiotomy is made or if a laceration needs to be sutured.
- Paracervical blocks. Local anesthetics can be injected through the vagina into the nerves of the cervix to decrease the pain of cervical dilation. Because paracervical block frequently leads to a drop in the fetal heart rate, it isn't used much any more.
- Pudendal blocks. Local anesthetics can be injected into the walls of the vagina, to numb the nerves that sense stretch within the birth canal and vaginal opening. Pudendals aren't used very often, but are quite safe and can be effective for pain as the baby descends.
- Complementary pain therapies. Several types of alternative medicine treatments can modulate pain sensations before they reach the brain. Acupuncture has been used for labor, but I haven't seen data on its effectiveness. Transcutaneous electrical nerve stimulation (TENS) units, which attach over your abdomen, confuse the nerves' signals and may

diminish pain. Lastly, sterile water injection into the skin of the lower back has been shown in research studies to help with back pain during labor.

I regret that I tried intravenous pain medicine during labor. It just confused me. I felt weak and not myself. Next time I'll just get an epidural. (Kate R., financial analyst)

Planning Ahead

Many first-time moms approach labor unsure of what will be best, and plan to keep an open mind about epidural anesthesia. Because the transition phase of labor is so difficult, though, most of these open-minded moms lose their resolve and take an epidural with only minutes or at most a few hours of labor still to go. If you really like the idea of natural childbirth, don't keep your mind too open—set everything up so that you are most likely to succeed. Surround yourself with support for natural childbirth. You may be able to tell early on that natural childbirth isn't for you, but if you make it as far as transition, stay strong. Remember that you are almost there!

It is a privilege to have a baby today, with so many choices to help you cope when the going gets tough. Learn about all your options, look into your heart to decide what will probably work best for you, and then be flexible, since labor never goes exactly as anticipated. As I have advised, you'll want to choose your birth location and team by what you think you'll want, then enlist support—from your partner, friends, family, and/or a doula—to help you cope with the unexpected.

Remember, too, that although worrying about birth is normal, labor is but a day or two of your life, and no matter how challenging, the result will be a new family member you will love for a lifetime. Some women have easy labors, and some have awful experiences—but most moms are absolutely willing to do it again in order to bring another baby into the family. Women have given birth for millennia; you can do it too.

When they gave me Pitocin it was my first baby and I didn't realize it would make the contractions so strong. I didn't know when enough was enough. I appreciated that epidural, even though I had planned on natural child-

birth. For the next two babies I just planned on an epidural and it was comfortable and it wasn't stressful. I could just focus on having the baby and not worry. (Jennifer A., secretary)

I'm less adamant about not having an epidural this time around. Since I did it natural the first time, and I enjoyed that (as much as anyone can enjoy it), I'm leaning that way again. But I'm not opposed to the epidural this time either. (Elizabeth S., online producer)

I tell the story of her birth over and over. I am not going to be a crazy hippie telling everyone to have natural, but it worked for me. I felt tired afterward but so strong. I could have gone home that day. She was totally alert right after birth and interacting with us, and my recovery was easy. (Danielle R., trust analyst)

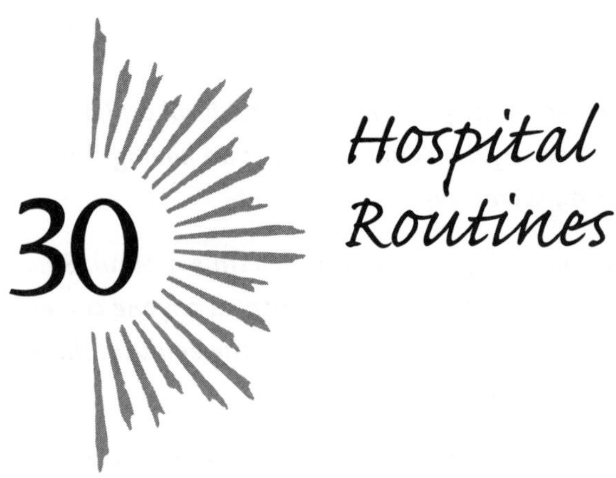

30 Hospital Routines

In the Monty Python movie *The Meaning of Life*, modern birth took place in "the fetus-frightening room." Although that scene seemed pretty funny to me at the time, it also pointed out how procedures that feel routine to hospital personnel can be unfamiliar and even intimidating to patients and their families. This chapter will explain commonly used technologies for hospital birth, including external and internal fetal monitoring and Pitocin augmentation of labor. While all of these measures may not apply to your labor experience, becoming familiar ahead of time will help you understand why interventions may be suggested, so you can make informed decisions about your care.

Admission Procedures

For centuries, babies were born without monitoring the heartbeat or labor pattern. They came when they came, however they came—and most of the time emerged healthy. But the uncommon complication was tragic: no one wanted to risk a long, obstructed labor that threatened the health of mother and infant, for example, or an oxygen-deprived baby who hadn't tolerated labor contractions. Many of the technological advances in childbirth that have become routine over the past few decades were initiated to prevent these rare disasters.

When you arrive at the hospital in labor, you will probably be asked to change into a hospital gown. The doctor or nurse (or both) will ask about your medical history and any allergies, and do a brief physical examination. You will most likely have an intravenous line (or a capped-off IV called a heparin or saline lock) placed in a vein in your hand or forearm, and some blood will be drawn to send to the lab. The nurse will place a fetal monitor on your abdomen for at least twenty minutes, so the medical team can check on your contractions and the baby's heartbeat. In most hospitals these practices are routine and expected. It is your right to ask about any procedure beforehand, of course, and, to decline treatment after getting information about the risks, benefits, and alternatives. Birth centers typically have fewer routine procedures than hospitals do.

External Fetal Monitoring

Most hospital birthing units use the electronic fetal monitor to continuously track the baby throughout labor. With belts around your belly that hold two sensors in place (one to listen to the heartbeat and one to feel the hardness of your abdomen), the monitor creates a graph of the heart rate and contractions, and beeps with each heartbeat.

Healthy babies typically have heart rates between 120 and 160 beats per minute; their heart rates accelerate when they move, just like your heart speeds up when you climb stairs. The increase in pace when the baby moves is a sign that the baby is in good condition, getting enough oxygen. Although contractions can be a stress on a fetus, most babies tolerate labor well. External monitoring accurately discerns contraction timing, too, but because the measurements are influenced by how tight the belt is and whether you are thin or heavy, it doesn't quantify the exact strength of each contraction—so don't feel discouraged if your contractions feel big but look small on the monitor.

Before I got the epidural the external monitor fell off right before my strongest contraction. I was upset—I wanted credit for that contraction! (Galit A., tax attorney)

Continuous Monitoring versus Intermittently Listening

The fetal heart rate is one way that we can rest assured that the baby is doing well, but as I mentioned earlier, research has shown that continuous fetal monitoring is not necessary in healthy pregnancies, and actually increases the chance of getting a cesarean. Listening to the heartbeat at intervals, or "intermittent auscultation," is an effective alternative to continuous fetal monitoring in uncomplicated pregnancies, and is designed to keep the baby safe during labor

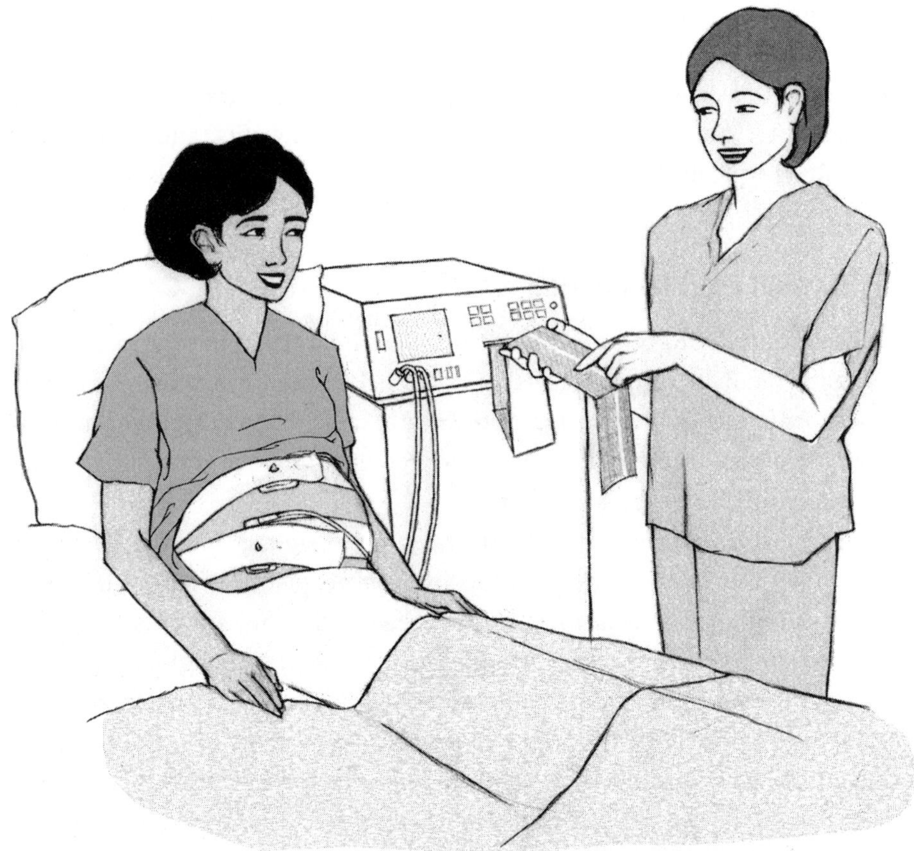

The fetal monitor's belts measure the baby's heart rate and your contractions.

without tethering you to the monitor. Typically the nurses will listen to the baby on a strict schedule: once every half an hour in early labor, every fifteen minutes during active labor, and every five minutes when you are pushing.

You may find that you are most comfortable staying in bed and feel safest hearing the continuous ticking of the baby's heart. But if you want to walk around, go in the shower or tub, or just create a less medical environment, feel free to ask if intermittently listening to the fetal heart rate is an acceptable alternative for you and your baby. Ambulatory wireless monitors are available in some hospitals, too, allowing you to be monitored continuously without restricting your mobility. Whatever type of monitor is used, it is standard procedure to leave it on constantly after epidural anesthesia, or if the pregnancy becomes medically complicated. Many OB units use continuous monitoring any time the laboring mom is in her bed.

The nurse temporarily connected me to an external fetal monitor, explained how it worked, and announced that all looked fine so I was free to roam the halls. (Rebecca M., senior vice president, financial corporation)

Following the Progress of Labor

In addition to watching the baby's heart rate, the fetal monitor tracks the frequency of uterine contractions. By the time you pass four or five centimeters' dilation and enter the active phase of labor, contractions are typically two to three minutes apart. Cervical dilation accelerates to at least a centimeter an hour for first-time moms and even faster for women who have given birth before. If progress stalls after the active phase has started, the chance of needing a cesarean increases unless actions are taken to get labor back on track.

Cervical dilation and fetal descent into the birth canal are affected by factors that we call the "four P's":

Power. The strength and frequency of the contractions
Passage. The width of the birth canal (mom's pelvic bones)
Passenger. The size and position of the baby
Psyche. The mother's emotional state (anxiety can impede labor, probably because of the influence of stress hormones)

If cervical dilation isn't advancing after active phase has begun, your team will consider where the problem might lie: in the strength and timing of contractions, the size of your pelvis, the size or position of the baby, or the fear-tension-pain-anxiety cycle. Based on which of these "P's" is thought to be the culprit, they will recommend strategies to help get labor back on track: changing your position in order to shift the baby; using the medication Pitocin to strengthen the contractions; or even taking some pain medicine or having an epidural.

I got stuck at nine centimeters and was advised to get the epidural (I had been stuck for about three and a half hours at that point). Once I got the epidural I dilated to ten quickly. However, they had given me too much and

WHAT IS PITOCIN?

Pitocin is a synthetic form of the natural hormone oxytocin, which makes the uterus contract. Intravenous Pitocin is used for labor induction, and to make contractions stronger if labor isn't progressing. Because sensitivity to Pitocin varies, the initial dose is small and then increased periodically while the medical staff monitors its effects on the contractions and on the progress of labor.

It can be hard to accept a medicine to make labor stronger when you feel that you are barely getting through your contractions. You may find it difficult to believe that more powerful contractions are necessary. But research has shown that the longer a labor stalls out, the less likely vaginal birth becomes. So if the active phase has begun and your progress is slow, try to think of Pitocin as something that may help you avoid a cesarean.

I started to not feel the contractions. So we stopped the epidural and they started me on Pitocin. (Sandy B., social worker)

Measuring Labor and Its Effects on the Baby

Although the external monitor does a good job of measuring the baby's heart rate and your contraction pattern from the outside, internal monitoring may be recommended if your medical team wants to more accurately assess the strength of your contractions or listen more precisely to your baby's heartbeat.

Internal monitors are placed through the vagina in a procedure that typically feels like a slightly longer and deeper vaginal examination. If the bag of waters hasn't broken yet, the doctor or midwife will need to puncture the sac first (amniotomy). The internal fetal heart monitor will be attached to the baby's scalp with a small wire, which will register the baby's heartbeat more directly. The internal pressure monitor will measure the strength of the contractions with a pressure-sensitive tube that lies next to the baby. Neither of these monitors will harm your baby, although after birth you may see a little nick on the baby's scalp from the heart monitor. Once the internal monitors have been inserted, a wire and/or a thin, soft tube will come out of your vagina and attach to the monitor. Sometimes switching to internal monitoring actually increases your mobility, because, unlike with external monitoring, readings don't depend on position-sensitive belts. But internal monitoring does keep you within a few yards of the base unit, usually in bed.

Internal monitoring is usually required when:

- Labor isn't progressing normally. In this situation, internal monitoring can help your medical team decide if your contractions are strong enough or if stimulating your labor with Pitocin might move things along.
- Your baby's heart rate is worrisome or can't be followed easily with external methods. Internal monitoring may provide reassurance that the baby is just fine, or evidence that interventions are needed.

Common Concerns during Labor

It can be a relief for moms to realize that many labor "complications" are commonplace and easily addressed. These include:

- Fetal heart rate false alarms. It can be tempting to focus on the fetal monitor. Unfortunately, what you see isn't always reassuring. For example, it's not unusual for the baby to move away from under the sensor, so that the heartbeat doesn't pick up for a moment, or so that the mom's (slower) heart rate shows up instead. False alarms are quite common: don't panic. Your nurse will adjust the monitor and answer any questions you may have.
- Urinary retention. During labor urinating can be difficult, especially after an epidural, or if the baby's head is low in the birth canal. If your bladder gets full, the nurse may need to insert a catheter to let the urine out. Depending on how long labor is expected to last, the catheter may be inserted for a few moments when needed, or left in until the baby is born. If you don't have an epidural, you may feel a pinch when the bladder catheter is inserted. Once in, though, you should not be aware of it.
- Fever. If you get a fever during labor, the baby's heartbeat will go faster, as will yours. Fever may be normal, especially in women with epidurals, but

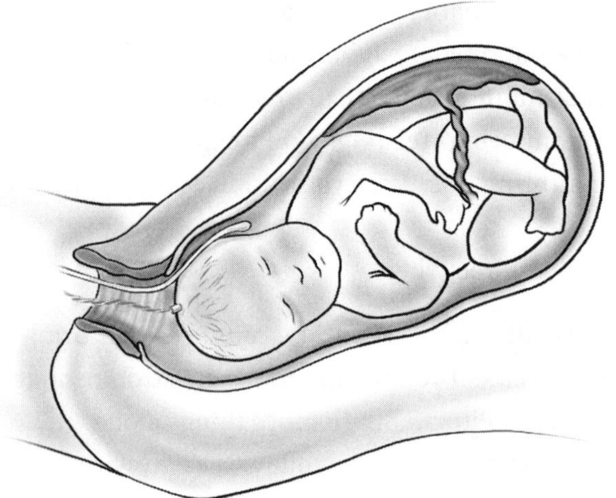

The internal fetal heart monitor attaches to the baby's scalp with a small wire. The internal pressure monitor measures the strength of the contractions with a pressure-sensitive tube that lies next to the baby.

it can also be a sign of an infection in the uterus that requires antibiotics. If you had a fever during labor, the pediatrician or family doctor will check your newborn for signs of infection. Sometimes antibiotics are given to the baby for a few days, until it is certain that no infection has developed.

- Meconium. Amniotic fluid is usually clear or pale yellow, but if the baby has pooped into the water it may look anywhere from apple green to a thick, dark greenish-brown. While it is true that a fetus may move its bowels during a time of stress, most of the time when a baby poops it's just confirmation that the intestinal tract is mature and functional. The bigger issue is trying to prevent the thick brown fluid from getting into the baby's lungs. Your team will talk to you about their routine procedures if meconium-stained fluid is seen when your membranes rupture.
- Cord around the neck. Many parents have heard stories of babies born with the umbilical cord around the neck and worry about choking. While the cord around the neck does sound terrible, it can be reassuring to remember that fetuses don't need an unrestricted neck to breathe—the necessary oxygen is delivered though the umbilical cord. When the cord is around the baby's neck, it may get stretched as the baby descends, causing noticeable changes in the baby's heart rate pattern, but the baby isn't getting choked, despite how it sounds to those of us who depend on our necks for breathing. We who deliver babies see "nuchal cords"

frequently and deal with them easily. After the baby's head delivers, the cord can be unlooped, or quickly clamped and cut, to allow for a safe delivery.

When it comes to labor and delivery, knowledge is power: the power to overcome your fears about any delivery complications, the power to wisely choose with your team the options that are best for you and your baby, and the power to feel proud and happy that you did your best when you finally hold your little one in your arms.

If your medical practitioners intensify their efforts to monitor your baby during labor, you may initially be frightened. But you should know that often the baby is just fine—and the goal is simply to find out for sure as quickly as possible. Every OB unit has standard procedures to follow if concerns develop. For example, if the baby's heart rate is worrisome, you may be asked to change position or breathe some extra oxygen to help the baby recover. If labor seems to be stalled, internal monitors may be offered to help understand why. If the baby needs to be born quickly, a cesarean or operative vaginal delivery with vacuum or forceps may be recommended. When disturbances like these arise, you should feel free to ask why recommendations are being made. But it also will help if you stay focused on the most important outcome: a healthy mother and baby.

Approximately ten minutes into pushing, my daughter's heart rate began to dip. My doctor explained what that could mean, and what the possible repercussions were if the rate dropped lower. She talked about the possible necessity of forceps, suction, and/or a C-section. She also told me that since my baby had been doing well up to this time, she wanted me to continue pushing to see if we could get the baby delivered vaginally. I agreed. The last thing I wanted was any of those interventions. No more than five or so pushes later, perfect Natalie arrived. (Rebecca M., senior vice president, financial corporation)

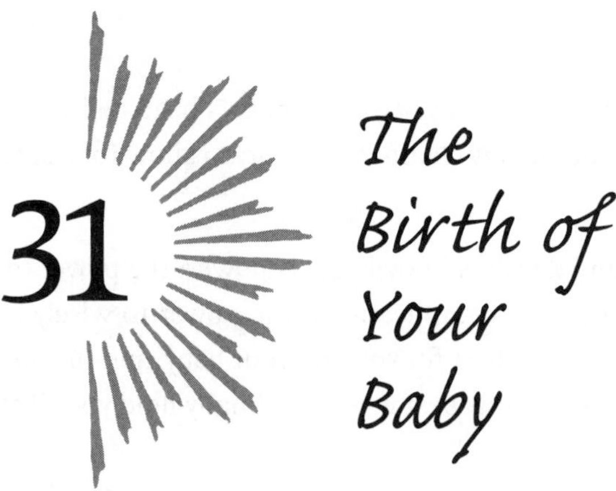

31 The Birth of Your Baby

And now for one of the most amazing moments of your life: the birth of your child. As the baby descends through the birth canal, the top of the head starts to show with each push. You may be able to see it if you ask for a mirror, or feel it by reaching down. One nice thing about a mirror is that it shows you when your pushing is most effective, so you can do more of what works. Pretty soon, the head will be visible even between pushes: this is called crowning.

With an epidural, crowning may feel like pressure or discomfort. Without an epidural, this part is often very intense and unpleasant. Most mothers-to-be want to speed things up and get the baby out. Warm compresses can be soothing, helping the muscles to relax as the baby descends.

Who Will Be in the Room When the Baby Is Born?

At this point, your visitors will be present, as well as your doctor or midwife, your nurse, and possibly a few others: the anesthesiologist, a student or resident, a nurse for the baby, a pediatrician. In a perfect world, anyone who didn't need to be there to help you would ask permission first, but this isn't always the case. It is your right to know who these people are, and what their role is in the care of you and your baby. Often, though, at this point you are so focused on what you are doing that you don't really care who is attending your birth.

While I was pushing it was just me, the nurse, and my husband, which was very nice. I went to my friend's birth and it seemed like there were fifty people in the room. (Galit A., tax attorney)

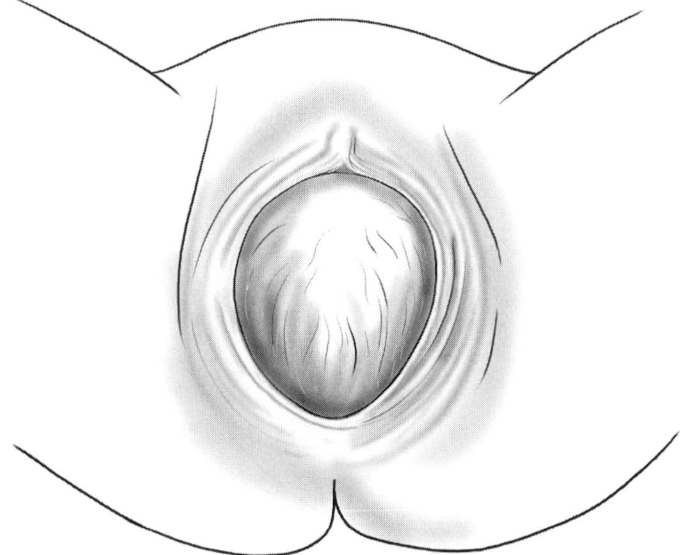

Crowning. As it crowns, the baby's head stretches the opening of the vagina.

William, my stepfather, was an unexpected surprise. When they said it's time to push, he came barging in the room and was there . . . the nurses looked all concerned . . . but at that point I couldn't have cared less . . . besides, he helped hold my legs while I was pushing and my mom got tired. (Zenia M., nurse's aide)

The Moment of Birth

When the baby is crowning, the midwife or doctor will be able to see how you are opening up to accommodate the baby's head. A slow, controlled birth allows the tissues to stretch instead of tearing. If the birth needs to be hurried along (due to concerns about the baby, for instance), or if it looks like there truly isn't enough room, a surgical incision or "episiotomy" may be done to enlarge the vaginal opening. Typically you would be numbed up with an injection of local anesthetic, unless you had an epidural that was keeping that area anesthetized.

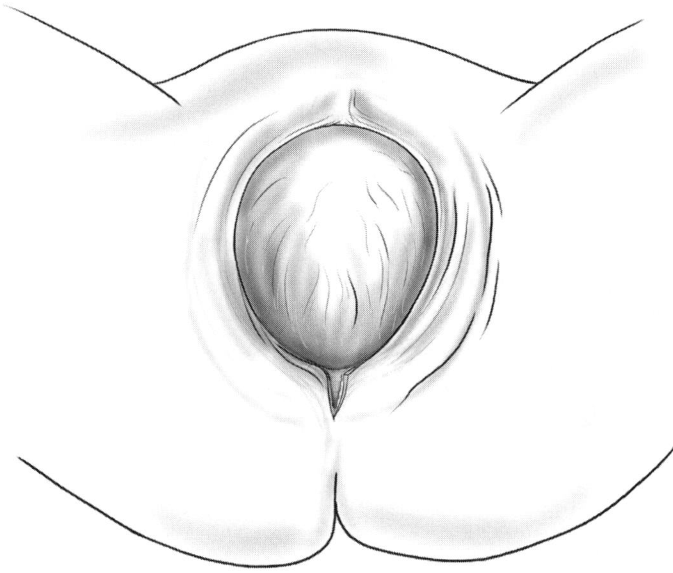

Midline episiotomy

Sometimes just the baby's head stretching the vaginal opening makes it numb enough so that the incision isn't felt.

After the baby's whole head delivers, the doctor or midwife may suction out the nose and mouth; then the rest of your warm, wet baby will slide out. Try to remember to open your eyes so you can see your little one emerge into the world.

After birth, two surgical clamps will be placed around the umbilical cord. Either a family member or your practitioner will cut the cord; it's a nice way for the dad or another important person to participate in the birth. Some families like the idea of waiting until the cord stops pulsing before cutting it, but medical research doesn't show any clear benefit from this practice.

Brian was very into cutting the cord. He grabbed the scissors out of my OB's hand. I think if Brian wasn't so into it, the baby's grandfather would have fought him for a turn. (Zenia M., nurse's aide)

The doctor cut the cord. My husband was standing there, and they asked him. He said no—I think he was just afraid. (Amanda O., meeting planner)

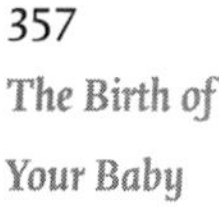

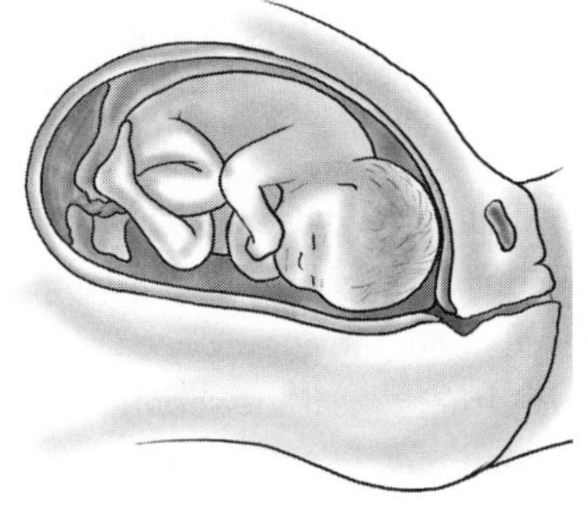

Early labor

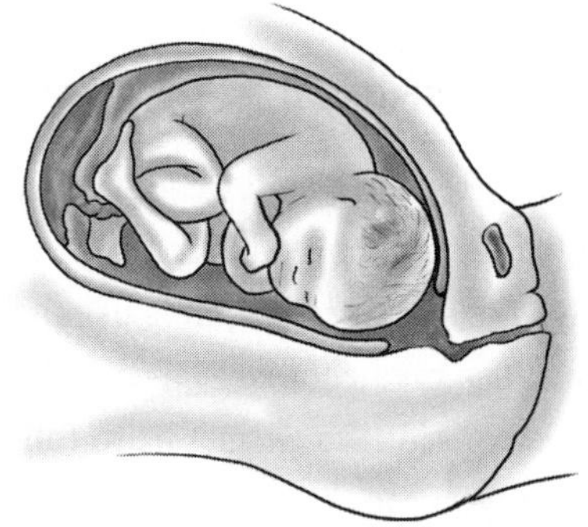

Almost complete dilation

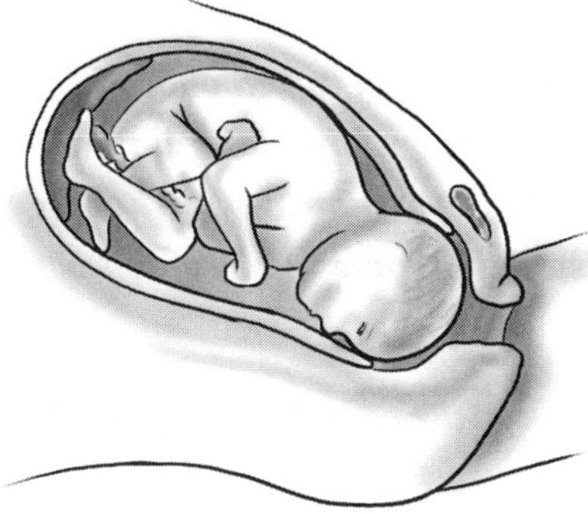

Pushing

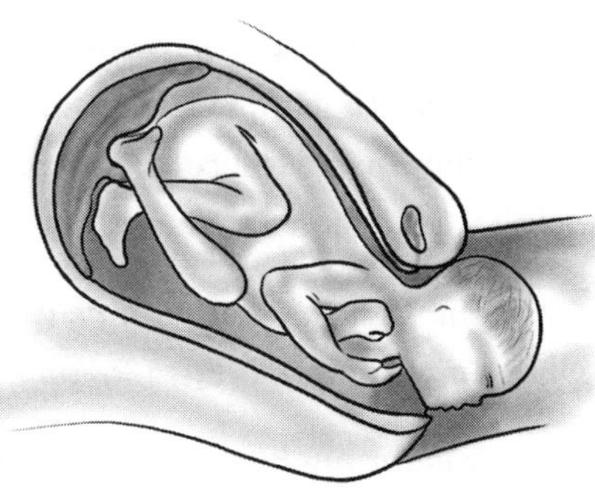

Delivery of baby's head

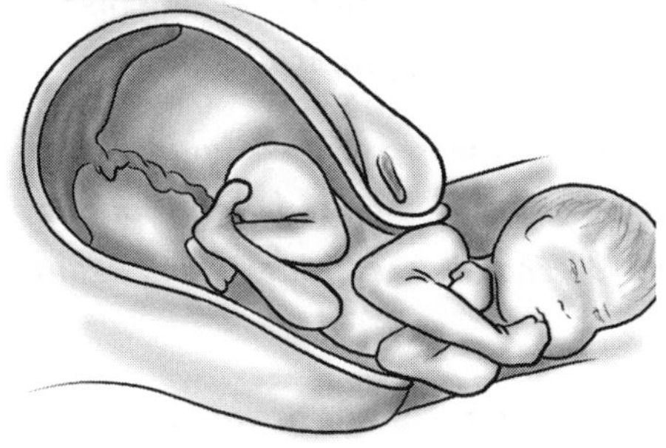

Delivery of baby's shoulders

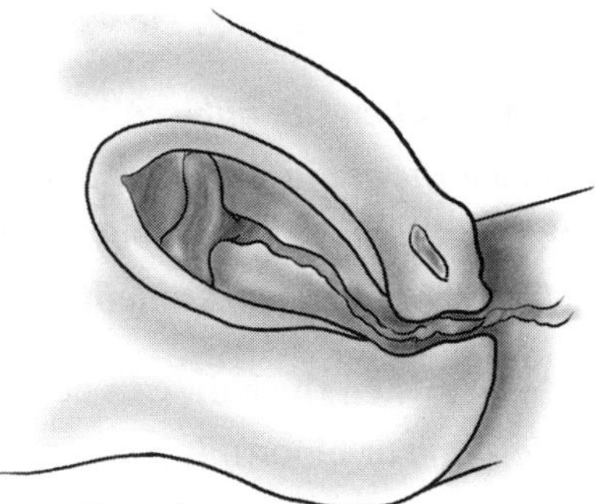

Placenta

Birth

WHAT IS SHOULDER DYSTOCIA?

Rarely, after the baby's head emerges its shoulders will become stuck in the vagina. Often simple maneuvers like drawing your legs up will help to dislodge the shoulder, which is usually wedged under the pubic bone in the front. The medical team has a series of steps they take if the shoulders get stuck. Your job would just be to follow instructions, and when asked, push as hard as you can.

They asked Ben if he wanted to cut the cord. We had talked about this in advance because we knew that he would be uncomfortable with that. He didn't want to get queasy or pass out. So he knew that they were going to ask him to cut the cord, and he had sort of prepared himself to say no. (Christi M., medical student)

One time I asked a father if he wanted to cut the cord. He said, "That's what I pay you for." (Elisa R., ob-gyn)

I didn't want my husband to watch down there, but he was totally amazing. He was so positive and excited and emotional and loving . . . it was all OK. He kept telling me, "You can do this" and looking me in the eye. I know I couldn't have done it without him. When I saw his reaction to seeing his son, it was mind-boggling. He was just fabulous. (Kate R., financial analyst)

At first, when the baby came out, Ben told me it was a girl. We hadn't known the sex in advance, but I was convinced, based on my gestalt about the world, that it was a boy. I said "really?" Then I asked him to look again. (Christi M., medical student)

I love it when the baby can be handed directly to the mom (if you don't mind a little slime or blood). It just seems nicer to me if the first things the baby sees are happy parental faces, rather than the nurse and the underside of the infant warmer. The newborn will need to be dried off and kept warm, either skin-to-skin with mom, wrapped in blankets, or on a nearby exam table under a warmer.

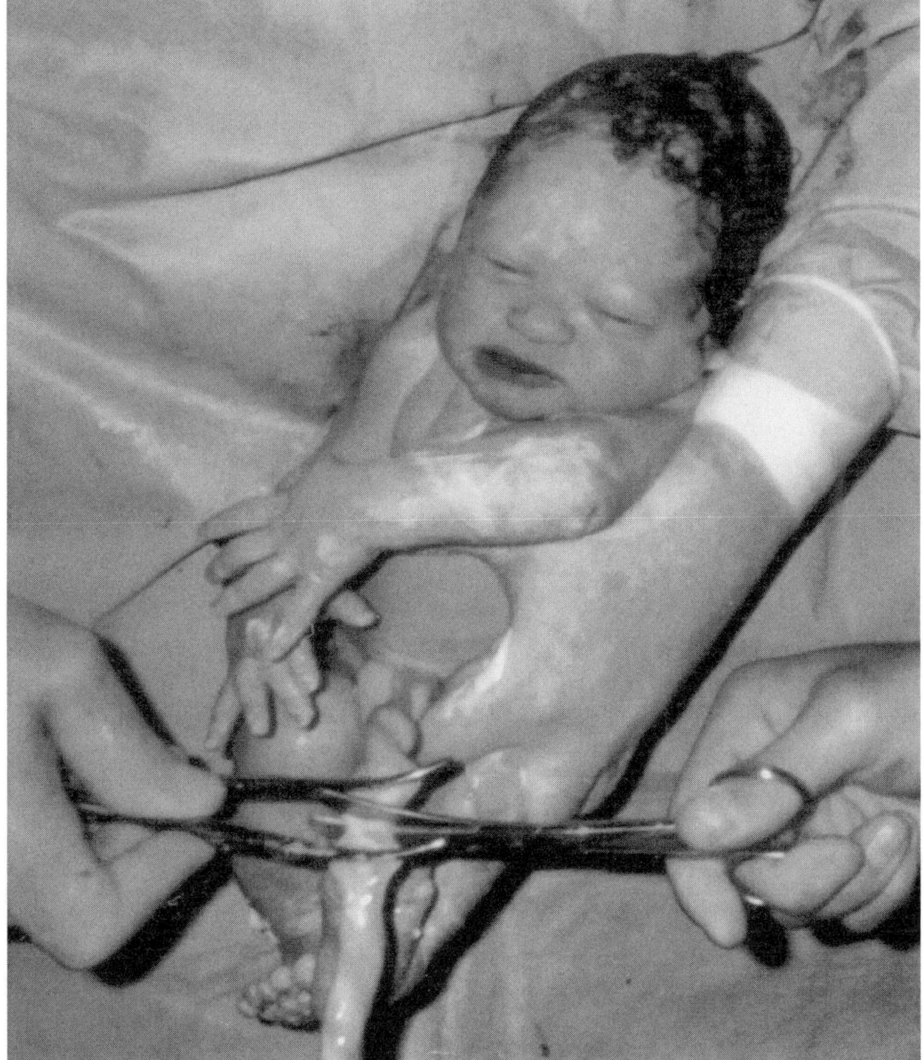

Zenia Marrone

Cutting the umbilical cord

Although the nurses have steps they must take by law, including eye ointment to prevent infection and a vitamin K shot, these can usually be delayed for an hour or so, for you to have time with your new baby. Any suctioning to remove mucus from the airways can usually be done in your arms. Of course if help with breathing or more intense medical attention is needed, the nurse or doctor will let you know.

FIVE POINTERS FOR THE PERSON WHO WILL CUT THE CORD

- If the birth becomes complicated in any way, the doctor or midwife may decide she needs to cut the umbilical cord—so try not to get your heart set on this aspect of your participation in the birth.
- Be sure to cut where the doctor or midwife indicates. The incision should be made *between* the two clamps.
- The cord is thicker than you might expect: don't be surprised at how much resistance you feel between the scissor blades. Cut forcefully!
- Don't worry: how the cord is cut doesn't influence how the belly button looks later in life. Innies and outies are determined by the structure of the abdominal wall.
- Enjoy! You are marking the miraculous transition from fetus to newborn.

The Afterbirth

After delivery your focus will probably be on your newborn, but the midwife or doctor still has some work to do. The placenta (afterbirth) must detach itself from the inside of the uterus before you can push it out. The placenta is softer and smaller than the baby, and this pushing is generally brief and easy. Some blood usually flows out with the placenta. Uterine contractions then close off the open surface inside the uterus where the placenta was attached, and the bleeding slows down. Typically the mom gets a dose of Pitocin immediately after the placenta delivers, to help the uterus contract, which lessens the amount of blood lost. Massaging the uterus through your abdomen or putting the baby to breast also causes uterine contractions. If you are saving the cord blood, collection can be performed from the umbilical cord before the placenta comes out, or immediately afterward.

After the placenta delivers, your doctor or midwife will examine your vagina to see if you need any stitches. If you aren't numb from an epidural, local anesthetic can be injected so the stitching doesn't hurt. Absorbable sutures are used so no stitches will have to be taken out. Because only the part of the stitch under the skin dissolves, however, you may notice string-like sutures or little suture knots in your underwear over the next several weeks, until all of the stitches are gone.

After the birth is all done, it's time to curl up and bond with your new baby.

I guess it was sort of a whirlwind because the labor and delivery was so easy, then she's out. I had them clean her up a bit, but then all of a sudden I'm holding this little baby and wondering how we'd gotten to that point so easily. (Amanda O., meeting planner)

I found, both times, the experience of birth to be awe-inspiring. There is a strange similarity between being at a birth and being with someone when they die. There's this sense that someone comes or leaves—from somewhere else—and an awareness of feeling that we're part of something so much greater than ourselves about which we really have very little understanding. I felt it was truly miraculous. (Anne O., director, nonprofit organization)

For both my husband and me, Natalie's birthday was a tremendously positive event in our lives—in part because we received an incredible gift, and in part because we had shared every step of the journey to creating that gift, from conception through delivery. (Rebecca M., senior vice president, financial corporation)

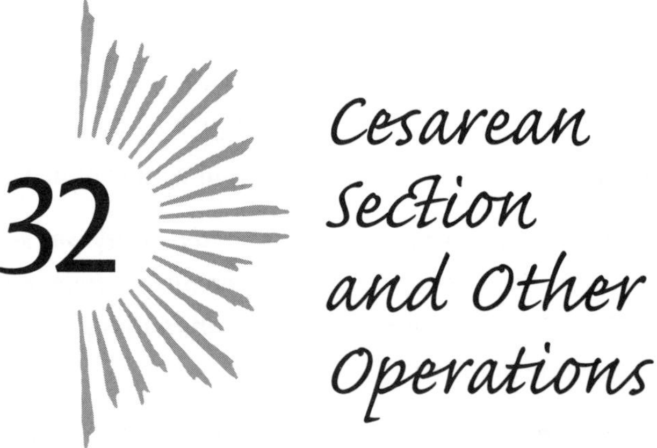

32 Cesarean Section and Other Operations

Although most women begin the labor process expecting to deliver vaginally, many labors end in cesarean section. In North American hospitals today, the rate of cesarean sections ranges from about 15 to over 35 percent. Operative vaginal deliveries, in which vacuums or forceps are employed, are also quite common. This chapter, then, is designed to give you the basic information you will need if surgical delivery is recommended.

Operative Vaginal Deliveries

Operative vaginal delivery with vacuum or forceps is used to hurry birth along, particularly if there is a worrisome slowing of the fetal heartbeat or if the mom is becoming exhausted and unable to push the baby out. These procedures can only be performed once the cervix has opened completely and the baby's head has descended into the birth canal. It is best to think of vacuum- and forceps-assisted deliveries as an alternative to cesarean, although if the baby still doesn't come down easily after using these techniques, a cesarean may become necessary after all.

The vacuum is a suction cup that attaches to the baby's head so that the doctor or midwife can pull as the mom pushes. Usually the baby has a swollen scalp after vacuum birth. Rare complications include bleeding into the scalp or head.

Forceps are metal tongs that slide in and surround the baby's head, allowing the doctor to pull as the mom pushes. Because they take up extra room in the vagina, the most common complications of forceps deliveries are tears or bruises in the birth canal. Also, most babies have some bruising on their cheeks or temples after a forceps birth.

Vacuum and forceps are not used lightly because they can lead to complications. When compared to the alternative of cesarean, though, they have been shown (when needed) to be reasonably safe and quite effective. The choice between the two is usually made based on technical aspects of how the baby's head is descending, and the doctor's comfort with each method. Forceps were used routinely until the 1970s, but the vacuum procedure is more commonly used today; consequently, physicians trained recently may feel more comfortable with the vacuum. Your practitioner will discuss the pros and cons of operative delivery and the alternatives. While of course you can decline these options, keep in mind that the alternative may be a bigger surgery—cesarean section.

Cesarean Section

Cesarean may be recommended during pregnancy, or may become necessary during labor. Some moms are terribly disappointed to end up with a cesarean; others don't care how the baby gets out, or even prefer the idea of surgical birth. Regardless of how you feel about the procedure, though, it is important to recognize that any pregnancy may lead to cesarean: every mom-to-be should prepare emotionally for this possibility.

Common Reasons for Cesarean

The decision to deliver a baby by C-section should not be made without thoughtfully weighing the benefits and drawbacks—but the surgery itself can be a powerful medical tool for preventing devastating outcomes for mother and child. Some reasons cesarean may be recommended include:

- Non-reassuring fetal status. The medical team relies on the baby's heartbeat to know how the baby is handling the stress of labor. If the heartbeat is a concern, other tests may be done. In the end, if the team is worried about the baby, or even if they just can't be certain that the baby is okay, cesarean will be recommended.
- Failure to progress in labor. Sometimes, despite good strong contractions in the active phase of labor, the cervix will stop dilating or the baby won't descend down the birth canal. Usually the problem is that the baby is

WHY ARE SO MANY BABIES BORN BY CESAREAN?

Cesarean birth is more common today than it was fifty years ago. There are many reasons for this trend. Babies are a little bigger (moms too, for that matter), and our ability to identify a baby who isn't doing well has improved. Induction of labor, done quite frequently nowadays, increases the chance of needing a C-section. Doctors also worry about lawsuits, and don't want to be accused of waiting "too long" before recommending cesarean birth. Finally, surgery has become much safer, so the criteria for cesarean have broadened.

too big for the mother's pelvis, or the head has tipped so that a larger diameter is trying to come through. In such cases, cesarean may be the only option.

- Failed induction. Sometimes labor induction just doesn't work: medications are given, but the cervix never opens up. Cesarean then may become necessary if going home and waiting for natural labor isn't an option (for instance, if the membranes have already ruptured and infection is a concern).
- A poorly positioned baby. Babies who are "breech"—positioned so their feet will come first through the birth canal—can sometimes be turned by exercises late in pregnancy or by external cephalic version, in which the doctor rotates the baby by pushing on the mom's abdomen. If this procedure is declined by the parents, though, or doesn't work, the baby must be born breech. Research indicates that it is probably safer to deliver a breech baby by cesarean, especially if the doctor isn't experienced in vaginal breech births (which most doctors and midwives aren't, since nearly all breech babies have been delivered by cesarean since the 1970s). Babies lying sideways (transverse lie) can't deliver vaginally. If your baby is not headfirst and your due date is approaching, your practitioner will talk to you about the risks and benefits of external version, vaginal birth, and cesarean.
- Multiples. Triplets and more are typically delivered by cesarean. It is just

too hard to keep track of how each baby is doing during labor, and usually at least some of them are positioned oddly for birth. Headfirst twins, by contrast, can usually be born vaginally, and some doctors will deliver twins vaginally as long as the first baby is coming headfirst. Rarely, the first twin comes out vaginally and the second one requires a cesarean.

- Placenta previa. You may remember from an earlier chapter that placenta previa is when the placenta is located at the opening of the cervix. In complete placenta previa, the placenta spans the opening, preventing the baby from coming through, and cesarean is required for delivery.
- Active genital herpes. Babies may catch herpes if they deliver through an infected birth canal. The greatest risk occurs if the mother is experiencing her first episode of herpes around the time of birth; in this case, she hasn't yet had time to make protective antibodies and pass some to her baby through the placenta. Rarely, recurrent herpes, where antibodies are present, may still make a baby very sick. The standard recommendation, then, is to have a cesarean if a herpes sore is present near the vagina at the time of birth.
- Previous cesarean. Through the 1960s, the rule was "once a cesarean, always a cesarean." The risk of the uterus rupturing at the previous incision site was deemed too great to allow labor. In the 1970s and 1980s, however, research showed that in most cases the risk of such a rupture was only 1 percent, and that depending on the reason for the original cesarean, the odds of having a successful vaginal birth could be as high as 60 to 80 percent. Consequently, the trend was to attempt vaginal birth after cesarean, or VBAC. Now the pendulum has swung back somewhat, because doctors and parents have become nervous about risking uterine rupture, no matter how rarely it occurs. Moreover, some hospitals don't provide the back-up emergency surgical and anesthesia teams required to safely offer VBAC. If you had a prior C-section and want a vaginal birth, be sure to talk to your practitioner early on to find out whether VBAC is available and appropriate for you.

I pushed for two hours and then had to have a cesarean. I was frustrated with myself. I am kind of a competitive person, and I was frustrated that other people had easier experiences. (Sherri M., sales rep)

I think I will have an elective repeat cesarean next time—second babies are usually bigger than the first, and my recovery was really hard from such a long labor and then the cesarean. (Kendra F., civil litigator)

I got stuck at nine centimeters and they were thinking I was going to need a cesarean, but the anesthesiologist was tied up, so they allowed me to try to push and I got to deliver vaginally. (Galit A., tax attorney)

About a month before my due date I started asking for a cesarean. I had my spleen out, so I knew what it was like to recover from surgery, but I was very worried about labor. (Kate R., financial analyst)

Choosing Cesarean Section

What about having a cesarean without a medical reason—just because you want one? Many mothers-to-be are afraid of labor because it sounds uncontrollable, potentially long, and painful. Elective surgery may seem preferable: you schedule a date, get your anesthesia, and your baby is born. No watching the baby's heartbeat on the monitor, no anxiety about episiotomy or vaginal lacerations, no stretched-out private parts, and in the long run, maybe a lower chance of bladder incontinence and pelvic organ prolapse. But consider these important facts before requesting a cesarean:

- Recovery from cesarean is typically more painful and prolonged than recovery from vaginal birth. Most new moms are in the hospital for three nights and require pain medication for weeks. Successful breastfeeding is certainly possible, but may be more difficult after cesarean; many moms feel unable to provide full care for their newborns for a week or two after surgery.
- Serious complications are more likely to occur in cesarean deliveries. Although untoward events aren't common, surgical injury to the bladder, excess bleeding, blood transfusion, postoperative fever, uterine infection, and incision complications are all more likely with a cesarean than with a vaginal birth.
- Any of your future pregnancies will have about a 1 percent risk of uterine rupture, a potentially catastrophic event in which the uterine incision

WHY DO CESAREAN RATES VARY SO MUCH?

Cesarean rates can be quite different between individual practitioners and between birth locations. In general, patients of midwives are less likely to have a cesarean than are patients of physicians. The mother's risk level plays a role: medically complicated pregnancies are more likely to require cesarean delivery. But the practitioner's personal philosophy about birth, beliefs regarding the safety of surgery, concerns over lawsuits, and time constraints also play a part in the likelihood of recommending a cesarean. Overall, the percentage of births by cesarean varies because practitioners differ in their management of labor, how they diagnose these conditions, and how they weigh the risks and the benefits of surgery.

breaks open during pregnancy or labor. In the worst-case scenario, uterine rupture can lead to loss of the baby, excessive bleeding requiring blood transfusion, surgical removal of the uterus (emergency hysterectomy) if bleeding can't be controlled, and (rarely) maternal death.

- Surgical complications become more likely after multiple prior abdominal surgeries (including cesarean); if you are planning on having a lot of children, you may be setting yourself up for a difficult third, fourth, or fifth cesarean birth.
- I'd estimate that more than 90 percent of my patients who have given birth both ways say they would choose vaginal birth if given the choice. Reasons include a feeling of participating in the birth, easier recovery, and fewer surgical complications.

Medical journals are full of articles on the ethics of offering cesareans on the basis of "patient request." While some physicians are willing to provide this service as long as the woman understands the risks and benefits, others feel it is not good practice to offer a riskier procedure based just on patient preference. If you desire an elective cesarean, talk to your practitioner early on.

In other countries, women are allowed to choose a C-section. I mean, doctors schedule them all the time out of convenience. The schedule is packed all day with C-sections on the Friday before the holiday weekend. I think a lot of women would choose a C-section if given the choice. (Jane J., advertising executive)

When it comes to the postpartum recovery, comparing the C-section and the vaginal delivery, I have to say, it's six of one and a half dozen of the other. I mean, you don't sit on your C-section scar, but you sit on your episiotomy. (Linda S., creative director)

After my cesarean I just wasn't interested in breastfeeding. I was too uncomfortable. The whole experience was traumatic for me. (Sherri M., sales rep)

My first was born vaginally, and my second by cesarean. Vaginal delivery, while exhausting, was a far more memorable experience. I felt like an active participant in my daughter's birth. While equally grateful for a second healthy baby, the C-section was disappointing in that I felt like a passive participant. (Anne C., radiologist)

I was elated after the cesarean. Steve was by my side most of the time and was immediately given our children upon their birth. It was a pretty overwhelming feeling of love. (Edie U., school psychologist)

What Exactly Is a Cesarean?

Cesarean section is a way to deliver a baby surgically, through the mother's abdomen. The term comes from the Latin "caedere" which means to cut. No, Julius Caesar didn't have one—despite that legend—in those days a mother wouldn't have survived a surgical birth, and history has it that his mother lived to old age. The skin incision is usually a "bikini" cut, made across the abdomen just above the pubic hair; the nurse may clip or shave the top of your pubic hair before surgery. (When a very rapid delivery is needed, a faster vertical incision extending down from the belly button may be chosen.) After the abdomen and uterus have been opened, the surgeon will reach in and lift out the baby. The umbilical cord will be clamped and cut by the doctor, and the baby will be handed

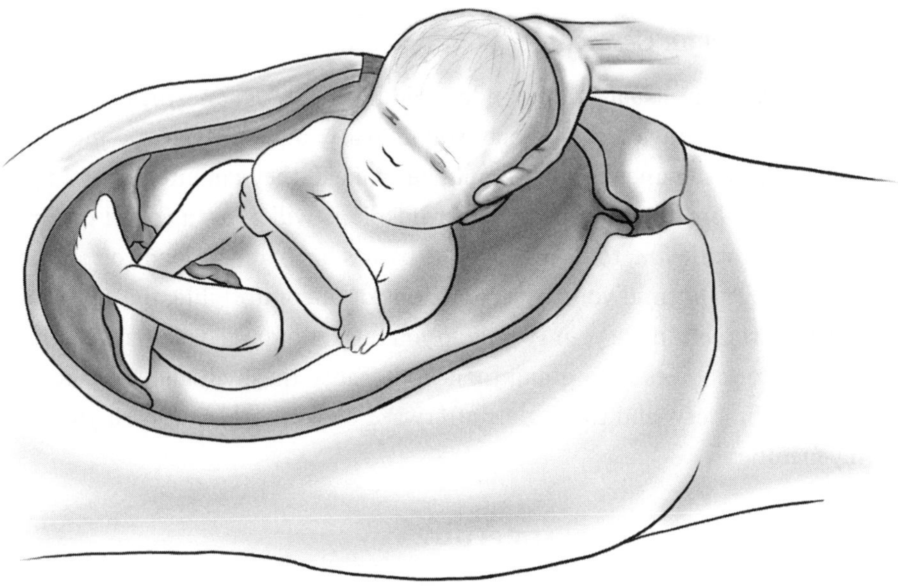

Cesarean section is a surgical procedure in which an incision is made in the mother's abdomen and then into her uterus, so that the baby can be lifted out.

off the surgical field to a nurse or doctor to dry off and examine. Then the placenta (afterbirth) will be delivered, and the incisions closed in layers.

The baby may be brought to the parents at this time, or kept warm by the nurses until surgery is over. The skin incision may be sutured, or closed with surgical staples. From start to finish, a cesarean can take anywhere from twenty minutes to several hours, depending on the urgency of the situation and technical factors in the surgery.

I decided that if I needed another C-section, I preferred to not be strapped down, not receive oxygen, and to be able to hold my child immediately upon delivery (barring any medical issues). When my try at VBAC didn't work, the medical team honored my request, which made that C-section a bit better. However, the best experience was simply scheduling the third C-section a week before my daughter's due date, arriving at the hospital an hour before the surgery and not having to endure an exhausting labor! (Edie U., school psychologist)

Anesthesia for Cesarean

Cesareans are usually done under epidural or spinal anesthesia. Lying on the operating table wide awake may sound scary, but the systemic medicines that would keep you unconscious should be avoided: they can interfere with your baby's drive to breathe after birth. Most hospitals will allow a friend or family member to sit with you, to experience the baby's birth and to lend you support. Once the baby is born, if you are very anxious or uncomfortable, the anesthetist can give you something in your IV to help you relax. Epidural or spinal anesthesia are also better choices than going to sleep because they will allow you to hear your baby's first cry, and to be alert afterward so you can bond with your new family member.

REGIONAL ANESTHESIA: EPIDURAL

An epidural for a cesarean is placed just as for labor, but more anesthetic is given so the mom will become numb from her waist to her toes. If you have an epidural for surgery, you won't be able to move your feet, and in some cases you won't feel yourself breathe, even though air will be moving in and out just fine. The sensation of pain will be blocked, but it is normal to feel touch: you may sense a lot of pressure as the baby is being delivered. It is also fairly common to feel nauseated or even throw up during surgery.

Many hospitals leave the epidural in for a few days after the birth, which provides wonderful pain control without the drowsiness and other side effects of common postoperative pain medications. The dose of medicine in the epidural is reduced after the surgery, so that you won't experience pain but will have strength and feeling in your legs—this way, you should be able to get up and walk around after giving birth.

REGIONAL ANESTHESIA: SPINAL

Getting spinal anesthesia feels somewhat like getting an epidural. The anesthetist places a long thin needle between the bones of the mother's spine, all the way into the spinal fluid, and injects pain medication. Then the needle is removed, and the medicine begins to take effect. Spinal anesthesia is quicker to

TYPES OF CESAREAN SECTIONS

The incision that is made in the uterus is important for future risk: a *low transverse* incision heals best, with the lowest chance of rupture in a subsequent pregnancy. Fortunately, low transverse is also the most common type of cesarean. The weaker types of incisions, called *classical* or *vertical* cesareans, run up and down along the front of the uterus, and are generally only needed for babies that are in unusual positions or very small. The risk of uterine rupture after a classical cesarean may be as high as 10 percent, so labor is prohibited and all future babies are born by cesarean. The direction of the incision on the skin has nothing to do with the incision on the uterus, so looking at the skin scar doesn't tell us anything: asking the doctor who did the surgery or reading the operative note from the hospital chart is the best way to find out which type of cesarean was done and if vaginal birth is an option for the future.

place than an epidural, and the effects start sooner, so it can sometimes be used in emergency situations where the alternative is going to sleep for surgery. One dose of spinal anesthesia typically lasts about ninety minutes. After the delivery is over, and the effects of the spinal wear off, intravenous or oral medicines are taken to ease the pain. Some hospitals use a combined spinal-epidural, for the intensive and quick effects of the spinal and the ability to leave the epidural in for a few days for postoperative comfort.

GENERAL ANESTHESIA

Medicines that make you go to sleep are not as safe in pregnancy as regional anesthesia methods are: they are only used when alternatives are not appropriate, typically when the baby must be delivered very rapidly. During general anesthesia, intravenous and inhaled drugs are given, and a tube is placed into the mother's throat to help with breathing. Normally a family member will not accompany the woman to the operating room if general anesthesia is planned. After surgery, intravenous or oral medicines are provided for pain relief.

Given that I had the epidural, I felt little during the actual C-section—a bit of tugging, but no pain. (Edie U., school psychologist)

If You Are Scheduled for a Cesarean

One problem with scheduled cesareans (and scheduled labor induction) is that the baby hasn't yet given the signals to start labor. On rare occasions, the due date was calculated incorrectly, and an elective cesarean or induction brings a slightly premature baby into the world. If there are medical reasons for delivery, such as high blood pressure in the mother, this small risk may be justified. But if the timing is purely by choice, the American College of Obstetrics and Gynecology recommends that, in order to be sure your baby is ready, your pregnancy has lasted a full thirty-nine weeks (as documented by the dates when you had your positive pregnancy test or heard the fetal heartbeat the first time, or by measurements taken during a first or second trimester ultrasound). If cesarean or induction is scheduled earlier than that, or if dating parameters aren't clear-cut, amniocentesis is recommended: substances in the amniotic fluid will help indicate whether the baby's lungs are mature enough to breathe well in the outside world.

I was set up to have an amnio one day before my C-section was scheduled. I was very nervous and scared about the procedure. I did a lot of reading about it on how painful it would be. But I must say I barely felt any pain, nor did I have any cramps afterward. My experience was very good. (Natasha G., respiratory therapist)

For a scheduled cesarean, the most important instruction to remember is not to eat or drink after midnight the night before surgery. Although in an emergency a cesarean can be done when the mother has a full stomach, elective surgery is never offered under those conditions. The anesthesia team will cancel your surgery if you've had anything to eat or drink. If you take routine daily medications, ask ahead if you should swallow them with a sip of water or skip the dose. Also, leave the lower abdominal pubic hair shave to the professionals: the bacteria count on the skin goes up for a few days after shaving, and increases the chance of infection in the incision. Talk to your doctor for individualized recommendations.

Emotional Responses to Cesarean or Operative Vaginal Delivery

The range of responses to surgical birth continually amazes me. Some women really grieve when the birth doesn't go as they imagined—they mourn an anticipated rite of passage that went all wrong. Others feel relieved when a cesarean or vacuum birth is recommended after a long and difficult labor. And some moms would choose cesarean birth if given the option. In general, it is easiest to adjust to an unexpected surgical delivery if you feel totally clear about why surgery was needed, and if you had a part in the decision-making. In my experience, the birth situation that causes the most disappointment is the unscheduled C-section for the mom who had never considered the possibility and didn't feel included in the decision.

People around a new mother may not understand the feelings of loss brought on by cesarean, or by other disappointing aspects of the birth experience, especially when the baby is healthy. No one chooses to start parenthood feeling deeply disappointed, but those emotions can be hard to shake. For some women, the birth experience is truly traumatic, and counseling is necessary to come to terms with the events. Thinking ahead about the possibility of C-section may help you to cope, should a cesarean be needed. And if you had a traumatic birth experience and you are really struggling, be sure to get help.

I felt very sad that I'd had a C-section, that I hadn't had a regular birth. I felt sort of like a fake mom because I wanted so badly to push him out, to have that final exertion into life. (Linda S., creative director)

It may also be a relief to know that other women who have experienced surgical deliveries had mixed feelings too—but that in the end, the overwhelming love they feel for their newborn overshadows their concerns. For no matter how your baby emerges, this is still your baby's birthday, a date that will be important for the rest of your life, a day to celebrate every year.

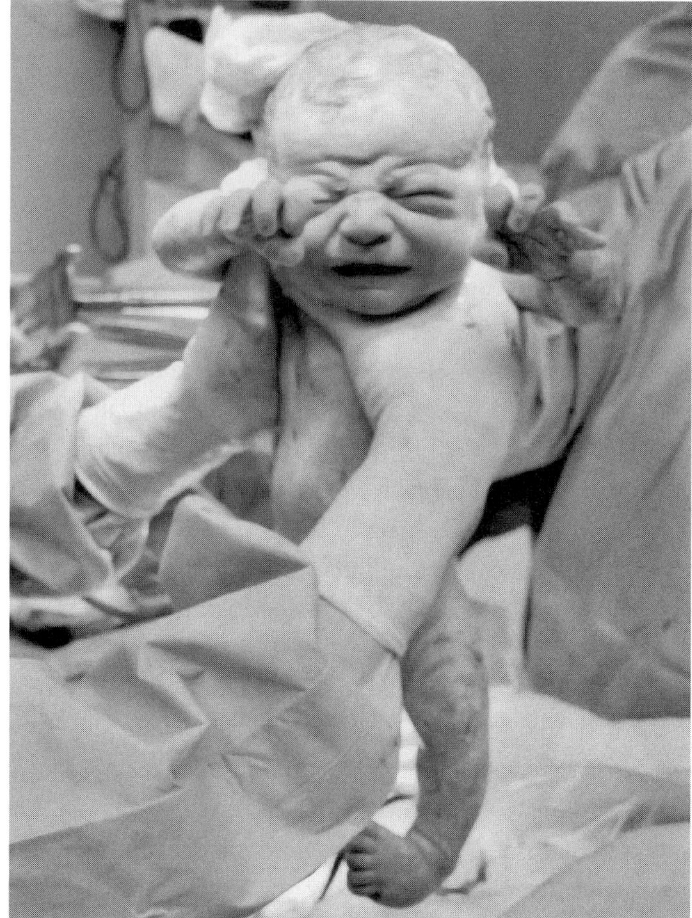
M. Landis

A newborn is shown to his parents during a cesarean.

I had some concern about a C-section because I was worried it wouldn't be as emotional a birth as a vaginal birth, but that wasn't the case. I found it to be just as emotional. The only thing that was frustrating is that they took Ronan away to clean him and clear his lungs out for a minute or two so I didn't get to see him immediately. (Jane J., advertising executive)

I felt like a failure by needing a second C-section and sent the doula home prior to going into the operating room. (Edie U., school psychologist)

You think that the delivery is going to be this emotional, touching experience and that if you have a C-section you'll miss out on that because surgery isn't really the place for it. Really, I think it's the same. You just don't get to hold him right away. And it's a lot less messy! (Jane J., advertising executive)

My first was an emergency cesarean, and it was scary. My second baby was born by repeat cesarean, and it was one of the happiest moments of my life. When I want to feel good, I go there as my happy place. (Eileen M., weather reporter)

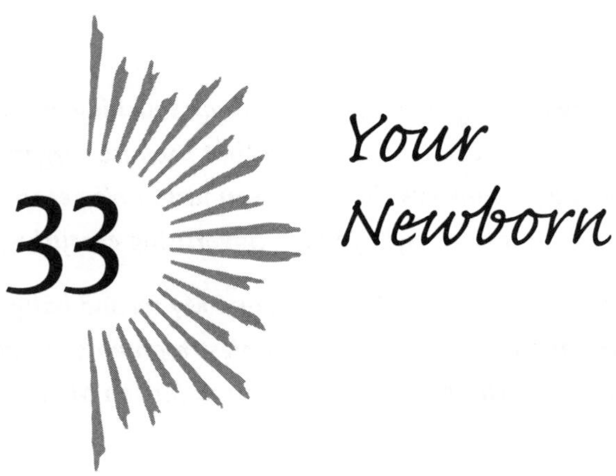

33 Your Newborn

Labor is over and your baby has finally arrived! It may be hard to believe that this marvelous little person came out of your body. Mark this moment in your mind—and look around at your visitors to commemorate their responses as well. Life will never be the same.

> ***The day after my first baby was born, my sister wrote down everything she could remember from that day and gave it to me. She included the weather, my labor, everyone's reactions to the baby. I was so happy to have all those details later on. It was the best gift she could have given me. (Eileen M., weather reporter)***

> ***She had been crying continuously since her first breath. The moment her father held her and spoke to her, she instantly quieted and became completely still. What a sight to behold. (Rebecca M., senior vice president, financial corporation)***

Your Newborn

Right after birth, the medical team will assess your baby. An Apgar score—which assesses the baby's well-being—is usually assigned twice, at one and five minutes after birth. If the score is low, the nurses and doctors will help the baby along by suctioning mucus from the airways or giving oxygen. We don't spank newborns like the old-timers did, but we do dry them off, and sometimes rub them to encourage them to start breathing. Although this all can be done while the baby is with you in your bed, hospital routine may dictate that the baby be

THE APGAR SCORE

Virginia Apgar, an anesthesiologist, developed a scoring system to help the obstetrical team judge if a baby needs any special help right after birth. Heart rate, breathing effort, color (blue or pink), muscle tone, and response to stimuli are each assigned 0, 1, or 2 points, creating the Apgar score. Any score 7 or over means the baby is doing fine. Lower scores indicate that medical interventions are necessary. The score is determined at one minute of age and then again at five minutes. Most babies score 7's, 8's, and 9's. No one gets a 10, because all newborns have poor circulation to their hands and feet, so they look a bit blue. If a baby still needs a lot of help at five minutes, another score may be determined at ten minutes. Babies often require assistance at first, so try not to get too worried if your medical team fusses over your newborn. Generally by ten minutes babies are perky and breathing on their own, with no harm done if it took a few minutes to get going. (And contrary to urban legend, your children's SAT scores will not be related to their Apgars!)

brought over to a warmer in your room where there is suction, oxygen, and good lighting. Babies get cold very easily—newborns need to be in a warmer, under the blankets with mom in bed, or bundled up.

During my cesareans, I listened as they measured, weighed, counted fingers and toes, and did the Apgar testing of each child. (Edie U., school psychologist)

A little meconium came out when he was born, and they wanted to take him away. Ellen (my midwife) said, "No, she's been in labor for thirty hours, and pushed for six hours, she's getting her baby." (Kristen S., public relations)

I had four family members with me during the birth. Then they all left me when the baby was born and went to him! (Zenia M., nurse's aide)

That Unique Newborn Look

You may be surprised to learn that newborns, brand-new ones, don't look like the babies that you see on television. Not that you won't love your baby—or think this little one is the most beautiful person you have ever seen—but objectively speaking, newborns may show the ravages of their journey for a few days. To be specific:

- They come out slimy. A new baby may be coated with mucus, blood, vernix (a thick white cream that keeps them from getting waterlogged), and amniotic fluid. If a slippery baby grosses you out, ask to have yours dried off before being handed to you.
- They may have hair in weird places. Lanugo is the name for the hair that some babies have all over their bodies, especially on the face, shoulders, and back. It goes away within a few weeks.
- They often have "cone heads." After a vaginal birth, particularly if pushing took a while, the head will be molded—shaped to fit through. This is an amazing adaptation of humans to squeeze our big brains through our mothers' pelvises—our skull bones are in separate plates that can scrunch together and change shape as needed. By a few days after birth, your baby's head will be round again.
- The scalp or face may look swollen for several days, especially after a vacuum or forceps delivery.
- The stump of the umbilical cord will hang off the belly button for days or weeks, until it shrivels up and falls off.

After birth my daughter looked like an old man—a shriveled-up thing. I wasn't expecting that. (Anne O., director, nonprofit organization)

I had a C-section. When my husband proudly plopped her on my chest, my arms were still tied down and she was rolling toward my face! I screamed "Grab her!" And then added, "and wash her off!" because she still had green meconium and red blood and white vernix on her. Nice first words, huh? (Elisa R., ob-gyn)

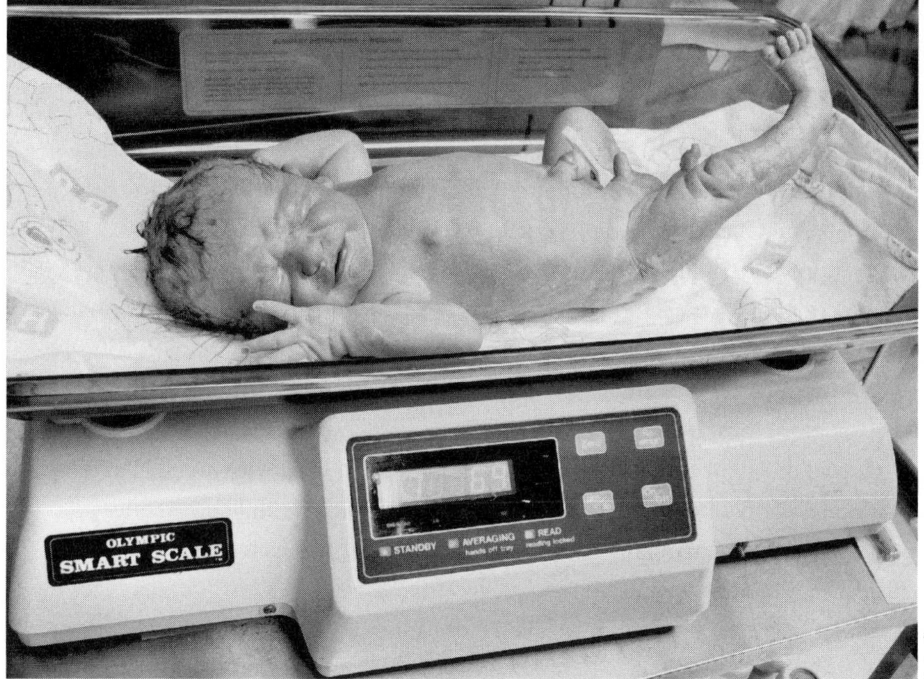

M. Landis

Newborn Procedures

Before you start the phones ringing, you will probably want to know the baby's weight and length, so you'll have something to tell family and friends. The nurses have a few things they will need to do for your new baby as well:

- Medical treatments. The nurses I work with refer to the procedures they perform at birth as "eyes and thighs." Antibiotic ointment is applied to the eyes to prevent blindness from infection, and an injection of vitamin K is given in the leg, to help the baby's blood to clot. Both procedures are required by law for all newborns. In most states, treatment can wait up to one hour, but nurses are often encouraged to check them off their to-do list right after birth.
- Newborn physical examination. Soon after birth the nurse or doctor will briefly check over your baby.

NEWBORN TESTS FOR METABOLIC AND GENETIC DISEASES

Some time ago, hospitals began testing newborns for common diseases and syndromes. The first state-required metabolic test was for PKU, a very rare disease in which a baby can't break down phenylalanine, an amino acid. If left untreated, PKU can cause severe mental retardation, but with early detection and a special diet, babies with PKU develop and function normally. For this reason, even though PKU is rare, the effects of early detection are so beneficial that testing is considered cost-effective. Today, using this same reasoning, most babies in the United States are tested for at least PKU, thyroid deficiency, sickle-cell disease, and hearing loss, with some hospitals automatically screening for more than thirty disorders, and some states only requiring testing for about ten. The March of Dimes website has great information on newborn testing at www.marchofdimes.com. Talk to your doctor or nurse if you want to learn more about your hospital's routines.

- Weight, length, and head circumference. Your baby will be weighed and measured within the first few hours of life. A photo of the newborn on the scale is a fun way to document the weight for posterity, so keep your camera ready.
- Baby bands. While your baby is still in the room with you, the nurse will place hospital identification bracelets on the wrist and ankle. You will wear a copy of the same bracelet, so that you and your baby will be known as mother and child while you are in the hospital. A third bracelet can go on the baby's father or on another person of your choice, if you want. The hospital staff will only give the baby to someone with a matching bracelet. Some hospitals also put on baby ankle tags that activate sensors near the doors and elevators just like at a department store, in the very unlikely event that someone would attempt to walk off with a newborn.
- Blood sugar testing. Smaller babies, extra big ones, and infants of diabetic mothers receive special attention at birth. These newborns may

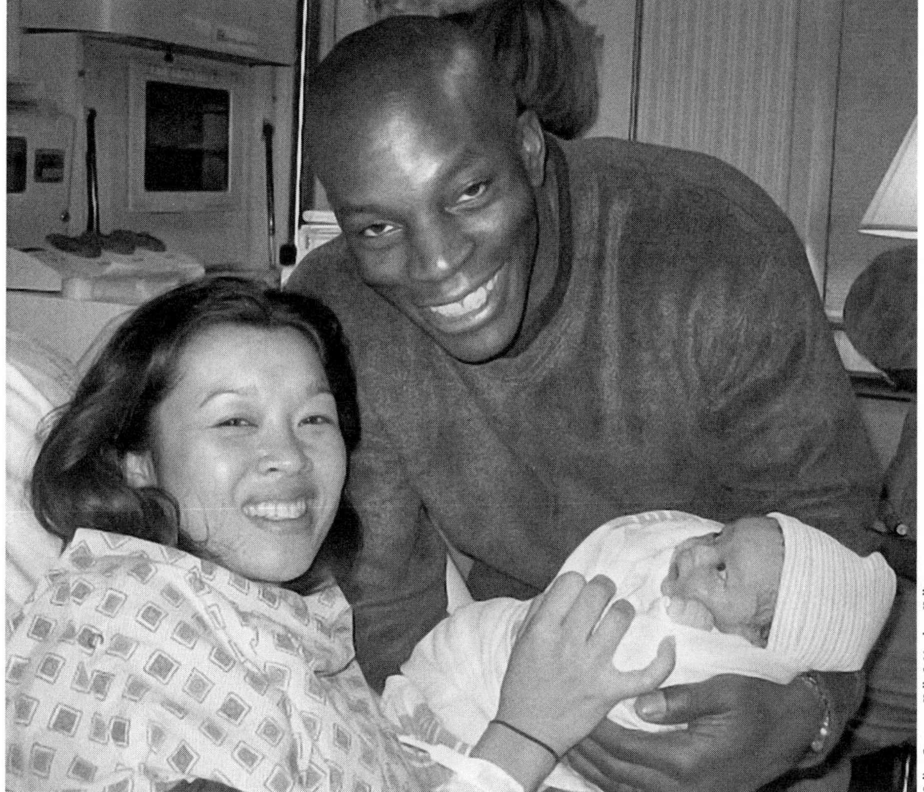

Celina Cunanan-Kelly & Matthew Kelly

have difficulty maintaining their blood sugar levels after they are no longer being fed through the placenta. Small samples of blood are taken from the heel to measure the glucose level after birth. If low, the baby is usually fed quickly, and the blood sugar level is retested at regular intervals until normal.

Family Bonding

Now that your baby is here, it's time to share the news. If you have other children, you may want them to be at the birth, or close by so they can be part of the togetherness right after the baby is born. Conversely, you may feel you need some quiet time with your baby before the troops arrive. Now is the time to snuggle up and get to know this little one who has been growing inside you for the past nine months. Childbirth is over and a life has begun.

Part 7

A Sea Change (Parenthood)

The moment your baby is born, your life—as an employee and colleague, individual and spouse—changes forever. This section will help you anticipate the delights and challenges of taking your new baby home. The transition to becoming a confident parent will be an achievement that rivals anything you have previously accomplished. But how will you strike a balance between your different roles? In the next chapters, I will discuss those first few days and weeks, addressing in particular your physical and emotional recovery, caring for your baby, and having a personal life. I will also go into aspects of reentering the workforce, breastfeeding at work, and strategies to help you achieve that elusive goal: a full and balanced life.

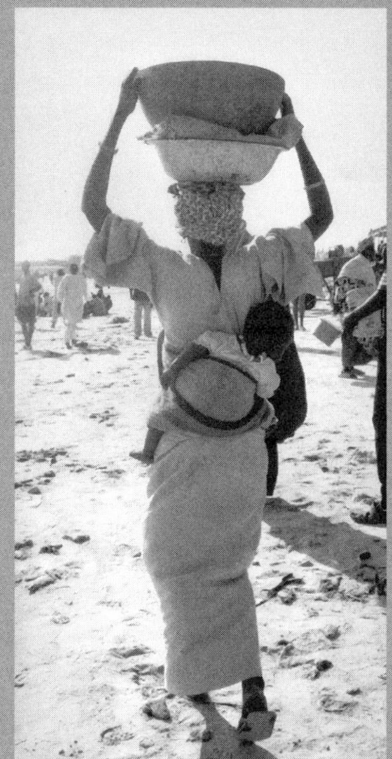

Ana Golpe

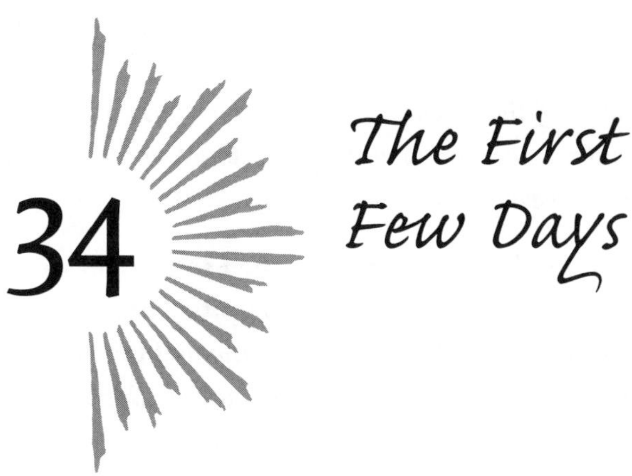

34 The First Few Days

Your first few days after childbirth may be exhausting, but most new moms also are elated and energized by their feelings of pride and love for the new baby. With each touch of a tiny hand or sleepy sigh at the breast or bottle, your life is richer, sweeter, and more vivid. You did it—you brought your beautiful little baby into the world!

> ***It is so empowering to create a life. The accomplishment makes you feel like superwoman. (Annie F., classical violinist)***

Family-Infant Bonding

Bonding is the sense of connectedness between parents and children. It starts with your first contact with your baby and continues over time. Holding and feeding your newborn and spending calm and quiet time together are important ways to build this strong family tie. But bonding isn't a one-time get-it-or-not phenomenon. Adoptive parents bond with their children, and parents of premature or ill babies find ways to bond as well. If all goes as hoped, those first days in the hospital will provide ample opportunities to connect with and enjoy your newborn.

> ***He has his Daddy's toes and he makes very funny faces. I think I love him more every time I look at him. You will have to excuse me, my hormones are a little raging! (Jen B., dance teacher)***

> ***Her dad was really surprised that he was attached. He was surprised that it was important to him since he thought he didn't want any kids. (Cheryl L., lawyer)***

I have very fond memories of the loveliness of my son in those days and the wonderful warm and calm feeling I had with my husband and extended family. (Jane J., advertising executive)

My daughter did not want to be put down for the first six to eight weeks of her life. It was hard on the second night in the hospital because she kept waking up and crying in her bassinet. I kept calling the night nurse for help, but she didn't have any suggestions. Basically, my daughter decided to co-sleep from the start, even though the night nurse wasn't too happy about that. (Cheryl L., lawyer)

The nurse's aide wanted me to keep the baby in the room with me all night. This was my sixth child. I told her, "I'll bond at home; I need to sleep." (Tammy L., accountant)

My husband doesn't function well short on sleep. Natalie and I were doing fine, so I had him go home after we moved to the postpartum floor. I needed that time for Natalie and me to get to know each other. I was also nursing, so there wasn't a whole lot he could do anyway. (Rebecca M., senior vice president, financial corporation)

A friend brought my older daughter to the hospital after Benjamin was born. We had bought this big Winnie the Pooh balloon and tied it to his bassinet in the nursery. We brought her into the nursery and said, "Look at all these cute little babies. Which one do you want?" Of course, she looked around, pointed to the one with the balloon, and said, "I want that one." So we said okay and took him back to our room. (Heidi R., law professor)

Healing after a Vaginal Delivery

Physically, you may be sore, particularly if this is your first delivery.

- The muscles of your shoulders, back, and legs may ache from pushing—after all, you probably never used those muscles quite like that before. If you had an epidural, you might be tender at the site of insertion. These aches and pains usually resolve within a few days.
- For a tender perineum (vaginal opening): ice is your best friend. The

hospital will probably have special sanitary pads that can hold ice chips, or those little packets that if crunched will turn cold. Use them! Ice diminishes swelling and inflammation and numbs the area. After twenty-four hours, sitting in a tub of warm water, called a sitz bath, may be soothing, and helps prevent infection. Oral pain medicines can also be taken to alleviate the pain. For many moms, ibuprofen (Motrin) and acetaminophen (Tylenol) offer enough relief; more rarely, narcotic pain medicines like codeine or oxycodone (Percocet) are needed. Narcotics are constipating, though; wise new moms limit their use. Because episiotomies and birth lacerations often extend close to the rectum (making mothers worry about their first post-baby bowel movements), a stool softener may be prescribed.

- Hemorrhoids, swollen veins near the opening of the rectum, are quite common after vaginal birth, due to the mechanical aspects of pushing. Ice and stool softeners are helpful here too, as well as witch-hazel soaked pads (under the brand name Tucks) and, after the first twenty-four hours, warm sitz baths.
- Pain with urination can be offset by pouring warm water over the area as you urinate: the diluted urine is less irritating to abraded skin. You may also choose to spray the area with an anesthetic like Dermoplast, or urinate directly into a sitz bath. (Urine is sterile, and won't cause infection of the sitz bath water.) The hospital can supply you with anesthetic spray and a squirt bottle for warm water; just ask for what you need.
- Bleeding is often surprisingly brisk for the first few days. Blood loss after birth tends to be heavier than a normal menstrual period, and because tampons shouldn't be used during this time, those who are accustomed to wearing tampons may be especially concerned about the amount of blood that is discharged after birth. Big disposable diaper-like pads are often useful for the first day or two, then maxis. The hospital will supply pads, and either a belt or stretchy mesh underwear that you can use to hold them in place. Small clots are normal. Bleeding should be down to the level of a period within a few days, but a brown to yellow discharge called lochia may persist on and off for six to eight weeks, sometimes mixed with some blood.

- Afterbirth cramps are usually mild with the first baby, and (for unknown reasons) become more severe the more children you've had. These contractions help to diminish bleeding, and shrink the uterus back down to normal. Many moms notice cramps most when they are nursing. Ibuprofen tends to be more effective than acetaminophen for crampy pain.
- Many new moms have swollen feet for a few days after birth. Within a week or two, you'll start to urinate a lot as the fluid moves into your blood vessels and is eliminated through the kidneys—and your feet should feel a lot better.
- Exhaustion after birth shouldn't come as a surprise. You may not have slept for a night or two, and your newborn may not respect your need for sleep. In addition, postpartum hospital units are not necessarily the most restful places. If you are having a hard time, talk to your nurse about limiting visitors and other disturbances, and turn off your phone, so you can rest when your baby sleeps.

The first night on the postpartum floor, someone came in every hour. They came in to check my vital signs, check my sutures, make sure I was okay. When the picture people came back for the third time that night, I seriously almost belted them. Finally, in the morning the pediatricians took Natalie to the nursery, so I thought I would take a shower. I was on the toilet, and the cleaning lady came in! I swear I almost lost it. I turned into the queen bitch and told everyone to stay out of my room. Eventually, they put a sign on the door that said do not enter without checking at the nurses' station. (Rebecca M., senior vice president, financial corporation)

Even though we'd planned to deliver in the birthing center, getting transferred to the hospital worked out okay. If you deliver in a birthing center, you leave in twenty-four hours. I didn't realize what a mess things would be. I just had no idea that stuff would keep coming out of me. I was really grateful to the nurses for cleaning me up. And for the breastfeeding help. We kept Adam with us the whole time. (Elizabeth S., online producer)

Recovering from a Cesarean Birth

Cesarean section is major surgery. The abdomen and uterus are surgically opened and closed; full healing takes months.

- If you had an epidural for delivery, pain medicines may be given through the epidural catheter for a few days, delaying the need for shots or pain pills and their potential side effects. Many hospitals use patient-controlled analgesia, in which you push a button to give yourself more epidural or intravenous pain medicine. (A lockout period and dosage limits will prevent you from overdosing.) Expect some pain, but for a few days be generous in keeping yourself comfortable. Postoperative pain may prevent you from exerting yourself in basic ways like deep breathing, moving around, and coughing—actions that are needed for recovery. For the first few days it is better to load up on pain relief than be afraid to move.
- The intestines are often slow to recover from the surgery, and gas may build up inside. Walking around, lying on one side and then the other, and limiting narcotic pain medications will help the gas to move through. Typically, you also won't have an appetite until a day or two after surgery.
- Your feet may be swollen because of the high sodium content of the intravenous fluids that are received during surgery and normal redistribution of body fluids after birth. Within a week or two your kidneys will clear the excess fluid and the swelling will resolve.

In addition to these discomforts, you will have a catheter in your bladder after the birth. The urinary catheter is typically inserted before the cesarean, to keep your bladder from filling up and getting in the way during surgery. This catheter and its attached collection bag are usually left in until the next morning, saving you a night of getting up to pee.

The nurses got mad at me because I advanced my diet really quickly after my cesarean. I had Ben go get me take-out from Chipotle. The nurse said you can't go from ginger ale to burritos. (Christi M., medical student)

Establishing Breastfeeding

The first few days are key for getting the baby to latch on properly and initiating your milk supply. Right after birth, babies are often in a quiet alert state, which makes it a wonderful time to introduce breastfeeding. Your baby may nuzzle around the breast or even latch right on. It's nice to get a good feeding in right away, because many babies are pretty sleepy for the next twenty-four hours, and getting them to nurse while groggy can be a challenge. After that, most newborns nurse quite frequently, usually eight to twelve feedings a day for the first few weeks. (Which means that much of your first month together will be spent nursing.)

Colostrum, the first milk, is thick and full of antibodies to help your baby. It may be hard to believe that the small amount of colostrum is all your newborn needs, but this is what nature intended. In addition to supplying colostrum to the baby, the most important aspect of nursing in the first few days is communicating to your body that a baby has been born, and that milk needs to be produced. The greatest stimulus to milk production is lots of time spent skin-to-skin with the baby, and the baby's sucking. To make sure you are touching as fully as possible, dress the baby just in a diaper, and either take off your bra, or leave the flaps down on both sides while you cuddle together. Your body heat with the two of you under a blanket will keep your newborn warm. If your baby isn't latching well by about the second day, pumping can help your milk supply to get going, which will then give the baby the reward she's seeking—and lead to more nursing. With excellent breastfeeding support, confidence, and patience, virtually all women can successfully breastfeed. Even so, those three factors can require some work.

- Breastfeeding support. Try to surround yourself with people who champion your desire to breastfeed, a group that ideally will include your nurses, doctors, spouse, family, friends, and any acquaintances who put their two cents in. If you are struggling, spend lots of skin-to-skin time with the baby, and seek out a lactation consultant.
- Confidence. It can be hard to dig up confidence, especially if you have heard lots of stories of breastfeeding "failures." But breasts are made for feeding babies! The best way to feel like you're on the right track

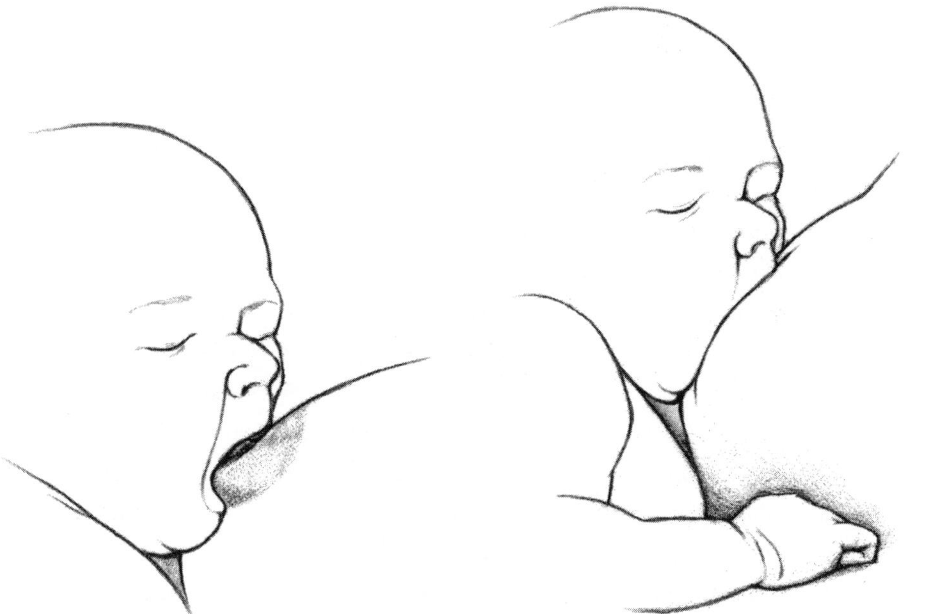

Breastfeeding works best when you don't make the baby latch, but rather allow him to position himself on the breast (with some encouragement, if needed). An effective latch is off-center and pain-free. For more information, see the website of the La Leche League at www.lalecheleague.org.

with breastfeeding is to stick with it and find others who make you feel supported and confident about your choice. For instance, a large number of moms in my practice are part of a local religious community and almost never "fail" at breastfeeding. Are they biologically different than my other patients? I doubt it. But they have tremendous support from their community, and confidence that all women are meant to nurse. Consider joining a breastfeeding support group for the opportunity to create a community of support for you and your baby.

- Patience. Remember that a crying hungry baby cannot learn to latch, and when you are tired and sore yourself, both you and your baby may get immensely frustrated. A mother can help her baby learn to nurse by keeping her little one calm and focused, so the baby will have more controlled movements. If your baby is crying too hard to nurse, move her into an upright position between your breasts. Make eye contact with

PACIFIERS

There are pros and cons to using a pacifier. Some believe that because sucking helps bring in your milk, you shouldn't have the baby suck on a pacifier; when the baby needs to suck, the breast should be offered. Others acknowledge that babies use sucking not only for food, but also to calm themselves—and although some babies find a thumb or fingers to suck, others don't. If you do decide to use a pacifier, I have heard the recommendation to get the type that doesn't have a "wrong side up." This way, when you are trying to give your baby a binky in the car, or when your hands are full, you won't have a 50–50 chance of putting it in wrong. Another blessing about pacifiers in years to come is that they are easier to limit than if your child sucks his thumb. The binky can be allowed only in bed, for example, but your baby's thumb, for better or worse, will always be available for comfort.

her, and talk quietly. Let her suck on your finger, with the soft side up toward the palate. If you feel frustrated, get help from a nurse or lactation consultant, or a calm friend who has nursed successfully. The general rule for the first few days: if half of your feedings are going well, you are doing fine.

I wasn't sure I could breastfeed, and I knew I wouldn't want my husband to see me nurse the baby, but after we had the baby it all seemed just normal and natural. I love being a mom. (Kate R., financial analyst)

When you are nursing, trying to get the baby to latch on, all these nurses keep coming in and grabbing your boob trying to help. I just needed some time alone with the baby to work it out. (Rebecca M., senior vice president, financial corporation)

It took me four days to get him to latch on properly. At one point I think a nursing state of emergency was called, and four nurses surrounded me,

trying to help. It was very frustrating, but once we got going, I loved it. I breastfed for a year. (Maggie P., administrator)

I would emphasize to women who want to breastfeed, to get as much information about it as possible before the baby is born, because you have no idea (a) how tired you'll be, and (b) that you and the baby will have no idea what you're doing. (Kristen S., public relations)

Pain with Nursing

Sometime between the second and fifth day after your baby's birth, your milk will increase from the smaller volumes of colostrum to the larger volumes of mature milk. At that point, you will begin to hear the baby swallowing while nursing, and your breasts may suddenly feel quite full. To prevent them from becoming painful and rock hard (engorged), it's important to nurse a lot on the day this happens, to stay ahead of the milk production and to give the baby a chance to learn how to handle these larger amounts. Feeding more frequently can help tremendously with breast fullness. Look for early cues that the baby is ready to eat, rather than feeding by the clock. If you get behind and are producing more than you are giving the baby, engorgement can lead to hard, painful breasts and a low-grade fever. Heat (using warm washcloths insulated under a baby diaper soaked in warm water) before feeding, and ice packs or cool cabbage leaves (with their perfect shape) afterward, may provide some relief. If the baby has trouble latching on because your breast is too hard, try expressing a little milk first to soften the nipple. After several days, supply and demand will balance out, and your breasts will be more comfortable.

Many new moms experience nipple soreness. Most commonly, this is caused by a poor latch, in which the baby only takes the tip of the nipple in her mouth. This poor positioning is not helpful for you—or your baby. Because the ducts that your baby needs to compress are farther back on the areola (the darker part of the breast surrounding the nipple), she won't get any milk when she sucks on the tip of the nipple, so she will suck harder, compounding the problem. Prolonged or repeated breastfeeding with an incorrect latch can lead to bruising, blistering, or cracking of the nipples. If the nipple bleeds, some blood may get into the baby's mouth, which does no harm to the baby, but it clearly indicates that she was on too shallowly. The first secret to pain-free nursing is getting the baby latched on properly. Breastfeeding is a learned behavior for mom and baby. If you can't manage to get your baby in a position that is comfortable for both of you, don't hesitate to ask for help.

PREVENTING SORE NIPPLES

We used to think that you could "toughen up" the nipples by rubbing them with a washcloth every day for a few weeks before the baby came. Unfortunately, nipple stimulation like this can lead to huge contractions that may stress the fetus, causing heart rate slowing—and it doesn't even prevent sore nipples.

Thinking that it is normal to have pain and putting up with pain instead of doing something about it is the main cause of sore nipples. Don't allow the infant to stay on the breast if you feel any discomfort. Move your breast or nudge your baby into a new position until you are comfortable. If necessary, you can painlessly break the suction of a nursing baby by inserting a clean finger between your breast and the baby's mouth, and pushing down on the breast.

If you already have sore nipples, try these tips for a quick recovery:

- Allow the nipple to get some air between every feeding. This can usually be accomplished by leaving the flaps of your nursing bra down.
- Avoid nursing pads that contain a layer of plastic, which may keep the nipples damp.
- Put a little colostrum on your nipples and allow it to dry after nursing. This can be quite helpful during the first few days, because colostrum is so anti-infective and healing. Mature milk, by contrast, is sweet and may aggravate sore nipples.
- Use purified lanolin cream on your nipples. Purelan, which is specially formulated to soothe raw skin, is safe for your baby.
- Have the baby nurse on the less sore side first, when her sucking is most vigorous.
- Feed the baby more often, so that she will be less ravenous (and maybe gentler) when starting to nurse.

If you find you are using these techniques and products longer than a day or two, get help—to achieve a more comfortable latch as soon as possible.

POSITIONS FOR BREASTFEEDING

A good nursing position is one in which you and your baby are both comfortable, and the baby is oriented so that she can latch on well. The baby needs support for her rump and her neck. Holding the baby in your lap, or lying down and nursing on your side, can both work well. The football hold can be helpful if you had a cesarean and need to keep the baby off of your abdomen for a few weeks.

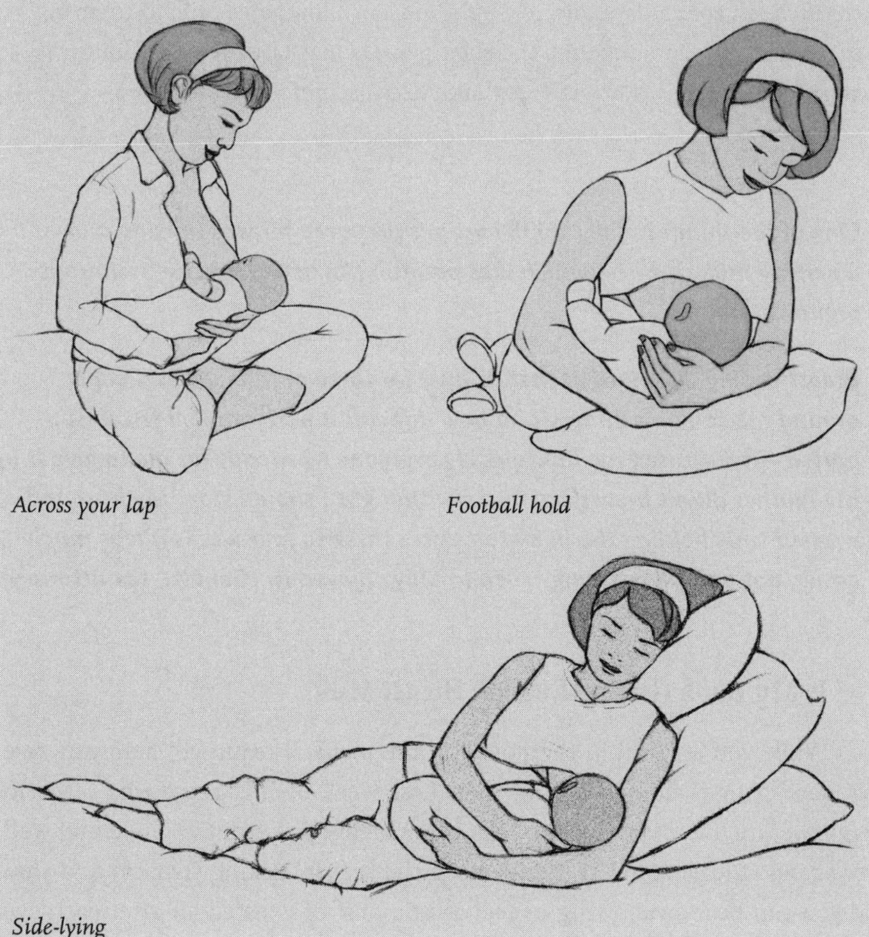

Across your lap

Football hold

Side-lying

BREAST PROBLEMS FOR MOMS WHO ARE BOTTLE-FEEDING

Even if you are bottle-feeding your baby, you may still make some milk. Stimulation of your breasts will only increase your milk production and engorgement. Instead, if you get engorged, wear a snug bra (like a sports bra) twenty-four hours a day, and don't express milk. Many bottle-feeding moms have no problems with engorgement, but if your breasts do become full, ice packs or cold cabbage leaves and oral pain medications should get you through any rough days. Alternatively, you can allow some milk to come out in a warm shower—although the engorgement may last a few days longer if some milk escapes, you will experience less discomfort.

One of the things I really think I wasn't prepared for was nursing and when my milk came in, which was painful. (Anne O., director, nonprofit organization)

Breastfeeding was hard at first. It hurt for three or four weeks. People around me couldn't understand how difficult it was for me. I felt unsupported—it surprised me how quickly everyone was ready for me to give it up. My mother didn't breastfeed and she thought I should stop. My husband wanted time holding the baby too. After three to four weeks it was much easier, not painful or trying. Then I really enjoyed it. (Galit A., tax attorney)

Is My Baby Getting Enough Breast Milk?

While you are still in the hospital, the medical team will help you assess how your baby is doing. During their first week of life, newborns often lose weight before they start to gain. This is not a concern; babies are feeding well if they spend at least some of their time at the breast sucking strongly and slowly and you can hear swallowing or feel a little puff of exhaled air after each swallow. Your breasts may feel softer after your baby eats, and she will seem more relaxed. The first poops—called meconium—will be thick, sticky, and black or dark green. After that, the color will change, gradually lightening to greenish yellow. Once your milk comes in and your baby is actually drinking it, she will make at least six wet diapers and three to four yellow, seedy stools a day. Particularly during the first two weeks of life, when your baby is learning what to do and your milk production is just getting started, pay careful attention to diapers. If your baby is not having at least two stools on any one day, or goes twenty-four hours without a stool, take her for a weight check, since good weight gain is the gold standard for whether your baby is thriving.

Your Emotions

You may feel like you are crossing an emotional minefield after your baby arrives. One minute you are proud and excited; the next, terrified and exhausted. This is normal. On day two or three you may even find yourself crying for no apparent reason, as you experience what is referred to as the baby blues or postpartum blues. This condition has nothing to do with postpartum depression, which is more severe and long-lasting. Usually with the baby blues you know underneath it all that you are fine; you actually can't comprehend why you are behaving so strangely. Thankfully, the baby blues typically last less than two weeks.

Given my "raging hormones," I simply needed to look at my newborn and the tears would begin to flow! (Edie U., school psychologist)

How do you feel about your experience giving birth? Because childbirth can be so intense and tiring, new moms often don't remember key details, and wonder about their labor or birth. Some feel unsettled with decisions that were made, or embarrassed about their behavior. (Of course that's ridiculous—there are no rules for behavior in labor, and your entire medical team understands that you have to get through it however you can.) If you had a doula, she can help you remember the sequence of events—she may even have taken notes for you. If anything about your birth experience is troubling you, ask your doctor or midwife to clarify why things went the way they did, and exactly what happened.

Your partner may have questions or concerns as well. Dads' emotions can run the gamut during these first few days. Talk together about how you each are feeling about the birth, and about the new baby. Even though your roles during the birth were certainly different, having a baby together is a shared experience like no other. If possible, it is nice if both parents can stay in the hospital with the baby. This tends to be less feasible when there are other children at home, but can be a wonderful bonding experience the first time around.

Many mothers expect to feel immediate love for the baby, but not every mom falls in love with her infant at first sight. Try to give yourself some space if you're feeling overwhelmed or full of doubt. You can't make yourself feel differently, even if you are disappointed about your response. Be reassured that within a few months you will most likely feel head over heels in love with your baby—but the first few days may seem more like you have just gotten on a nonstop roller-coaster. Take your time, share your infant with those you love, and get to know this new family member as you nurture her. Maternal feelings don't always turn on like a faucet—and really you don't even know this child yet—it may take days or weeks for you to feel settled with your new baby.

Spreading the News

You may feel like hunkering down with your family and shutting out the world. But remember that your friends, family, and coworkers have been waiting for this day too. They likely felt like they were pregnant with you and will want to be included in your celebratory calls. Yet you may become exhausted if visits aren't limited during the first weeks after birth. Consider inviting nonessential visitors for a short stopover during a specified, limited time span, leaving the rest of the day to get to know and enjoy your new family.

We said anyone could come to visit, but not to stay longer than thirty minutes. I'm glad we set that up beforehand. At the beginning, you're excited, but at the same time, you're just exhausted and need some time to rest. (Christi M., medical student)

Taking Your Baby Home

Before you leave the hospital, ask for advice about how to take care of yourself and your baby at home. The nurses will probably have some written instructions to give you, and they can be a valuable resource for general information:

don't be shy about asking all of your questions, large and small. Obtain prescriptions if you need pain medications and check in with your doctor or nurse for guidance about birth control options. Be sure, too, that you know when you are supposed to see your practitioner again in the office, and when the baby is due to be seen. You may even want to make those appointments from your hospital phone.

For great additional information on the care and feeding of your new baby, check out *Breastfeeding Made Simple: Seven Natural Laws for Nursing Mothers* by Nancy Mohrbacher and Kathleen Kendall-Tackett; the classic *Dr. Spock's Baby and Child Care*, by Drs. Benjamin Spock and Robert Needlman; and the informative and charming *Heading Home with Your Newborn: From Birth to Reality*, by Drs. Laura Jana and Jennifer Hsu.

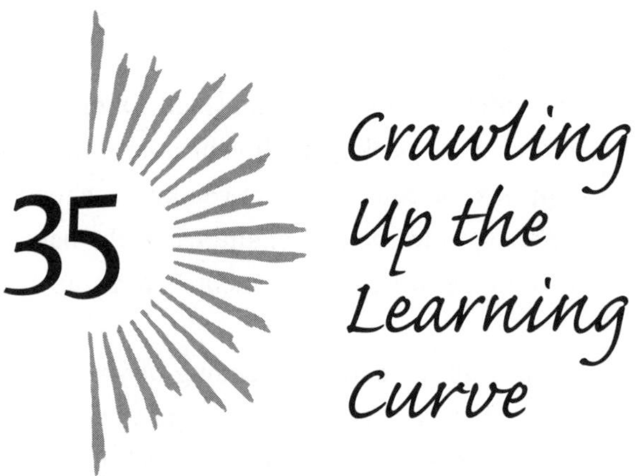

35 Crawling Up the Learning Curve

Arriving home with a first baby, though thrilling, usually feels a bit strange. When you left home to give birth, life was familiar, predictable—even if there were rumblings of changes to come. And now here you are, with this helpless little being in your care, and your world has been transformed.

I think professional women are used to feeling very capable. The day we were taking our first child home from the hospital, I couldn't help being surprised they were going to let me take this home without any special training. Where's my checklist? (Susan G., commercial airline pilot)

The first night at home, she screamed all night. She would fall asleep only when we held her. We had planned not to let her sleep with us for safety reasons, but the only place she calmed down was in our bed. (Danielle R., trust analyst)

Bringing the baby home was a learning experience. Neither of us have our mothers, so we really didn't have anyone to ask: is it normal to cry like this, or is this vomiting a sign of a serious problem? That was scary. (Kate R., financial analyst)

The first night we were home was really hard. You go from being treated like a queen in the hospital to having all the responsibility of this new person. I was knocked off my feet by the love and the fear that I felt. I didn't sleep that first night listening to make sure he was still breathing. The next day I was exhausted. (Annie F., classical violinist)

Introducing the baby to a big brother or sister also represents a sea change in family relationships. You may identify so much with your older child that you feel anxious about disrupting his perfect world, or you may be worried how you will have enough love (and time) for them both. But children do adjust and benefit from having siblings, and most parents of more than two children say that by the time you have your third, taking home a new baby brings pure joy.

I'll never forget leaving our son (who was almost two) to go to the hospital to have our second. I knew that I was going to turn his young world upside-down in just a few short days. He had been our first-born and obviously had our utmost attention and needed to share nothing. I left home in tears. (Edie U., school psychologist)

The second time around, you have a toddler running around, and they want to touch the baby. We were keen on wanting the kids to get along, so I was willing to let him touch the baby, poke her, put her fingers in his mouth. He just seemed so loud and jerky and dangerous around this perfect little newborn that this was really hard to do, even when it was my own child. I don't know if this strategy made any difference, but I have to say that they truly adore each other now. (Linda S., creative director)

They just say, here's your baby, and with the first one you think, oh crap. The second one, you totally know what to do; you're totally confident. (Susan G., commercial airline pilot)

Bringing home our third child was much easier. The boys were best buddies and they were sure that they were getting a sister. Sure enough, we had a girl. The best part about that for the boys was kissing her, playing with my hospital bed, wearing masks, and making balloons with surgical gloves. Ellie was welcomed with open arms. (Edie U., school psychologist)

Challenges

Here's one dirty little secret that no one warned you about: maternity leave isn't "time off." Unless you are outsourcing the care of your new baby, your immediate assignment is to let go of any fantasies about reading books, taking long baths, and catching up with friends during your "vacation." Caring for your newborn is a more-than-full-time job. The two greatest challenges for most first-time parents are time management and dealing with sleep deprivation.

I [now] forgive my friend Gina, who had a baby last year, for all of the times it took her forever to email me back. I figured all babies do is sleep—why can't you email me? I figured it out. They do a lot more than sleep. They cry. A lot. Then they sleep for twenty minutes, eat, and then cry for another two hours. Repeat. For three weeks. I'm kidding. Kind of. I love being a mom—it's just been a long day. (Jen B., dance teacher)

People always tried to tell me how it was going to be to bring the baby home, but I thought I could be in control of the situation. It was terrifying. I thought I fully comprehended how it would be to have a baby. But I was so tired! (Kendra F., civil litigator)

SLEEP DEPRIVATION

Most newborns don't know day from night at first. Eating every two to three hours generally translates to getting up at least twice each night for feedings during the first few weeks. And not all babies go immediately back to sleep. Typically the time between at least a few of the feedings will lengthen out to four hours within a couple of weeks—and if you're really lucky, this might occur in the wee hours, with fewer disruptions of your sleep. Many babies cluster-feed in the evening, tanking up on richer milk that allows them to stay asleep longer. (Formula-fed babies tend to stay full longer, and eat slightly less frequently.) If you are breastfeeding, you're the only one who can feed the baby right now. Your partner, though, can do other things—bring your newborn to you to nurse; change diapers; and resettle the baby so you can just go back to sleep. If you start to get totally exhausted, having someone else give the baby a bottle of pumped breast milk or formula so you can get a bigger block of sleep for a few nights may make all the difference in the world. The most efficient time to pump milk for later use is first thing in the morning, or an hour after a daytime feeding.

I had a lot of trouble at first with breastfeeding. She was a slow eater and I wasn't making much milk. So I would feed for one hour, then pump, then give her a bottle of formula. This left me only a fifteen-minute break before starting over again. This went on all day. After two weeks of this, my pediatrician referred me to a lactation counselor. (Christi M., medical student)

Even with breastfeeding, I recommend the bottle once a day, after the first few weeks. What worked best for us was cluster feeding at night. I breastfed the baby at 7 PM and 9 PM and put him to bed. Soon after that, I went to bed for the night. Then, my husband got him up at about 11:30 PM, gave him a bottle, and put him right back to bed. That way, I got a longer stretch of sleep. My milk production adjusted very easily. After five weeks, the baby was sleeping from 11:30 to 6:30 and I was getting nine hours of sleep. I felt great. (Mary Ellen M., pediatric nurse)

The most important step in protecting your sleep is to rest during the day while your baby naps. This may mean ignoring other things that need to be done—but it is crucial that you get a break, because adequate sleep is necessary for a sense of well-being, and extreme fatigue can contribute to postpartum depression. During these first few weeks, sleep should be one of your highest priorities.

TIME MANAGEMENT

My mother says the secret to happiness is having low expectations. Keep your expectations of what you are going to accomplish in a day lower than you think is possible. I tell all my new moms that if you can get one or two of your physical needs met by 5 PM, you are doing well. That might mean you have had time to eat and brush your teeth, but you are still in your nightgown.

How can a newborn take up so much time? First, feeding takes ten to sixty minutes each time, and at least during the first week, the baby may feed as often as twelve times in a twenty-four-hour period. If you are bottle-feeding, you will have all those bottles to mix up, warm for the baby, and wash up afterward. Then there is diapering (six to twelve times a day), changing clothes when they get poopy or spitty, calming the baby, giving a bath, playing together, and then your own physical care, including eating, keeping up with your fluid needs, and sleeping. Notice that my list doesn't include laundry, dishes, shopping, meal preparation, thank-you notes, entertaining guests, cleaning the house, making phone calls, paying bills, emailing, or taking calls from work. You have to give yourself permission not to be "supermom." Rally friends and family to help you during this time. For at least the first week or two, try to have another supportive adult with you as much as you can. It really helps to have someone to answer the door while you are feeding or changing the baby, give you time to take a shower or nap during the day, and troubleshoot with you when the baby is crying and you don't know why.

Superwoman was just a person who didn't know how to delegate. (Susan G., commercial airline pilot)

The biggest surprise for me when I had my first baby was the consumption of time. I had to schedule in anything that I wanted to do. It was even hard to find time for a bath. I didn't want to deprive the baby of anything so the baby always came first. (Jennifer A., secretary)

The lactation counselor was sort of harsh when I complained about how exhausted I was after two weeks of feeding the baby every two hours, then pumping to improve my milk supply, then giving the baby formula. When I told her that I couldn't get anything done, she said, "What do you have to get done that's more important than your daughter?" She made me feel like a bad mom. The pediatrician was much more understanding—he couldn't believe I'd even lasted two weeks like that. (Christi M., medical student)

I do have mascara on today but not clean socks. You can't have everything. (Jen B., dance teacher)

I don't think I'm depressed. It's not like I don't care about the laundry; I just can't get to it. (Katherine B., psychiatrist)

When I was home on maternity leave after our second, my son went to his daycare because that was my only time to really bond with the baby. Also that way, when he came home, he was able to occupy all of our attention. So he didn't have to feel like he lost his only-child status right away. (Linda S., creative director)

Baby Nurses and Postpartum Doulas

Why get help after birth? Throughout recorded history, in all cultures, new mothers have been relieved of all duties except caring for their newborns. In our modern society, however, many families are spread out geographically and so grandparents or other extended family members may not be able to assist the new mom. For this reason, many parents hire help for those first few weeks at home.

I had a baby nurse because everyone in my family had one. It was expected. (Debbie S., lawyer)

A baby nurse is not a licensed nurse, but more like a nanny, with extensive experience with newborns. Baby nurses generally live in around-the-clock for the first two weeks at home, but in some circumstances may be hired for day or night shifts, or for longer or shorter periods. The baby nurse can teach you about baby care, including bathing, diapering, feeding (breast or bottle), cleaning the cord stump, and care after circumcision, and will help you get your new baby on a schedule. She provides all aspects of care for the baby, including doing the baby's laundry and straightening up the nursery area, allowing you more rest. Baby nurses typically don't do household chores unrelated to the newborn, or errands. The cost for a baby nurse varies depending on her experience and geographic location. Some families find that reimbursement can be drawn from a flexible benefits health plan from work. You can find a baby nurse by asking at your hospital or searching for "baby nurse" online.

Having a baby nurse gave me a sense of security, but when she left I was terrified. In a way, it was just delaying the inevitable. I cried all day. (Debbie S., lawyer)

Postpartum doulas, in contrast, work by contract with you, generally a few hours a day, or overnight. They help in any way necessary—offering education, emotional support, protected time for sleep, and breastfeeding help. They also do errands and light housekeeping, prepare meals, and provide sibling care. Postpartum doulas typically have formal training or certification in newborn care and breastfeeding support. To locate a postpartum doula, ask at your hospital, or search the Doulas of North America website www.dona.org or the Childbirth and Postpartum Professional Association at www.cappa.net.

Most new parents who hire a baby nurse or doula are grateful for the help, instruction, reassurance, and rest. If you plan to hire a baby nurse or postpartum doula, make sure that you have documentation of her training and experience, and allow enough lead time to interview her and check references before you give birth.

When we brought our first baby home I was really freaked out about being home with this creature. So I hired a postpartum doula to help out, which was not a good experience. I'm not very comfortable having someone in my house, paying them to do things for me. (Janet G., attorney)

I would suggest hiring a baby nurse for a shorter time, and then having her come back just for nights a few times a week so you can catch up on sleep. (Debbie S., lawyer)

When he was awake he wouldn't stop howling unless he was moving. My father offered to walk around with him so we could sleep. It occurred to me then that we were going to have to let people help us. I was reluctant to allow help—I wanted to hold him all the time—in hindsight I should have let people help us more. (Annie F., classical violinist)

Emotions

Emotions during those first few weeks can be all over the map. It is important to be aware of how you are doing and to acknowledge your feelings. Almost any feeling you could be having is normal during this time—from ecstatic to overwhelmed and miserable.

I was euphoric after he was born. I just wanted to hold him. I didn't want to drive because I only wanted to hold the baby. The only thing I needed was some sleep. (Annie F., classical violinist)

The postpartum part was the most challenging part for me since my whole pregnancy was so easy. You're bleeding nonstop, so it's just really gross for a while. It's physically painful, but also very emotionally challenging. You have this baby to take care of, and you're sort of waiting to feel like your normal self again. (Amanda O., meeting planner)

Many new moms seem to bottom out emotionally at around two weeks. The novelty of the new baby wears off, and exhaustion from disrupted sleep catches up. Be vigilant in protecting your time and energy for at least two weeks, and then reassess. If you are doing okay, you can add in some other responsibilities and relieve assistants of their duties if you want to. You will get the hang of this, and it will become much easier as you become more competent, and as the baby gets older with less constant needs.

POSTPARTUM DEPRESSION

Many new moms worry about postpartum depression. You hear stories of women harming their children, and you may wonder if that is where your distress is heading. Unlike the "baby blues," which usually last less than two weeks and are characterized by tearfulness and feeling overwhelmed, postpartum depression is a true depression, occurring in about 15 percent of new mothers. Women who have struggled with depression in the past are particularly at risk, as are women with limited social supports, but anyone can develop this disorder of mood and thought. Signs of postpartum depression include hopelessness, apathy, lack of appetite or eating all the time, anxiety, agitation, sleeping constantly or not being able to sleep, and/or feeling disconnected from your loved ones. Some women with postpartum depression have thoughts about hurting themselves or the baby, which may be terribly frightening. Moreover, shame and guilt about these feelings can keep new moms from getting help. But postpartum depression is both common and treatable. Call your doctor, midwife, or mental health professional if think you may have postpartum depression or anxiety. Another resource is Postpartum Support International at 1–800–944–4773 or www.postpartum.net.

POSTPARTUM PSYCHOSIS

Postpartum psychosis is the form of postpartum mental illness that makes headlines. Women with postpartum psychosis may hear voices, have intrusive thoughts, or harm themselves or others. About one in a thousand new moms develop postpartum psychosis, but those who do are at risk of serious consequences, including suicide and infanticide. Postpartum psychosis is more common in women who have been diagnosed as schizophrenic or bipolar, or who have these conditions in the family. Husbands and other family members of new moms should be aware of this condition and seek help immediately if the mom is feeling or behaving in an unusual way. Postpartum psychosis is treatable.

I was afraid to go back to work three months after the cesarean. I still wasn't feeling that great. Different doctors told me they thought I was depressed, but I had never been depressed before and didn't recognize it. Eventually I took the prescription for Zoloft and it did make me feel better. (Sherri M., sales rep)

In some ways the second birth was easier because I had more friends to help and I knew the postpartum depression would be coming, so it didn't hit me like a brick as it did the first time. (Anne O., director, nonprofit organization)

I had some depression as I weaned each of my daughters at about a year. The first time, I didn't recognize it, because I thought that postpartum depression only occurred in the few months immediately following birth. When I had my second, and I felt the depression coming on again, I took antidepressants. I'm now enjoying early toddlerhood with my second daughter much more than I did with my first. (Brenda W., lawyer)

Your Continuing Physical Recovery

If you had stitches, you may be sore for weeks. Most moms don't need pain medications after a week or two, except an occasional ibuprofen or Tylenol. Even after a cesarean, by a few weeks most new moms only need over-the-counter medications. This doesn't mean, though, that you will feel totally back to normal. While healing, you need extra sleep, and rest. Once you feel okay, walking will be a perfect way to get exercise. Heavy-duty training like sit-ups, leg raises, weights, running, and other major aerobics, by contrast, should wait for clearance from your doctor or midwife; ask about exercise at your six-week checkup.

COMMON PROBLEMS

- Vaginal bleeding. Bleeding usually slows down by two weeks after birth, but intermittent spotting or light bleeding is normal for six weeks or more. Passing clots larger than a quarter, recurrent heavy bleeding, or discharge with a foul smell isn't normal and should be reported to your practitioner.

- Nipple soreness. Any soreness of the nipples should resolve by a few days after birth. Persistent problems may be a sign of trouble with the baby's latch or might indicate a breast infection, and should be brought to the attention of a lactation consultant or your doctor or midwife.
- Breast engorgement. During the first weeks of lactation, your breasts may feel quite full when you need to feed the baby, and then soften with each feeding, until the process of supply and demand evens out. Once breastfeeding is fully established, moms typically don't get that overfull feeling, even when it's time to nurse.
- Painful nursing. Breastfeeding should be painless. Deep breast pain during nursing can be a sign of an infection in the breast. A sore area on one breast may indicate a blocked duct or mastitis. Call your practitioner or lactation consultant if you have breast pain.
- Leaking from the nipples. When the breasts are full, it is normal to leak from the nipples. Wearing a soft bra even while sleeping can help prevent dripping during the night. Absorbent pads are usually necessary inside your bra, to prevent major leaks. Change them frequently so that your nipples will stay dry.
- Constipation and hemorrhoids. Hemorrhoids are dilated veins located under the skin by the rectum, or just inside the anal opening. They can itch and burn, and may bleed during a bowel movement. Pregnancy, pushing, and constipation all aggravate hemorrhoids. The best treatments for hemorrhoids are to avoid constipation, take sitz baths, and use topical hydrocortisone ointment or suppositories. Constipation can be prevented by limiting narcotic pain medicines, taking an over-the-counter stool softener like Colace, drinking lots of fluids, exercising, and not taking too much iron. Talk to your doctor or midwife if your hemorrhoids or constipation don't resolve after a few weeks of these simple treatments.
- Leaking urine. After vaginal birth, the muscles and nerves near the opening of the bladder can be stretched out, leading to poor bladder control. Strengthening those muscles with Kegel exercises will usually help. If you are still leaking by the time of the six-week checkup, talk to your practitioner. Leaking urine after a cesarean isn't common and should be reported to your doctor.
- Hair loss. After the baby, a sudden drop in hormone levels synchronizes

HOW TO KEGEL

If you are having stress urinary incontinence (leaking with a cough or sneeze), Kegel exercises can get those muscles toned and strong again.

- Identify the muscles that stop the flow of urine. Those are your pelvic floor muscles, which Kegel exercises are designed to strengthen.
- Contract your pelvic floor muscles for five seconds.
- Continue clenching them for another five seconds (at first you may not be able to get past one or two).
- Release your pelvic muscles slowly while you count to five again.

Do sets of five or ten Kegels multiple times a day. Use common repeated activities to remind you to Kegel—when you are on the phone, anytime you are waiting (red lights, at the store), whenever an advertisement comes on television . . . whatever works for you. With one hundred to two hundred Kegels a day you should see a real difference within a few weeks.

the hair follicles so they all go into their aging phase simultaneously. This can lead to hair loss, which you may notice as a clogged shower drain and thinning hair. While such hair loss may be disconcerting, it is not permanent. This shedding is called telogen effluvium and typically lasts one to five months.

DRIVING

It may be hard to believe that you can't drive right away after having a baby. But think about this: in order to drive safely you must be off of all narcotic pain medicines, not be overly fatigued, and feel comfortable enough to turn around and look behind you to back up, work the clutch (if you have a manual transmission), and react in an emergency. Typically this takes a couple of weeks after a vaginal birth, and three or four weeks after a cesarean.

Visitors

Visitors can be a great help, but not if they expect to be entertained like guests. If someone offers assistance, ask for what you need—run to the store, empty the dishwasher, hold the baby while you get a break. If you are worried about germs, have a bottle of hand cleanser (like Purell) near the front door—and offer it freely.

Visitors who act like company can pose a problem. Most new parents do not have excess energy for entertaining guests. Your doctor or midwife can help here—ask for advice on how long guests can stay, and use that rule when your guests arrive: "I am so glad to see you. My doctor says I can have visitors for up to an hour, so come on in and visit for a short while. I can't wait to show you the baby." It is hard to limit visits when people have traveled from afar, so discourage people who won't be helpful from traveling long distances to see the baby right away. Again, quoting your doctor's recommendations can help a lot in this situation. Your partner, as well as other close friends and family members, may also help by protecting your family from any invasion of unhelpful guests. Talk ahead about what you will need in order to limit stress during this challenging time.

Sharing the Load

The baby's father (or other co-parent) can take on many important roles when the new baby comes home. Although he can't breastfeed, he can bring you the baby to nurse, change diapers, take charge of the bath, shop, give you a break for a shower, and run interference with visitors. Some new moms want to do it all—and feel that they are more competent or more suited to newborn care than their partners—but you have to realize that if you take over all of the baby care, you will always be more competent, setting up a situation in which he won't feel comfortable taking care of the children. If you really want to share parenting, you need to start right away. Optimally, the dad should take some family leave at this time, so he can share childcare duties right from the start.

My fiancé bet me 150 diaper changes that I'd get an epidural. He's still paying. (Danielle R., trust analyst)

They graciously gave my husband two weeks of family medical leave, and it was so nice to have him around in the beginning. I remember his first day back to work, I was a wreck. I cried all day. (Jill H., gynecologist)

The baby and I didn't mesh very well at first. He needed to eat constantly and my nipples were torn up. I consider myself to be a very together person. I thought I ought to be able to handle this. But when my husband had to go back to work after a two-week paternity leave, I thought NO, you can't. (Kendra F., civil litigator)

If there are older children at home, the dad may need to take over some jobs that might have been the mother's, such as bath time or food preparation. He can spend time with the children when the new mom is tied up with the baby, helping to buffer the effects of all these changes, or bond with the baby while mom enjoys the older kids.

If there is no other parent in the picture, friends and family members will need to pitch in. A postpartum doula or baby nurse may also help ease this transition.

Because I had a C-section, I couldn't carry her up and down the stairs. My husband Ben had to go back to school, so my mom stayed with me during the first week, then Ben was there on the weekend, then his mom stayed the next week. It was so nice to have someone there to cook meals for us and help me so I wasn't stuck with the baby on one floor of the house. (Christi M., medical student)

When it's your fourth or fifth child, people seem to forget that the birth even happened. When it's your first child, family and friends come to visit to help out, but after that they think you can do it yourself, that you're some kind of expert. (Carolyn S., parenting educator)

Relationship Stresses

The arrival of a new baby can stress the parents' relationship. If the dad is back at work, he may be tired when he gets home, especially since he too may be up at night. He can't understand what the mom's day was like, and may want her to take care of *him*, especially since she "isn't working" now. Meanwhile she has been with the baby nonstop. She is exhausted and wants to be rescued. She has been waiting all day for help. You can see how this might lead to conflicts. Now is a crucial time for good communication. *Babyproofing Your Marriage*, by Stacie Cockrell, Cathy O'Neill, and Julia Stone, is a terrific resource on communication. Partners need to express their concerns and listen to the other's reality. A sense of humor helps a lot as well. This isn't easy! Who needs more sleep at night: the new mom who is with the baby 24/7, or the dad who has to work the next day? Negotiating a fair balance is a key part of parenting.

My husband and I did not fully realize how brutal the first year of having a new baby could be. The sleepless nights led to exhaustion, which led to bickering, blaming, and decreased satisfaction with our relationship. Someone told us that their first year with their first child was the most difficult year of their marriage. This comforted us tremendously. Sure enough, sometime during our daughter's second year, things began to improve. (Brenda W., lawyer)

Sex

A new mother will typically find that her sex drive is very low. Hormonal changes, fatigue, discomfort, distraction, and (for a breastfeeding mom) constantly sharing her body with the baby all may play a role. After six weeks, when sex is attempted, vaginal lubrication may be poor, due to the hormonal changes after birth and the low estrogen levels during breastfeeding. Sex can be quite uncomfortable from these hormonal changes and from tenderness due to birth trauma, which may last for months. Needless to say, a sore bottom (or a sensitive abdomen from a C-section) doesn't make sex more alluring. Dads too may find that they are so tired or distracted that sex isn't on the agenda for a while.

It took a long time to have the desire for sex simply due to exhaustion. It took a good six months to really enjoy sex again. Once I felt better, we were fine. (Edie U., school psychologist)

Even if you are the rare new mom who has the urge, it is advisable to wait until the bleeding has stopped before resuming intercourse. Many doctors recommend holding off until after the six-week medical appointment—so that your practitioner can be sure that you have healed, and that your cervix has closed down, diminishing the risk of infection. Until your six-week checkup, too, you should use only pads, not tampons, because tampons may increase the chance of developing a uterine infection.

Your first period after having a baby can be weird. It may be heavy or light, short or a bit long. If you're nursing, you probably won't get a period for months, though a bottle-feeding mom may get her period by eight weeks postpartum. Keep in mind that your first ovulation may occur before your first period; bottle-feeding mothers have been known to already be pregnant at their six-week doctor's appointments. Breastfeeding itself is a pretty good contraceptive for a few months, but it is not 100 percent effective. If you are going to resume sexual activity before seeing your practitioner, be sure at least to use a birth control method like condoms or a spermicide.

While sex may not seem too tempting to most new moms, closeness is still important. Some women become so involved with the baby that their partners are barely on their radar. Fight the urge to focus only on your little one: your relationship needs attention too. If sex seems to have taken a back seat, don't be surprised—you are not alone. But if you and your partner are finding that your sex drives are mismatched, or that you aren't feeling close, talk together about what you can do to meet each of your needs. Get in the good habit now of setting some time aside for each other.

After about three weeks of nursing a hungry baby, it was incredibly wonderful to have my husband kiss and appreciate my breasts without rooting or latching on! (Deb L., writer)

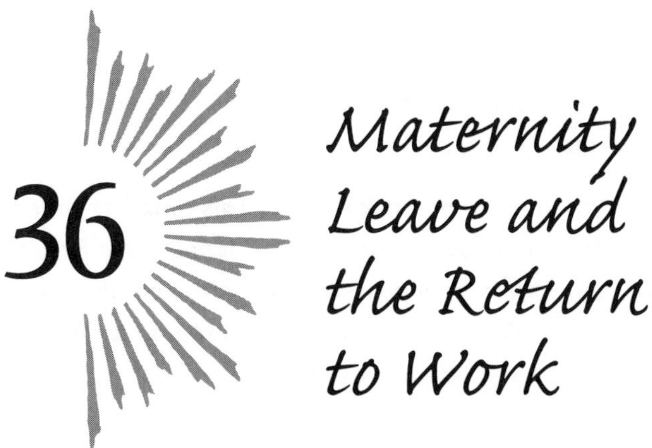

36 Maternity Leave and the Return to Work

It may not seem so at first, but eventually you will get into a rhythm of taking care of your infant and getting through the day. Your little one should start sleeping better, and you will learn to read her signals and feel more confident in your responses. Feeding, too, will be less of a struggle—ultimately either the breastfeeding will work out, you will bottle-feed, or you will figure out some sort of combination of approaches that satisfies your baby. In short, you will discover what works best for you and your family.

Making the Most of Your Maternity Leave

Many working moms feel out of their element when they are first home with their babies. They are used to waking up each morning and getting out of the house, having a structured and social day, and tackling a to-do list full of measurable accomplishments. Against this backdrop, the adjustment to the somewhat unpredictable rhythms of a newborn can be difficult.

Because social isolation amplifies these challenges, finding a group of other moms can make all the difference in the quality of your maternity leave. Connect with friends, neighbors, a parent center, a playground, a breastfeeding support group, a community center, baby-and-me classes—whatever kind of group feels right for you. The important thing is to find a way to meet other moms home with babies who can offer you companionship and support (as well as a reason to get out of the house now and again).

The hardest weeks don't last forever: over time, babies become a lot more fun. By two months, your infant will start to respond to you, smiling, laughing, and (best of all) obviously recognizing you. Caring for your little one will feel more rewarding as your baby starts giving back.

Only one more week 'til I have to go back to work. This time has gone by so fast. My little man is laughing now and looks right at you when he smiles. If you spit your tongue out at him he'll do it back. He also had his first major explosive bowel movement. Don't worry—I took a picture of it for Daddy so he wouldn't feel left out. (Jen B., dance teacher)

Interacting with Your Workplace

Some new moms are able to put their jobs totally behind them. But many women must continue to meet some work demands during their "leave."

One benefit of waiting to have children until later in life is even though I had more responsibility at work and couldn't really take time off, I also had more flexibility and could adjust my schedule to fit my reality. (Jane S., state governor)

I was responding to emails regarding work issues within three or four days of getting home from the hospital. Had it not been for the fact that I had a C-section, I could have been at work comfortably. (Jane J., advertising executive)

I was the ONLY employee, so I had to hire someone to replace me while I was gone. I went back to work with Joe when he was about three weeks old. I put up a crib in my office and started coming in sooner than I had planned because what was needed just wasn't getting done. I worked from nine to three o'clock four days a week. (Anne O., director, nonprofit organization)

If you must interact with your workplace during your maternity leave, try to:

- Designate one person for all communications with you—so you don't have to deal with multiple contacts. (And don't forget the thank-you present if that role is burdensome!)
- Use email as much as possible, so you can respond according to your family's schedule.

- Be the one placing the call, if you must be in phone contact (and hopefully only one call each day). Unless your baby's naptime is totally predictable, you will be less stressed if you choose when to put on your work hat.

I really felt like my boss sort of wrote me off. The human resources department would say things like "If you come back . . ." I would think, "IF? My husband doesn't have a job; you mean WHEN I come back." It was like they expected me to change my mind and not come back to work. And I wondered what opportunities they were letting others have under the presumption that I wasn't coming back. The idea that I might be missing out on opportunities just killed me. (Jane J., advertising executive)

Preparing for Reentry (or Not)

Many new mothers are not paid at all during their "family leave" and financial pressures hasten their return. Others feel a personal need to get back to the workplace, and still others have a strong desire to stay home. Factors that typically play a role in the decision about when and if to return to work include:

- The family's need for the income
- Costs of childcare
- The belief that the mom should be home with the baby
- Worries about someone else watching the baby
- The desire to be with the baby more hours a day
- A personal need to remain in the workforce
- Commitment to the job
- Enjoyment of working
- Enjoyment of being home
- Baby's sleep habits and health

I went back to work after five weeks. I did miss my daughter, but I had to go back for financial reasons. I used a lot of my time before I even had her. I used the five weeks that I had left of paid personal time. (Mihsah B., factory worker)

I remember walking to the mailbox to get the mail, and it was just exhausting. I had friends who had given birth around the same time, and they wanted to meet at the mall for lunch. I felt sort of defeated, like I should have been stronger. (Susan G., commercial airline pilot)

The downside of being the boss is that things may not happen when you aren't there at work, so I had to go back. Katie adapted very well to daycare, but then she was only seven weeks old. I cried; she didn't. (Juanita G., research scientist)

I did not have a choice because my husband is out of work, but I would have returned quickly anyway because in general I really like my job. (Jane J., advertising executive)

It was very hard to leave [my children], but I was looking forward to returning to some adult interaction. (Stephanie B., FedEx courier)

I only took four months off in part because I am not an infant person and was eager to get back to work, and in part because I didn't want to take too much time off when I had only started at the job eleven months earlier. (Janet G., attorney)

I have noticed that people who love their jobs go back no matter what the maternity leave policy is. My job only gave me ten weeks. My baby was colicky and when I asked for more time they said no, so I quit. (Brenda W., lawyer)

While I was very reluctant to return, after being back I really feel it is good for me to have a focus in addition to my son. Many women I have spoken to say that working out of the home makes them better moms. There is still a great deal of guilt that accompanies working, and I hear from others that this just continues as your child grows, but I have to admit that after being an independent working woman for some time, at least part of my sense of self and value is tied into my work. (Loren W., vice president of marketing)

Not planning to return to work—I don't really make enough money to cover the cost of daycare. Plus you worry about a not-so-great daycare.

I think eventually I'll go back, just not for the next couple of years. (Zoe B., inventory manager)

Many parents find that their plans change: they feel differently than they expected once their baby has arrived. You have the right to change your mind. Be aware, though, that if you don't go back to work, you may owe your employer the cost of any benefits, including health insurance payments, paid on your behalf during family leave (but not those paid during disability leave).

When I was pregnant with my first child, I expected to return to work full-time and continue my career as I had it planned. Once I held that incredible baby in my arms, I no longer wanted to work as many hours. (Jenny K., internist)

We had thought my husband would stay home with the baby, but after she was born, he felt these new responsibilities to support his family and wanted to work more. Meanwhile, all I could think of was how to organize my life around this baby. I was shocked by my change in feelings about how important my job was. (Emily H., executive director, nonprofit organization)

When the babies came along, I thought I would like to stay home; I really wanted to be a mom. But I realized pretty quickly that I became bored and irritable and that I missed being with adults. I was just a better person to be around when I was working. (Jill H., gynecologist)

Even with the small amount of time I was out (six weeks), I feel as if it hurt my career. Part of my job was given to someone else during my time out of the office, and I have not gotten a single high-profile project since I have been back. I wish I had gone back after three or four weeks because I think I would not have lost as much ground in my career. (Jane J., advertising executive)

Whenever I was not working, I felt I should be working. I fit in better with moms who work. But when I tried to go back to work, it didn't feel right. (Debbie S., lawyer)

I'm a financial analyst—I plan, that's what I do. But I shouldn't have planned to go back to work. It wasn't right for me. I didn't realize how I

would feel. I used to be all about my job and being one of the boys. But I love my new role in life as a mother. I feel like my values are better; I know what is important and I am less stressed. (Kate R., financial analyst)

The transition back to work made me question my career (which I loved and still do). Yes, work was important, but nothing would ever be all encompassing again. It just couldn't be. (Rebecca O., librarian)

The decision about when and if to return to work may be subject to external pressures as well. Family members, coworkers, employers, friends, and acquaintances may all weigh in on your decisions. Once you think it through, and feel like you know your own mind, have confidence that you are the best judge of what's right for you and your family.

People really questioned me about going back to work when she was only eight weeks old, but I had been off since five months into the pregnancy and I wanted to get back to work. I needed to reconnect with that self. I missed the structure from work, compared to a day with a two-year-old. (Julie M., veterinarian)

When I went to mommies' groups, I didn't want to say that I was ready to get back to work because that's not really the accepted way to feel about it. (Cheryl L., lawyer)

Women feel strongly about if you should work after you have the baby. It is aggravating—such a sense of self-righteousness about the choice to stay home. They suggest that women who work don't provide the same quality of mothering, when studies show that working women and stay-at-home moms spend about the same amount of time with their children. The home moms just do other things. Friends who worked full-time advised me not to slow down my career, or [I would] take a pay cut and end up working just as much. In the end you just have to make your own decisions. (Naomi B., attorney)

Some of my female colleagues had expectations that I would "pave the way" on a variety of things such as working shorter weeks or taking the twelve weeks off, and I was seen as not being very helpful since I only took six weeks

THE LONG-TERM FINANCIAL IMPACT OF LEAVING THE WORKFORCE

Although staying home with the baby is clearly the best choice for some women, I worry that many parents are not taking the years ahead into account when they make these decisions. Even though childcare costs may consume most of a mother's salary when her children are young, the tradeoffs may be worth it. For one thing, although traditionally female jobs like teaching and nursing often have programs to help women reenter the workforce, many other jobs are not so accommodating—so the lost time may permanently derail a promising career. And while no one expects divorce or a major financial reversal, these misfortunes do occur. Staying away from paid work for years typically makes it harder for a mom to cope with such challenges because it compromises her earning capacity (not to mention her 401K account) and her self-confidence in the working world. I hate to see women stay in terrible marriages because of the effects that divorce would have on their (and their children's) financial stability.

after my son was born and went right back to a full-time schedule. I think in some ways the women in my office felt I betrayed them because I didn't push for more motherhood time. (Jane J., advertising executive)

I have slowed down my career to do both—in my firm you are essentially off the partner track while you work part-time. I often feel that both worlds get short shrift, but at least I have it set up so that I can ratchet my career back up later. (Naomi B., attorney)

We used to talk about how our salaries just barely covered the childcare expenses, but we still wanted to stay in the workforce, accumulate retirement benefits, keep current in our professions, and have a source of self-esteem that wasn't entirely wrapped up in our kids. (Jean B., editor)

Planning Ahead for Your Return

If you are planning to return to work, get back in touch with your colleagues as your return date draws near, so you won't be blindsided by changes, and so they can get used to the idea that you will be back soon. Don't forget to thank those who have been covering for you—sincere appreciation can help diffuse any simmering resentment. Consider bringing your baby for a visit the week before you return, too, both to ease your way back in and to get any return-to-work paperwork out of the way. Choose a time that won't disrupt the workplace too much, so that people will have a moment to say hi.

If you plan to breastfeed, talk to your boss or coworkers ahead of time if that will help you make the arrangements that you need. On average it takes ten to twenty minutes to empty the breasts, and you will have to allow time to set up the pump and clean up afterward. You will need privacy, as well as a way to keep the milk chilled until you get home. Plan ahead for how you will manage, and present your strategy in a matter-of-fact way. Some women find it more comfortable when they use the most clinical terms and keep their breasts out of the discussion: "milk" rather than "my milk," "pump" instead of "breast pump," and "nursing" rather than "breastfeeding." For more tips on breastfeeding and returning to work, see Chapter 38.

Find out the policy on pumping and storing milk before the baby is due. Make sure you have a plan in place if breastfeeding is something you think you want to do. Also, make sure you are going to be able to take the breaks that you need to pump. (Mary Ellen M., pediatric nurse)

As you prepare for your return, look through your wardrobe. Most likely, you are not exactly the same shape as you were before you had the baby. Be sure you have some clothes for those first few weeks back—your early pregnancy clothes may do. If you'll be pumping breast milk at work, loose tops that can be lifted up, or clothes with vents in the front made for nursing, will help you avoid exposing a lot of skin when you pump. Bright or dark print tops are least likely to show if milk leaks during the day; a blazer over will offer extra security. Cottons and synthetics stain less than silk, and dark colors are better than pale. Above all, avoid one-piece outfits—you would have to get nearly naked to pump!

Childcare Options

Childcare arrangements should be made as early as is practical, but the timing varies depending on your plans. Some daycare centers have yearlong waiting lists. Nannies, by contrast, usually can't be hired months ahead unless their current job is scheduled to end or you are willing to pay them for their time before they start working for you.

Think about what sort of structure will meet your family's needs: in-home with a nanny or au pair, daycare in someone's home, or care in a daycare center? The costs of childcare vary depending on the sort of arrangement and what you negotiate. In calculating what you can afford, remember the childcare tax credit, and check if your employer provides a flexible spending account. In a flexible childcare account, your workplace withholds several thousand dollars from your pay, then reimburses you for eligible childcare expenses using pre-tax income.

The greatest challenge may be figuring out which daycare will provide the best experience for your little one. Daycare centers and some family-run daycares will be licensed, which means that they meet minimum state requirements. Accreditation through organizations such as the National Association for the Education of Young Children is voluntary, and usually holds the daycare to a higher standard than licensure does. (You can check whether your favorite center is accredited at www.naeyc.org.) Get recommendations from friends and family members who have used daycare; your human resources department may also know of centers that have worked out well for other employees. Visiting the setting a few times before sending your child is also important, to see for yourself how the staff interacts with the children. Consider convenience factors as well as quality of care—picture yourself back at work, using the arrangements you have made.

Children need to know they are loved. They don't get scarred because you go away as long as they are cared for by other loving adults. (Annie F., classical violinist)

DAYCARE CENTERS

Daycare centers tend to be large facilities that group children in rooms by age. Some employers offer daycare on-site. Many daycare centers have long waiting lists: if you think you will choose this option, start your research early in pregnancy.

What Parents Like

- Daycare centers are more regulated and scrutinized than care in a private home or with a nanny would be: they must be licensed by the state and may be accredited by national organizations, and other parents come and go throughout the day.
- Daycare centers have predictable, reliable hours that are not dependent on one care provider's availability.
- A good daycare center is professionally run and structured around age-appropriate educational activities.
- As your child gets older, she will especially enjoy socializing with the other children.
- If you only have one child, a daycare center may be less expensive than hiring a nanny.

Drawbacks

- Some daycare centers don't take young infants.
- Strictly enforced hours may not coincide with your work schedule and can put pressure on the end of your workday if you must pick up by a certain time.
- Exposure to lots of children may lead to frequent colds and other infections. And because centers have strict rules about sick children, and will not allow your child to come with a cold or fever, you may be left without childcare even when your child is only mildly ill.
- Fees are per child, so if you have several children, hiring a nanny actually may be less expensive.

Our daycare center was great. I loved the fact that the owners and teachers at the school treated my children like they were their own and shared in the joy of watching my children grow; that my kids were doing fun, creative, and educationally sound activities in a very safe environment; and that they loved going to school each day. (Laura J., writer)

FAMILY DAYCARE

Childcare in someone else's home is called family daycare. A family daycare provider may be a stay-at-home mom who is supplementing her income by taking in an extra child or two, or someone who runs a business of providing in-home care for children.

What Parents Like

- The setting is smaller than a daycare center and the atmosphere may feel more similar to home.
- Older babies benefit from socializing with the other children.
- Family daycare is often less costly than a daycare center, and if you only have one or two children, also less expensive than hiring a nanny.

Drawbacks

- In-home family daycare is not as regulated or supervised as daycare centers are: many family daycares operate below the radar of accrediting organizations.
- With family daycare you may be more dependent on the availability of one person—if the caregiver needs surgery, for instance, childcare may not be available for several weeks.

NANNIES

A nanny cares for your children in your home. Some nannies have professional training in early child development; others are women with experience with young children but little formal education. For this book I will use the term nanny for anyone in the spectrum of personnel who come into your home to provide childcare, even though some reserve that term for professional caregivers trained at a nanny school.

What Parents Like

- Having someone in your home is very convenient: you won't need to get the baby up, fed, and dressed while you are getting out in the morning.
- Professional nannies are trained in infant care and child development.
- If your child has a cold or other mild illness, childcare will still be available.

NEGOTIATING WITH A POTENTIAL NANNY

Your nanny is a very important person in your family—ideally, she is part of a parenting team. The best way to make sure that your style and expectations match is to discuss the important details of the job completely and honestly, and right up front. If you are hoping for some housekeeping services along with childcare, or have strong feelings about television watching or vacation time, negotiate before hiring your favorite candidate. Be clear, too, about how taxes will be withheld and what your nanny's Social Security contribution will be.

- For care in your home, you set the house rules.
- If you have a few children, a nanny may be less expensive than daycare.

Drawbacks

- You are totally dependent on the person you hire. If she calls in the morning to say she can't come to work, a parent will need to stay home or scramble to make other arrangements.
- Nannies are mostly unregulated, and have no supervision while on the job.
- Nanny-school nannies are screened and trained but typically limit what they do to help your family: they are only there for childcare. They may do the baby's laundry or some baby food preparation, but may not be willing to tidy up the house or run to the store.
- As time passes, the child and sitter both may feel isolated at home.
- To pay your sitter legally, you must contribute to worker's compensation and unemployment insurance, withhold federal taxes from her salary, withhold her half of Medicare and Social Security taxes (or pay her half) and then, when you submit your federal taxes, pay what you withheld and what you owe on her behalf. Each January, you will need to provide her with a tax reporting form.

Hire a nanny so you don't have to worry about daycare drop-off and pick-up. (Lisa H., community planner)

When I was hiring our first nanny, I wanted her to clean up the kitchen after breakfast and empty the dishwasher, but I was embarrassed to ask because I thought she might be insulted. When I broached this with the agency, they suggested that I just describe what the job entailed, and then offer her the job. It worked out great; she cared for our son (and us) for five years. (Maggie P., administrator)

AU PAIRS

An au pair is a young woman (or man) from another country who lives with your family for a year. In exchange for room, board, and a stipend, she will take care of your children for a number of hours each week. Au pairs are not employees; they live as part of your family, taking meals with you and sharing your home. The agency will screen and interview the applicants, although you will be able to briefly interview several by phone before one is placed with you.

What Parents Like

- Au pairs are convenient and less expensive than nannies, and provide the added benefit of acquainting your children with other cultures.
- Their hours tend to be flexible because they are living in.
- They always show up for work because they live there.

Drawbacks

- Au pairs are usually young, and may not have experience in infant care.
- The forty hours of care a week they typically provide may not meet the needs of parents who work full-time and commute.
- Many au pairs have never been away from their families before and get homesick.
- Au pairs sometimes behave like the young adults they are, and may have active social lives when off duty (like going out to bars and coming in late).
- Changing caregivers annually can be emotionally hard on the family.

HAVING A FAMILY MEMBER OR CLOSE FRIEND CARE FOR YOUR CHILDREN

Care from a family member may seem like the perfect solution—a person you know and trust, with whom the children will have an ongoing relationship, provides childcare at no cost or at less cost than hiring outside help. Although this sort of arrangement can work well, be aware of several potential drawbacks: without an employer-employee relationship, you may not be able to ask the person to help you in exactly the way you need help—be it varying their hours or helping with chores; she may have her own ideas about child-rearing that don't fit with your values; and if things don't work out, family relationships can become strained.

Get live-in help if you can afford it. (Jane J., advertising executive)

The difficult thing about having an au pair is that you aren't sure if you are the employer or the parent. Don't worry about sharing your home with a stranger, though. As soon as you walk in, the au pair will leave to go out with her friends. (Elisa R., ob-gyn)

I'm lucky because my mom lives with us and takes care of him most of the day. On the one hand, that's terrific because I know he's loved and cared for, but on the other hand, I can't really tell her how to raise a child. I mean, she raised me, and she thinks she did a pretty good job. (Jane J., advertising executive)

BACK-UP CHILDCARE

Be sure to take emergencies into account: what are your back-up plans if your baby falls sick or your caregiver suddenly becomes unavailable? Some communities have visiting nurse services that will arrange in-home care for a mildly ill child. Think ahead about contingencies, and try to have two or three alternative arrangements.

You really need to designate between the two parents who's going to be the backup parent during the day. One of you needs to have a job that's flexible enough to leave if there is an emergency. (Cheryl P., radiologist)

MAKING THE CHOICE

Leaving your child with someone else can be scary. Don't stop researching until you are comfortable that you have found a good option for your family. If you are breastfeeding and want to continue, be sure that your childcare provider wants to work with you to help you succeed. Talk to other parents, interview the care provider or daycare director, call references, and if considering a daycare center or family daycare, be sure to visit and see the caregivers in action before you make a choice.

FOR MORE INFORMATION

- Childcareaware.org is a nonprofit organization with information and connections to daycare.
- The National Association of Childcare Resource and Referral Agencies at www.naccrra.org provides lists of accredited daycare centers by location.
- For an excellent resource to help you think through all the options, check out Linda H. Connell's *The Childcare Answer Book.*

STARTING CHILDCARE

Once you have made your arrangements, consider beginning childcare before you return to work. If possible, ease in with an hour the first day, and then some longer stretches. Ideally you should leave the baby for at least one whole day before you need to be back at work. This will give you some time to get ready, allow you to observe the situation, and help you and your little one to adjust to the new arrangements.

If you are nursing, pump a bit more during the weeks before you resume work so that you will have a stockpile of bottles ready, and won't feel pressured to express a lot of milk at work while you are adjusting to your return. Try pumping before the baby wakes up in the morning, or an hour after nursing, or pump on one side while the baby feeds from the other. Some mothers find that if they can get the baby nursing from just one breast at each feeding, each breast gets used to only emptying every six hours or so, making it easier to pump less frequently at work.

Try to get the baby on a schedule from the beginning. The schedule will change several times in the first couple of months, but it is always easier to leave the baby with a caregiver if you can have some sort of schedule in place. It is better for the baby, you, and the person watching your baby. It helps everyone feel a little more secure while you are working. Even now, Sean feels security in knowing what is coming next and is really easy to leave with family or babysitters. (Mary Ellen M., pediatric nurse)

Getting Back to Work

Some workplaces will allow you to use family leave to phase back in, working part-time for a while before ramping up to full speed. If you must return full-time, try to start midweek, so that you will only have to manage two or three days before a weekend break.

I had to go back to work this week! Boo. Just a couple of dance classes then all hell breaks loose next week. I cried when I left. I had to tell myself that he doesn't even know I'm gone! It is nice to be among adults again. (Jen B., dance teacher)

On your first day back, try to arrive early to feel less frazzled. Do a test run beforehand, so you are realistic about how long it takes you to get up and out. New moms often describe their first days back to work as "wrenching." You may feel sad, anxious, or disoriented, but you will get back up to speed quickly if you stay focused. Remember that your colleagues and employer may be watching you to see how serious you are about working. If you are committed to staying in this job, the best thing you can do is try to be professional and efficient. Things typically get easier after a week or two.

The first day I went back to work, it felt like Velcro on my heart. (Elisa R., ob-gyn)

I was worried that he wouldn't know I was his mom once I went back to work. Someone told me that children always know their parents, because

the quality of the interaction is just different. That was a relief to hear—and it was true. Even though I returned to working sixty hours a week when he was seven weeks old, it was obvious that I was his favorite person in the world. (Marge G., obstetrician)

Know that no matter what or who takes care of her, when you walk through that door it is you, the mommy, that she wants and prefers. (Brenda H., pediatric resident)

Going back to work was hard for the typical reasons but nice to do adult things, use my brain, talk to more people. (Galit A., tax attorney)

The first day back to work is just the worst. I sent myself flowers both times and took myself out to lunch on the first day. I had to do all these little things for myself to remind me that I had this other part of my life that I enjoyed and that I could enjoy a leisurely lunch without having a newborn sucking at my nipple. The first week was very tough, but after that, I found my stride. And now that one's a preschooler and one's a toddler, I actually enjoy going to work. (Linda S., creative director)

I remember when I dropped off Jonah, I cried on the public bus all the way to work. The first one is just heart-wrenching. With the second and third, you're prepared for those emotions. (Carolyn S., parenting educator)

I was driving to my office that first morning and I was tearful, and there was a traffic jam. I felt irritated and had the "why me's" pretty intensely that morning to begin with. I finally saw up ahead what was detaining all of the cars. It was a mother duck crossing the street with all of her babies behind her. I had such a powerful urge to turn my car around and go home to my baby. (Rebecca S., program director)

Once at work, it was very much "business as usual," so much so that it felt a little strange to feel so normal, by which I mean not traumatized from being away from my son. (Loren W., vice president of marketing)

The first day back to work was awful. I cried on the way in, and I called my parents just to have someone to talk to during the drive. Then the second day was much easier. It's really hard to leave in the morning, but now I really enjoy the time at home and at work. (Christi M., medical student)

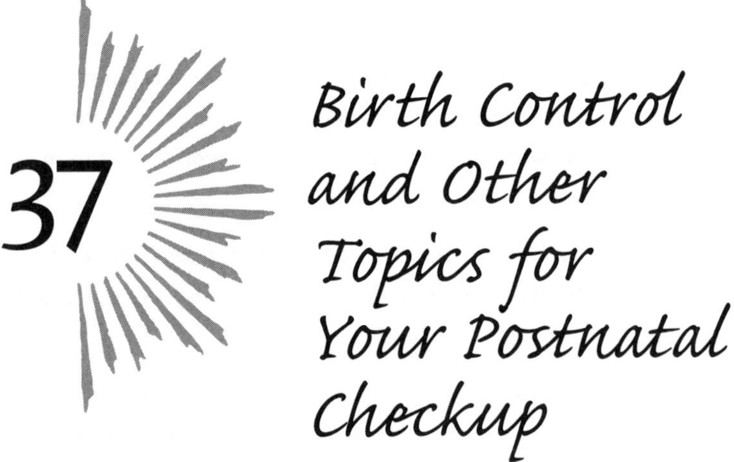

37 Birth Control and Other Topics for Your Postnatal Checkup

Your doctor or midwife will probably ask to see you for a routine postpartum checkup about six weeks after your baby is born. Your medical team wants to find out how you are recovering from birth, ensure that you have a contraceptive method (if you want one), and answer your questions. Often this visit is also useful for obtaining medical clearance for your return to work and for talking about when it's safe to have sex again. Most new moms bring their babies to their postpartum checkups, to show off their adorable bundle to the staff who helped make it all happen.

The Postpartum Visit

During your postpartum appointment, tell your doctor or midwife how you have been doing. Be sure to report any pain or bleeding, and bring up your concerns. Constipation, hemorrhoids, leaking urine, breastfeeding, hair loss, fatigue, resuming work, exercise, sex, and emotions are all common topics for this appointment. If you have questions about anything that happened during labor, raise them now so you can feel settled about your experience.

You will probably have a physical examination, including a breast check and a pelvic exam. Your uterus and cervix will be examined to see that they are getting back to their pre-pregnancy size and shape. A Pap smear can also be obtained if you are due.

If you had any vaginal stitches, your practitioner will see how the area is healing, and give you a green light when it is okay to restart sexual activity. Many new moms are afraid that sex will hurt. Talk to your doctor or midwife about what to do if you do have pain when you resume intercourse.

Contraception

Birth control is one of the most important topics for the postpartum appointment. Even if you don't have any sex drive yet or you're still sore, someday you may again want to have sex, and you will need to be prepared. In the table on page 442, birth control effectiveness is calculated in percentages that refer to the proportion of couples who would not get pregnant using that method for a year. The failure (pregnancy) rate is 100 minus the effectiveness. For example, if a method were 90 percent effective, 10 percent of couples using that method consistently for one year would be expected to get pregnant.

After the baby, my sex drive was so low. When my doctor asked what I wanted for birth control, I asked for something that would decrease my husband's sex drive! (Gita K., research scientist)

NATURAL BIRTH CONTROL METHODS

Some parents opt out of using store-bought contraceptives, and instead rely on more natural techniques such as:

Abstinence

- Advantages: Very effective, given that if sperm don't enter the vagina they can't reach the egg.
- Disadvantages: Generally not the most fun choice, and it eliminates one path to feeling close with your partner.
- Notes: Many factors conspire against an active sex life during the first few months after a baby arrives. Hormonal changes after birth and during breastfeeding may diminish a woman's sex drive and cause vaginal dryness; sex may also be uncomfortable due to vaginal healing or a cesarean incision. In addition, many couples are simply too tired during the first few months to focus on sex.

Natural Family Planning

Natural family planning (also called periodic abstinence or the rhythm method), uses the calendar, daily body temperature, and/or cervical mucus changes to identify ovulation; sex is then avoided during the fertile time.

- Advantages: This method is accepted by all religious faiths and is hormone-free.
- Disadvantages: Natural family planning requires fairly regular menstrual cycles—which may not regulate for months after having a baby. And your body's usual ways of signaling ovulation and an impending period won't be reliable during the first months after the birth.
- Notes: Natural family planning requires that you know your body well and are willing to carefully track your monthly cycle. Couples who use it successfully typically need to abstain from sex for more than a week each month.

Lactational Amenorrhea Method

To prevent pregnancy, the lactational amenorrhea method relies on the fact that breastfeeding suppresses ovulation. This method is 98 percent effective at preventing pregnancy if your baby is younger than six months and is only getting breast milk (no solids or supplements), *and* if you have not yet had a period. Otherwise, all bets are off.

- Advantages: This very effective method is accepted by all religious faiths.
- Disadvantages: For many couples, "98 percent effective" is not reassuring enough. In addition, most new moms supplement with food or formula before six months, so the lactational amenorrhea method will not be an effective technique for very long. And beware: after six months, the first period is likely to be *preceded* by ovulation, so a pregnancy can occur without the warning of a missed period.
- Note: I know of a nurse-midwife who became pregnant while breastfeeding, before she even had a period. She found out she was pregnant with her second daughter when she felt the baby move!

Withdrawal (Coitus Interruptus)

With the withdrawal method, the couple has intercourse, but the man pulls out before ejaculation.

- Advantages: Withdrawal works for some couples.
- Disadvantages: May be unsatisfying; requires self-control on the part of the male partner; and not always effective.

BARRIERS AND SPERMICIDES

Interfering with the sperm's ability to reach the egg is a common approach to contraception, especially postpartum, when nursing moms may not want to use hormones. The most common barrier methods are:

Latex Condoms (Male)

A latex condom is a sheath that fits around the man's penis to capture any ejaculated sperm. Male condoms are most effective when they are used before intercourse starts, not just before ejaculation.

- Advantages: A lubricated condom can add lubrication for sex, which may be lacking right after the baby and while you are nursing; it can prevent sexually transmitted infections; and it doesn't require taking a medication every day, which is an advantage if sex is infrequent.
- Disadvantages: Condoms are not effective if they stay in the bedside drawer—and their use requires that the couple interrupt their love-making. Some men complain of the decreased sensation, but other couples enjoy the delay in the man's orgasm that goes along with this slightly diminished sensation. If you are latex-sensitive, you may have a skin reaction from the condom.
- Notes: Latex condoms can be purchased at your drugstore. The best types say "reservoir tip," but with all condoms, be sure to leave room at the end for the ejaculate so it won't break. Condoms containing spermicide are no more effective than plain ones—there isn't enough spermicide on them to make a difference.

Female Condoms

A female condom is a polyurethane bag that is inserted into the woman's vagina before intercourse. A ring on the edge prevents the whole condom from falling into the vagina, and a ring inside at the end of the bag keeps the condom from falling out during sex.

- Advantages: The female condom prevents sexually transmitted infections. It also doesn't require taking a medication every day, which is appealing if sex is infrequent.
- Disadvantages: Requires that sexual activities be interrupted to insert the condom.
- Note: Some couples find the looseness of the female condom unpleasant.

Spermicides

Vaginal suppositories, foams, gels, or films that are inserted before intercourse to kill the sperm before they reach the egg are referred to as spermicides.

- Advantages: Spermicides do not require taking a medication every day, which is helpful if you are having sex only once in awhile. And although they are not that effective when used solo, when combined with lactational amenorrhea, spermicides can give you that extra protection you are seeking.
- Disadvantages: You may need to interrupt your sexual activities to use a spermicide.
- Notes: Spermicides can be found near the condoms at your local drugstore.

Diaphragm

A diaphragm is a latex dome that you fill with spermicidal jelly and then place into the vagina before intercourse—although it sounds like a barrier, the primary purpose of the diaphragm is to hold the spermicide over the cervix.

- Advantages: A diaphragm doesn't require taking a medication every day if sex is infrequent, and it is slightly more effective than spermicide alone.
- Disadvantages: Sometimes changes in the vaginal walls make it difficult to fit a diaphragm until a few months after the baby. Requires planning ahead or interruption of sexual activities.
- Note: Must be fitted and prescribed by your practitioner.

HORMONAL METHODS

Some women choose hormonal contraceptive methods after the birth of their babies. The most well-known of these methods are:

Estrogen-Containing Pills, Patches, or Rings

Whether the hormones enter your body through your mouth (pills), skin (patch), or vagina (ring), estrogen-based methods use hormones to suppress ovulation. Hormones are usually cycled three weeks on and one week off, allowing for a monthly period, although some formulations lead to less frequent periods.

- Advantages: These very effective methods do not require planning for sex.
- Disadvantages: Estrogen-based methods are not compatible with breastfeeding, at least for the first six months, because they will interfere with the quality and quantity of your milk. (After six months, they may be a good choice for nursing moms.) You also must remember to take a pill every day, change a patch weekly, or change a ring monthly.
- Note: Bottle-feeding moms can use estrogen-containing contraceptives starting around six weeks after the baby is born.

Progestin-Only Birth Control Pills (the "Mini-Pill")

Progestin-only birth control pills are taken every day of the month. They interfere with the cervical mucus and uterine lining so that the sperm can't get to the egg.

- Advantages: The mini-pill does not contain estrogen and is safe for breastfeeding moms and others who shouldn't take estrogen. It also doesn't require planning for sex.
- Disadvantages: The mini-pill is not as effective as standard estrogen-containing pills.
- Notes: Every pill in the pack has real hormone in it—you can't skip the last week like you may have if you took regular pills in the past. You should also be aware that the mini-pill doesn't bring on a period; you get your period whenever you were going to.

Depo-Provera (DMPA or "the shot")

Depo-Provera is a synthetic progesterone that lasts for three months after it is injected.

- Advantages: Depo-Provera is very effective and may lead to absent periods. It also is very simple: you just need to get a shot every three months, and you don't need to plan for sex. This method is a good choice if you should not take estrogen.

- Disadvantages: Depo-Provera can cause weight gain, irregular bleeding, and possibly an increased chance of osteoporosis (brittle bones) later in life. Its longevity is also a concern for some women. It may take up to a year to regain fertility after use, and there is no turning back: one shot remains in your system for six to twelve months.
- Notes: Many women receiving Depo-Provera injections will have irregular bleeding for the first six or twelve months; many have no periods at all after that. Not having a period while on hormonal birth control methods is safe (as long as you are certain you aren't pregnant). The uterine lining is just so thin that it doesn't need to shed.

Implantable Rod (Implanon)

Implanon is a thin plastic rod that is surgically inserted under the skin of the upper arm, where it slowly releases a version of the hormone progesterone.

- Advantages: The implantable rod is very effective and doesn't require any attention after insertion. Even though its contraceptive effects will last three years if left in place, fertility is regained immediately after removal. It may be used by women who shouldn't take estrogen.
- Disadvantages: Implanon will cause your menstrual cycles to be irregular or absent. It requires a minor in-office surgical procedure for insertion and removal, after which you may have swelling or pain at the insertion site. Many women also don't like that the rod may be felt or seen under the skin.
- Note: The Implanon is similar to Norplant, a six-rod system that was taken off the market due to problems with removal. The single rod is designed to be easier for the doctor to take out.

Emergency Contraception (The "Morning After" Pill)

Emergency contraception involves taking either progestin (Plan B) or both estrogen and progestin (Preven) hormones within seventy-two hours of unprotected intercourse to prevent fertilization and implantation.

- Advantages: Emergency contraception is very effective, and a good option if the condom breaks or you regret not having used birth control when you should have.
- Disadvantages: This method is not 100 percent effective, and it doesn't provide ongoing birth control.
- Notes: Emergency contraception reduces the chances of getting pregnant by 75 percent. If 100 couples have one act of unprotected intercourse and then use this method, only two will end up pregnant instead of the expected number of seven or eight. If you have not started your period by three weeks after you use emergency contraception, you should take a pregnancy test.

INTRAUTERINE DEVICES (IUDS)

For some women, the easiest, most reliable, and most comfortable method of birth control is the intrauterine device. IUDs are small plastic inserts that your practitioner can place into your uterus after the six-week checkup. A plastic string attached to the device is left protruding from your cervix about an inch into the back of the vagina. You can feel the string with your finger to check that the IUD is still in place. The intrauterine device used to be thought of as a post-conception method, but studies have shown that sperm typically don't make it to the egg when an IUD is in the uterus.

- Advantages: IUDs are very effective and long-lasting, and they don't require remembering a pill every day or planning for sex.
- Disadvantages: These devices are expensive when used only short-term. In addition, IUDs acquired a bad reputation in the 1970s because one type (the Dalkon Shield) had a string that wicked bacteria up into the uterus, causing severe infections. All of the IUDs that are currently available are much safer than their ancestors, although occasionally complications or infection can occur around the time of insertion.
- Notes: Two types of IUD are available. The copper IUD (Paraguard) may make your periods heavier or crampier than usual, so if you had bad periods before the baby, the copper IUD might not be a good choice for you. This IUD lasts for ten years and can be inserted after unprotected

intercourse as a "morning after" contraceptive. The other kind, the progestin IUD (Mirena), releases a small amount of hormone into the uterus and lasts for five years. Abnormal spotting or bleeding may be troublesome for the first few months, but once that window is past, most women have either no periods at all, or only light bleeding once a month—either of which is safe, and often a welcome side effect.

COMBINING METHODS

Two less-than-perfect birth control methods can be combined for excellent protection. If one method is 90 percent effective, but you use it with a method that is 70 percent effective, you have 70 percent protection on that 10 percent chance, improving the odds of contraception to 97 percent, with only a 3 percent chance of getting pregnant in a year.

- Advantages: Combining methods allows you to optimize their effectiveness.
- Disadvantages: You'll have to deal with the disadvantages of each method.
- Notes: Often breastfeeding moms can rely on the lactational amenorrhea method in combination with another simple method like a spermicide or the mini-pill. And as women age and their natural fertility diminishes, a method that you may not have felt safe with when younger, like withdrawal or spermicide alone, may become a reasonable choice.

PERMANENT METHODS

Sometimes a couple will know when their family is complete. In this situation, permanent contraception may be a welcome way to transition into a life stage when sex is just for fun.

Tubal Ligation

Tubal ligation is a surgical procedure in which the fallopian tubes are obstructed so that the sperm and egg can't meet. It can be performed at the time of a cesarean, immediately after a vaginal birth through a small incision near your belly button, or beyond six weeks postpartum using a laparoscope through one or two small abdominal incisions.

- Advantages: Tubal ligation is a very effective procedure; if cesarean is needed, the tubes can be tied after the baby is born without adding significant surgical time, risk, or discomfort for the mother.
- Disadvantages: If done with laparoscopy, tubal ligation typically requires general anesthesia. Also, although the procedure is considered permanent (and so you must be certain that you never want to get pregnant again before going ahead), for about one in a hundred women, tubal ligation fails and pregnancy occurs.
- Notes: Even though reversal procedures exist, they are very expensive and not covered by insurance. And because of the occasional failure of tubal ligation, if you think you are pregnant after having this procedure, take a home pregnancy test.

Hysteroscopic Tubal Obstruction (Essure)

During the hysteroscopic tubal obstruction procedure, coil-shaped plugs are inserted into the fallopian tubes through a telescope placed into the uterus through the vagina. The plugs can be placed six weeks after childbirth or later.

- Advantages: Hysteroscopic tubal obstruction can be performed in the doctor's office under local anesthesia. It doesn't require an incision or significant recovery time.
- Disadvantages: Only a limited number of doctors are currently trained in this technique, and it hasn't been around long enough to know for sure whether there will be any long-term issues.
- Notes: Hysteroscopic tubal obstruction requires backup birth control for three months, and then an X-ray dye test to be sure the tubes are occluded, before you can rely on it for effective birth control.

Vasectomy

Vasectomy is a surgical procedure in which the male partner's vas deferens (the tubes that carry the sperm) are tied off through a small incision in the scrotum. Vasectomy requires only local anesthesia.

- Advantages: Vasectomy is very effective, and among the permanent options, costs the least and has the lowest risk of complications (because of the minimal anesthetic and no entry into the abdomen).

Comparing the Effectiveness of Birth Control Options

Method	*Odds of not getting pregnant during one year of use*	*Compatible with breastfeeding?*
	Natural Methods	
Abstinence	100%	Yes
Natural family planning	80–99%	Once regular cycles resume
Lactational amenorrhea method	98% if all rules are followed	Yes
Withdrawal (coitus interruptus)	81–96%	Yes
	Barriers and Spermicides	
Latex condoms (male)	88–97%	Yes
Female condoms	75–95%	Yes
Spermicides	79–94%	Yes
Diaphragm	82–94%	Yes
	Hormonal Methods	
Estrogen-containing pills, patches, or rings	97%	No
Progestin-only birth control pills (the "mini-pill")	96%	Yes
Depo-Provera (DMPA, or "the shot")	99.7%	Yes
Implantable rod (Implanon)	99.6%	Yes
Emergency contraception (the "morning after" pill)	See text	Yes (Plan B preferred)
	Intrauterine Methods	
Intrauterine devices (IUDs)	99%+	Yes
	Combining Methods	
Any two methods	Multiply the two failure rates to calculate the new failure rate	Yes
	Permanent Sterilization	
Tubal ligation	99%	Yes
Hysteroscopic tubal obstruction (Essure)	May be as high as 99.8%	Yes
Vasectomy	99.8%	Yes

Note: The failure rate (chance of getting pregnant in a year) is 100 percent minus the effectiveness.

THE DOCTOR'S NOTE AND POSTPARTUM MEDICAL LEAVE

Your job may provide forms for your practitioner to fill out, stating when you gave birth and how much leave you need. In general, employers have standard amounts of medical leave allowed for vaginal birth (usually six weeks) and for cesarean (typically six or eight weeks). If you are truly not physically ready to return to work after that period, because of a medical problem or complications from birth, your doctor or midwife can confirm that in writing. Such a letter may provide you with prolonged disability benefits, which typically pay better than family leave. Conversely, if you want to resume work before the standard six weeks are up, your job may require a note clearing you for early return.

- Disadvantages: Although reversal procedures exist, they are very expensive and not covered by insurance.
- Notes: Because some sperm may remain "downstream" from where the vas deferens is tied off, additional birth control must be used until a semen analysis shows that sperm are no longer present.

After we had the baby, Tim was going to get a vasectomy. But one month after my third child was born, even though we knew this would be our last, I just didn't feel ready and he agreed, so we used condoms for a year before we felt ready for this permanent decision. (Deb L., writer)

After we had our second child, I wasn't ready to have any kind of permanent birth control procedure. Even though we knew we wouldn't have any more children, I didn't want to close that door and admit we were really past that phase. (Beth L., computer science researcher)

Our diocese offers a course in natural family planning, and now we know so much more about what happens to my body—even my husband does. The course lasts six weeks, and there's a book that goes with it.

What's nice is that they're always there to call if you need help or have a question, even years after you take the class. (Norma J., teacher)

Questions

Often new moms have saved a lot of questions about their physical and emotional health for the postpartum appointment. Making a list of all your concerns in advance can save time, and ensure that your needs are met during the visit. Remember, too, to take along any forms you need to have filled out for work.

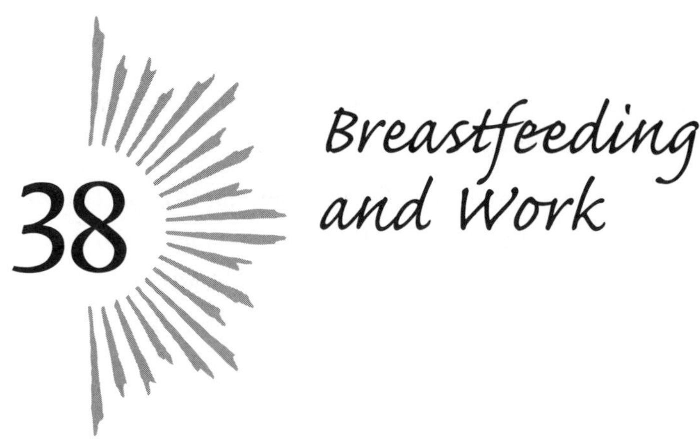

38 Breastfeeding and Work

Many mothers and babies really enjoy nursing, and the moms find a way to continue to nurse upon their return to work—whether by running out to the baby during the day or having the baby brought in, pumping milk, or breastfeeding during just the morning and evening. A lot of different arrangements have allowed mothers and their babies to enjoy the intimacy and wonderful health benefits of breastfeeding even around a busy work schedule. The information in this chapter will encourage you to think creatively about how you might continue to breastfeed (if you want to) and will provide information about the logistics of pumping, storing, defrosting, and feeding the baby your milk.

> ***I sincerely believed that my milk was best for my baby. I also thought that the closeness and contact of nursing would help to support the bond between us despite being separated during my work day. (Kari S., librarian)***

> ***I nursed for a year. That pump was more attached to me than my purse was. We'd be out on live shots and I would just lock up the live truck and plug into the generator. The windows were all dark. (Eileen M., weather reporter)***

> ***I scheduled my lunch hour at the same time each day so that I could go to my son's daycare and nurse him. (Kari S., librarian)***

> ***I didn't pump at work. I worked in a clinic five minutes from home and would run home to nurse during the day. I nursed my son for twenty months. I pumped at home sometimes to stockpile milk for when I wasn't there. (Karen D., veterinarian)***

If you travel a lot for work, arrange to bring your child and a caregiver or spouse with you. (Elizabeth S., online producer)

With my son, I was able to breastfeed for eighteen months, but I pumped constantly. I pumped at work, at home. I just pumped, pumped, pumped, pumped, pumped. With my second, pumping at home was just out of the question. Maybe on weekends, but I wasn't going to stay up until midnight to pump when I had two kids and had to be at work the next morning. (Linda S., creative director)

When you're breastfeeding and you come home from work, don't worry about a schedule. Your body will adjust—just feed the baby. You throw out the clock, and it works. (Carolyn S., parenting educator)

Planning for Your Return

Whether you plan to pump milk or provide formula, returning to work before your baby is six months old means she will probably need to learn to take a bottle. Most sources tell you not to introduce the bottle too early, so as not to disrupt breastfeeding. Others recommend one bottle a day starting ten days before going back. But research that looked at introducing one bottle a day at just two weeks of age found that babies continued to breastfeed just fine; and early initiation, at around three to four weeks, may have its benefits: for example, it will allow the mom to have a break while the dad or other caregiver has an opportunity to feed the baby. Keep in mind, though, that if the baby gets a bottle and you don't pump or hand express that amount of milk, your milk supply will probably diminish. And once you start giving a bottle, it is a good idea to continue to offer it most days—many parents tell stories of the six-week-old who took the bottle so well that they discontinued the practice, only to find that their four-month-old was totally unwilling.

IF YOUR BABY IS RELUCTANT TO TAKE THE BOTTLE

- Have someone other than you give your baby the bottle, and stay out of sight and earshot during the feeding.
- Make bottle-feeding fun and relaxed; try again later if your baby doesn't seem interested. If the bottle becomes a battleground, your baby will

develop negative associations with bottle-feeding and it will become more difficult.

- Offer a bottle containing breast milk or formula as a toy when the baby isn't ravenously hungry. Most babies like to put toys in their mouths and will find it interesting and pleasant.
- Experiment with different feeding positions, milk temperatures—and if using formula, with different brands. Ask your baby's doctor for recommendations.
- Don't panic if your baby isn't interested in taking a bottle. If all else fails, she can be fed with a rubber-coated or plastic spoon, eyedropper, feeding syringe, or from a small, soft plastic cup. Babies will not starve or dehydrate themselves out of stubbornness. For detailed instructions on these alternate techniques, see the website www.askdrsears.com or talk to your lactation consultant.

Make sure you or someone gives your baby a bottle before you start back to work. There is nothing worse than calling to check on the baby and hearing them screaming in the background because they are hungry and you are not there to feed them. For some babies, it takes a while to get used to doing both. (Mary Ellen M., pediatric nurse)

BOTTLES FOR THE BREASTFEEDING BABY

There are several bottle types, in different shapes and systems. You may have to try a few to figure out what works best for your baby. One benefit of the type with plastic bag inserts is that you can freeze milk in the sterile plastic bags that come with the bottles, and then when you defrost it, you don't have to transfer milk to another container. Some experts, though, believe that several of the beneficial properties of breast milk, including the antibodies, are better maintained when the milk is frozen in glass or polypropylene (frosted plastic) bottles, rather than in plastic bags.

Nipples vary in material, shape, and in the size of the holes, which determines how fast the milk comes out. Milk should drip out slowly when the bottle is held upside down, and should squirt if you squeeze the nipple. Preemie nipples may be too flimsy for an older baby with a strong suck—the tip can actually break off (a choking hazard). Start out with nipples that are appropriate for your baby's age, then figure out what your baby likes. Some babies do better with silicone nipples rather than rubber. Nipples marketed as "orthodontic" aren't particularly better for the baby than other shapes, but some babies prefer them.

To encourage continued successful breastfeeding, select a bottle nipple that is most responsive to how a baby nurses—deep latch-on, a lot of suction, a tongue that "strips" (sequentially compresses) the nipple—and most closely resembles the slow flow of milk from the breast. Try to find a nipple with a long shank, wide base, and small holes preferably on the top rather than the tip. Nipples that imitate nursing include Avent System Newborn Nipple, Munchkin Slow Flow, HealthFlow Stage I, and Gerber Nuk.

To mimic nursing, position the nipple fully in the infant's mouth (at least one inch in) so that the lower lip covers the broad base and the jaw is open wide. Some people suggest holding the baby as if breastfeeding, switching arms mid-feeding, but often babies do better with a bottle if they are seated in a more upright position. Position the bottle so that fluid just fills the tip of the nipple, keeping it nearly horizontal so that gravity does not cause the milk to flow too quickly. The younger baby (under three or four months or so) may need the adult to "pace" the feeding, watching the baby's face to pull the nipple back out so the baby doesn't gulp nonstop. Play with different nipple shapes and flow rates if feedings take too long. The baby should usually complete a feeding in fifteen to twenty minutes.

Once the baby has started a bottle, it should be finished within an hour, or the remaining milk should be discarded. Germs from the baby's mouth multiply rapidly at room temperature.

STOCKPILING BREASTMILK

Most breastfeeding moms try to store some milk before they return to work, which not only provides a stockpile for the baby but also offers the chance to learn how to work the pump before the pressure of making it happen on the job. Pumping one extra feeding a day can be started as soon as your milk supply is well established. Don't be too discouraged if you don't get much at first; it takes a while for most women to become comfortable on the pump, and to find a setup that works for them. The best times to try are in the morning before the baby wakes up, right after nursing (if your breasts aren't empty), or an hour later. Expect to produce more milk earlier in the day.

Pumping milk from the breast isn't like sucking fluid through a straw—more suction doesn't equal more milk. Instead, nursing depends on "letdown," the milk ejection reflex, which is triggered by touch and emotions, and mediated by hormones. When letdown occurs, muscles in the breast contract and the ducts widen, pushing milk toward the nipple. You may feel tingling or a sudden heaviness in your breasts. Unfortunately, anxiety, tension, and distraction can interfere with the flow of milk. In order to successfully pump, you will need to feel relaxed and in the nursing groove.

The art of pumping is so psychological. If I was stressed and running "just to do it" nothing would come out. Then I would relax, look at a picture of her, and then the milk would flow. Love is what will release your milk, not the machine itself. After a while my body became so used to the process, just the noise of the machine itself would start letdown. (Brenda H., pediatric resident)

To be successful pumping, I had to have a really strong imagination. I used "visualization" techniques. I would picture my baby happily feeding, warm and cozy and then falling off to sleep with a drip of milk coming out of his mouth and his fat little hand unfurled and relaxed. (Rebecca O., librarian)

Initially, I would look at pictures of my baby and listen to relaxing music as I pumped, but now that I am in a routine my letdown occurs even when I am multi-tasking, supporting my breast shields and bottles with one hand and working with the other. (Jennifer J., family practitioner)

I would highly recommend the hands-free pump bra so that if you have an office that locks you can continue to work on your computer or make phone calls while you are pumping. This is also a great way for women who get anxious while pumping to relax and think about other things, thus increasing the chance of letdown. (Rebecca S., program director)

What Kind of Pump Should You Choose?

Breast pumps vary tremendously: by cost, source of power, ease of use, and whether you pump one side at a time or can express from both at once. The options may seem bewildering at first. Lactation consultants can match your needs

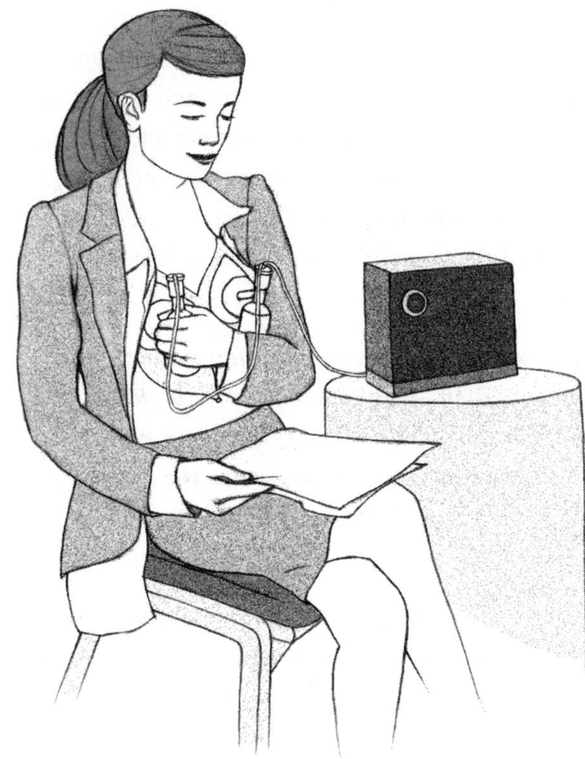

Double pumping at work

and resources to the right pump, but if you're choosing on your own, you'll want to consider these factors:

- Weight and size. Will you carry your pump to work? Where will you store it?
- Suction strength. What is comfortable for one woman is too powerful for another. Try to find a pump with adjustable suction.
- Cycle time. A pump with a quick suck-release cycle option may help with letdown.
- Speed. If you have only a short time available to pump, choose one that can pump from both sides.
- Noise level. If you need to pump discreetly, you will want to choose a quieter model.
- Cost. Manual pumps are usually available for less than fifty dollars, while a good electric pump can run you from seventy to over three hundred

dollars. Under some circumstances, health insurance or a flexible healthcare account will help pay for a pump; ask your human resources department.

- Ease of assembly and cleaning. If you will use your pump every day, you won't want to spend extra time putting it together and getting it clean.
- Rent or buy? Rentals are available for the most expensive, heavy-duty, hospital-grade types. You'll still need to purchase the personal parts: the breast flanges, bottles, and tubing (which total about fifty dollars). Pumps made for personal use, however, may not be sealed and milk particles, which can harbor viruses, may get inside where they can't be cleaned. To avoid infection, then, most experts don't recommend borrowing or purchasing a used personal-type pump. Ameda's personal electric double pump, the "Purely Yours," may be an exception: it is hygienically sealed and specifically designed to be safe for reuse from one mother to the next, as long as the second mother purchases her own new attachments.

Many mothers complain about the noise of the electric pump. They do not want other people to hear what they are doing. To that I say buy two of the manual Medela hand pumps! They work great and are very quiet. (Brenda H., pediatric resident)

I used to do patient callbacks while I was pumping. I worried a bit that it sounded like I was phoning from a dairy farm. (Marge G., obstetrician)

Manual (nonelectric) pumps are the least expensive, but some are tiring to use. The Avent Isis and the Medela Harmony are easier to use than other types, and may actually be preferable to electric pumps under some circumstances. Hand expressing by "milking" the breast can also be effective, especially if you only need to pump occasionally.

Battery-operated pumps tend not to produce as much milk as the plug-in electric kinds do, and although they are less expensive to buy than electric pumps, a significant expense is hidden in the cost of batteries. Most pumps take AA or C batteries; one set lasts through only two or three sessions. Warranties for these pumps typically run only ninety days.

Electric pumps are the most expensive, and typically have a one-year warranty. As you might expect, they plug into the wall socket, but may also provide a battery option or car adapter. A car adapter can be surprisingly helpful when all else fails and you are desperate for a place to pump. The battery option is good when the electricity fails, or if you don't have access to a wall outlet, but is not worth seeking out if it means getting an inferior pump. Having a manual pump available or learning to hand-express can address these situations.

While traveling, my husband didn't like to stop very often for feeding breaks, bathroom breaks, etc. So I had to pump while he drove. One time while zipping down route 77 South I had a feeling someone was watching me . . . I looked out my window only to find a truck driver maintaining a constant speed watching me pump my very full breasts. When he noticed he had been found out, he flashed me a big grin, gave me a thumbs up and sped away. I yelled, "That's what they're for," but I don't think he heard me. (Tina S., lactation consultant)

Because I work in the field and do not have an office to go to, I had to pump in my car. Twice a day I would pump at thruway rest areas or in the parking lots of my customers. After a while I developed a pretty efficient system. In order not to have to wash or sterilize anything outside of my house, I brought two sets of pumping supplies with me in the morning in Ziplock bags. I kept a cooler in the car to store the pumped milk. (Deborah S., sales rep)

Some electric pumps mimic the baby, sucking quickly at first to stimulate letdown, and then more slowly after a few minutes, in a process called "self-cycling." They typically have a button so you can manually switch speeds as well. Less sophisticated pumps run at a constant pace, but allow you to vary the suction.

A lactation consultant can help you find the pump that will be best for you. Whichever pump you choose, be sure it is easy for you to use, portable if you need to travel with it, and will serve your purpose—be it an occasional night out, or three times a day collecting at work.

Using a Breast Pump

Expect that the first few times you pump you won't obtain a significant amount of milk. Keep at it—your response will improve over time. Pumping both breasts at once often produces more milk. Try shields and inserts of various sizes to see which works best. If a pump makes your nipple hurt, the suction may be too strong, or the part your nipple draws into may be too narrow. Don't continue to use a pump that causes pain.

You may find that you can express more milk early in the day, and early in the workweek. Although your supply may drop off by the fourth or fifth workday, a day or two off with your nursing baby will help ramp it back up.

TIPS FOR SUCCESSFUL PUMPING

- Read the operating instructions before using your new pump.
- Wash your hands with warm soapy water or antibacterial cleanser before each use.
- Be sure you have all the parts you need, and clean bottles to collect into.
- Bring on your milk letdown reflex before you start, by thinking about your baby or something else relaxing and pleasant. Have an item with you that reminds you of the baby (like a worn T-shirt or blanket), or try listening to music that you associate with nursing. Some moms call their homes and listen to their babies' noises in the background while pumping.
- To physically assist with letdown, you can place warm washcloths on your breasts, massage from the edge of the breast toward the nipple, stimulate the nipple, or express a little milk manually.
- Moisten the edges of the funnel to make a better suction on your breast. Place the cup over your nipple and areola. Hold the pump firmly in place or use a pump bra or pumping band to fix the pump in place. Lean slightly forward so the milk will more easily enter the bottle.
- Pump about as frequently, and at around the same times, as your baby would feed so you keep up your milk supply. Ten minutes on a side after the milk starts flowing typically is enough. Pumping more times for short intervals generally yields more milk than one or two longer sessions. Stop pumping when the flow becomes minimal. Break the suction by inserting a clean finger between the funnel and your breast.
- Drink liquids when you pump to replace lost fluids, just as you should be sure to drink at home when you nurse.
- The color and aroma of the milk may vary day to day depending on what you have been eating. If your baby accepts it, it is fine to use.

- Keep the milk cold in a refrigerator or insulated bag (with freezer packs or ice). Transport the milk home in an insulated container. Milk that a baby hasn't begun to drink can be kept at room temperature (up to 78 degrees) for six to eight hours.
- Wash all the parts that have touched milk with warm soapy water or breast pump wipes. If you want to sterilize them, place them in the top rack of the dishwasher, in a bottle sterilizer, or in a specially designed plastic bag in the microwave.

The new microwave steam bags for the breast pump parts are essential. They make it so easy to keep everything clean and ready to use again. (Brenda H., pediatric resident)

The hardest thing about pumping in my truck was finding a way to make sure my hands were clean after working. I finally went and bought a box of rubber gloves. This way I just wear the gloves when I pump and then throw them out. (Stephanie B., FedEx courier)

I was able to use the lactation center downstairs, which was very convenient. I used the refrigerator in my lab for the milk. The main problem was that it took a lot of time—forty-five minutes a day. The lactation center had very nice pumps that let me pump both sides at same time. I would catch up on reading; it helped take my mind off of the fact that I felt like a cow. (Juanita G., research scientist)

STORING MILK

Servings of pumped milk can be stored for future use in glass or plastic containers. If you store your milk in bottle-insert bags, place those inside a freezer bag so they don't get freezer burned. Always write the date on your stored milk, and the child's name if you are going to bring milk to daycare. Milk stored longer than the safety guidelines should be discarded.

To avoid having to waste this "liquid gold," freeze breastmilk in single serving sizes. Some parents freeze the approximate amount the baby has been taking, as well as some one-ounce bottles for when the baby needs more. Remember that a used bottle must be discarded after an hour, even if the bottle isn't finished. It should not be stored in the refrigerator for another meal.

When only a small amount is pumped, chill it in the fridge before freezing. You can then combine a few cold samples and freeze into one serving. Never pour warm milk on top of frozen, because it can defrost the surface of the frozen milk. Remember, too, to always leave some room at the top because liquids expand in the freezer.

Frozen milk should be defrosted in the refrigerator and used within twenty-four hours. Defrosting in the microwave is not a good idea: it can create scalding pockets of milk within a container, and it destroys vitamin C and antibodies. If you need to thaw frozen milk more quickly, place it in a bowl of warm water. If the milk separates, gently swirl it to get the fat mixed back in. Always check the temperature of milk on the inside of your wrist before feeding your baby.

One thing that killed me was that the daycare was very strict with rules and would throw out unconsumed breastmilk. (Loren W., vice president of marketing)

I think the biggest obstacle for moms is the false impression that we need to sterilize everything that milk touches. I went crazy at first with a thin bottlebrush getting in every nook and cranny of the breast pump parts. But the truth is that is not necessary. Realizing that really frees up a lot of time, resources, and frustration! (Rebecca O., librarian)

Pumping versus Supplementing with Formula

If you are able to pump, you may find that you don't need formula even after you are back at work. This situation is ideal for your baby's health: pumped milk contains nutrients, antibodies, and other elements that formula just doesn't have. But pumping may be stressful: it can be difficult to find time at home when the baby isn't going to need to eat soon (so you can stockpile), and to make accommodations at work. Infant formula has been around for decades and does a pretty good job, so don't get too upset if your baby needs some formula when you return to work—especially if you are nursing while at home.

Be flexible and forgiving of yourself if things don't work out exactly as you had planned or hoped with regard to pumping and providing breastmilk bottles. (Kari S., librarian)

Guidelines for Storing Breastmilk

	How long to keep	*How to use*	*Notes*
Fresh milk	Six to eight hours at room temperature or up to five days in the fridge	Can serve cold, or warm up in bowl of warm water. Smaller babies may become chilled from drinking cold milk	Fresh is best, but not always convenient
Defrosted milk	Milk that has been frozen and thawed but not heated is safe at room temperature for up to four hours, or in the fridge for twenty-four hours	Can serve cold, or warm up in bowl of warm water. Once milk has been thawed in warm water, it is good for that feeding, or can be stored in the fridge for up to four hours	If the milk separates, swirl it to mix the cream back in. Never refreeze
Pumped milk in a cooler	Milk can be stored in an insulated cooler bag with ice packs for up to twenty-four hours	Can serve cold, or warm up in bowl of warm water. Smaller babies may become chilled from drinking cold milk	An insulated lunch bag with ice or freezer packs works well
Milk in refrigerator-freezer	If your refrigerator shares a door with the freezer, milk can keep for two weeks. In freezers with separate doors, milk stays fresh for three to six months	Milk should go into the freezer within twenty-four hours of pumping. Defrost for up to twenty-four hours in the fridge, or in a pan of warm water	Store toward the back of freezer, not in the door. Use the oldest samples first. Never defrost on the stove or in the microwave—you lose vitamin C and antibodies, and hot areas of milk can scald your baby

Guidelines for Storing Breastmilk (Continued)

	How long to keep	*How to use*	*Notes*
Milk in deep freezer	Six to twelve months	Milk for freezing should go into the freezer within twenty-four hours of pumping. Defrost for up to twenty-four hours in the fridge, or in a bowl of warm water	Put the newest milk toward the back of the freezer, so that older samples will be used first

Note: Once a baby has begun drinking from a bottle, it must be used within an hour or discarded.

I wasn't too upset about using formula, while I know some women hate the idea of it. Having this attitude made it easier by taking pressure off of myself. If I had felt pressured to exclusively offer breastmilk, I could have been very disappointed with myself or perhaps even given up entirely. (Loren W., vice president of marketing)

Some of my friends who were pilots pumped in the airplane bathroom and brought a cooler to take their milk home. That was too much for me. My son didn't really like breastfeeding anyway—he was impatient and wanted the quick, easy feed from a bottle. I felt a little guilty when I stopped breastfeeding as soon as I went back to work, but both my kids are healthy as horses, so I don't think it did any harm. (Susan G., commercial airline pilot)

Some tips for pumping at work: set mini goals like to get to three months or six months. If cleaning the parts is too hard during the day, buy four sets if you have to, and wash them when you get home. You need to find little tricks to make it easier on yourself. At first I was self-conscious about pumping in my car, but eventually I used the pumping time as a way to relax, read, listen to the radio, or talk on the phone. (Deborah S., sales rep)

Benefits of Pumping at Work

- More breastmilk for the baby.
- Less discomfort and leaking from engorgement at work.
- Continuing to burn extra calories.
- Maintenance of your milk supply. Mothers who give their babies formula during the work week may have less milk for their babies on days that they aren't working.
- The satisfaction of giving something to your baby that only you can provide.

Pumping was a pain in the neck, but I loved that it was something only I could do for him. Even though I was working, I could still nourish my baby. (Marge G., obstetrician)

If pumping is possible but you have no way to store the milk (for instance, if you are traveling), consider practicing "pump and dump"—that is, discarding the pumped milk, so you don't get engorged and your milk supply will stay strong. Prolonged engorgement can cause plugged ducts, and if recurrent, can decrease milk supply. If you are really dedicated to getting your milk to your baby, FedEx will overnight breastmilk stored with dry ice.

When my son was about ten months old I had to go on a two-day business trip without him and I discovered that airports typically do not have locations for mothers to pump. I had to pump and dump in a restroom stall. Eventually I switched over and every time I went to the ladies' room I just hand-expressed some milk until I was comfortable, rather than taking the time to pump. (Kari S., librarian)

Sometimes, too, pumping during the day just isn't possible or desirable. Ultimately, you will need to figure out what works best for you and your family.

With baby number two, I allowed myself an occasional weekend day off—away with my hubby, hiking the canyon, etc.—and practiced "pump and dump"—which I could never do with number one—too much guilt over wasting precious milk! (Jill H., gynecologist)

Finding a Place to Pump at Work

Workplaces vary tremendously in their accommodations for breastfeeding moms. The best scenarios are having your baby with you at work, a childcare center on site, or a pumping room with hospital-grade electric pumps provided, but unfortunately, these opportunities are only rarely available. To set up the best arrangements for your needs, it may be helpful to talk with your employer beforehand about pumping accommodations. An office with a door that closes is enough for some dedicated nursing moms. Some women still find themselves sneaking off to their cars or to the bathroom (the handicapped stall has the most room and often has a shelf for supplies)—though if you want to avoid using the public bathroom, try reminding your supervisor that you wouldn't prepare food there. Your colleagues may provide support by helping protect you when you are pumping or by loaning you a private location.

I pumped in our live trucks in the middle of crowded fairs, doors locked and windows blocked. God bless our photographers, they were so understanding and supportive to stand guard. (Eileen M., weather reporter)

I work in an old city building with big rooms divided into several offices. My office doesn't have a door, and I refuse to pump in a bathroom. My boss allowed me to use her office if it wasn't in use, or I would use the conference room, and put a note on the door "pumping in progress." (Brenda W., lawyer)

Despite state law and despite my efforts before leaving for my maternity leave, upon my return I discovered that I had been "assigned" an area inside a restroom (a stall with a chair instead of a toilet and a curtain instead of a door) for pumping. I was pretty horrified and asked for a different location. After several unsuccessful attempts at having human resources locate a private area for pumping that was not a restroom, I finally went to another department and obtained permission to use a clean, locked storage room for pumping. (Kari S., librarian)

My friend works at a school where there are a lot of new moms. Every day they go into the resource room, lock the door, and have a pumping party. (Tammy L., accountant)

I do have an office with a door in the land of cubicles, but it doesn't have a lock on it. I put up a sign on the door when pumping that said "Do not disturb." Five or six times, men ignored the sign and came on in. But I was committed to it, and the more I did it, the more I got over the embarrassment factor. I figured if they wanted to ignore the signs, they should be prepared for whatever they were going to see in there. (Rebecca M., senior vice president, financial corporation)

Once a mom has made the decision to pump at work, it is not a daily elective decision. It is a need . . . you need to pump at work for your breast's comfort, for your milk supply, and for your baby. (Brenda H., pediatric resident)

Finding Time to Pump at Work

Some jobs provide breaks and a lunch hour that can be used for pumping. Other jobs are less flexible or less predictable, but many arrangements that allow breastfeeding have worked out for moms with those sorts of jobs, too—from pumping just a minute or two multiple times a day, to formula feeding instead of pumping and just nursing nights and weekends.

Working in an emergency room, I never know what patient will come in the door. I can't breastfeed while a patient is having a heart attack, stroke, or other real emergency. I don't usually sit down at work. Sometimes I don't have time to eat or go to the bathroom. It is hard to imagine finding time to pump. But I would love to continue to breastfeed after going back to work so I will definitely try. (Melissa Z., emergency physician)

One of the challenges of breastfeeding while on the job was that I would be in depositions or trial situations where I didn't have control over the time. I just had to be assertive and say, "We've been at this for three or four hours, and I need a break." I just got used to making people accommodate. The men would get embarrassed, and the women (mostly) would be supportive. (Rebecca M., attorney and senior vice president, financial corporation)

I was a great pumper. I found that I could pump for a half hour once around 1 PM and get three feedings' worth of milk. I know that wouldn't work for everyone, but it was convenient! (Maggie P., administrator)

During the first six months back at work I had two out-of-town meetings. I did not feel comfortable leaving my son for multiple nights because I would miss him and I was concerned that his breastfeeding schedule would get messed up. For both meetings my husband came to take care of our son. I really had to stick my neck out with my company to make this happen. My husband had to stay hidden in the hotel room since no one else was allowed to bring spouses or families. (Deborah S., sales rep)

While some forward-thinking companies are becoming more accommodating, and some state laws guarantee time for women to pump on the job, many mothers still have difficulty continuing to breastfeed once they return to work. Breastfeeding advocates point out that nursing decreases maternal absenteeism on the job, because breastfed babies are less likely to get sick. If you want to try to persuade your employer to become more supportive of breastfeeding, sample letters that you can have your pediatrician or obstetrician sign can be found on the Internet. Try www.momobile.org/breastfeeding under advocacy and empowerment. Or use the letter on page 462 as a guide.

One night while I was pumping we got a call for an active burglary. I was throwing on my gear, my bulletproof vest—I felt like Wonder Woman. (Tracy G., police officer)

Ever since I was a medical student, I knew I wanted to be a cancer surgeon. But the surgeries are very long, up to five hours, and I couldn't leave to pump. I would soak through the ten pads I was wearing, my bra, my scrubs and gown, and the breastmilk would just run down to my feet. (Vivian V., oncologist)

I pumped every day at work, one to two times a day. Lately, I have been pumping in the back of my truck. One day last week I was sitting in Target's parking lot pumping. (Stephanie B., FedEx courier)

I used to pump at the animal shelter in the room where they kept the cats waiting for adoption. Each cat had its own cage, but they ran free in the room. Usually anyone who came in would be coming to play with them, but I was there to pump. I would set up my pump and sit on a bench, and the cats would come around and be very curious. (Julie M., veterinarian)

Sample letter to employer from your doctor or nurse

To: Date:

Company address:

From: Your employee's healthcare professional

Dear Employer:

________________________________ has chosen to breastfeed her new baby. I am seeking your support as this new mother returns to work.

Employers today face challenges in creating and maintaining work environments that balance the need for efficiency while supporting working families. Research suggests that nursing mothers take fewer sick days, because their babies have fewer illnesses. It is also likely that a mother's productivity will increase when she feels supported in her work environment and knows she is doing her best to provide for her child.

I am asking for your help in creating flexible arrangements that will allow this working mother to provide the best nutrition for her new infant.

Your employee will need to express (pump) breastmilk while at work, to provide nutrition for her baby and keep up her milk supply. This will require a twenty-minute break every ____ to ____ hours. She will need a quiet, clean, and private place with an electrical outlet to pump. (Restroom facilities are generally not considered adequate.)

Studies have shown that employers who support breastfeeding gain substantial benefits for their companies, including improved morale, increased productivity, lower employee turnover, and reduced absenteeism due to infant illness.

Thank you for your help in supporting your employee's decision to breastfeed her baby and for easing her transition back to work. Please contact me with any questions.

Sincerely,

____

Physician or Advanced-Practice Nurse

P.S. For more information on the benefits of breastfeeding to employers, and how to establish a breastfeeding-friendly workplace, please see the website of the Maternity Care Coalition at www.momobile.org (breastfeeding section).

I once soaked through my last breast pad at work and had the genius idea to put it in the microwave to dry it out and re-use it. The pad actually caught fire! (Eileen M., weather reporter)

I had this hands-free pump bra that attached to my battery operated pump so I could do other things while pumping. I even pumped when I was driving! (Heather H., real estate attorney) (Note from author: I don't recommend pumping while driving; it may increase your chance of having a car accident.)

Instead of getting an expensive pump bra, just cut slits in the front of an old sports bra. (Bonnie C., physician)

Pumping was a secret break for me. It helped me when the transition back to work was difficult; it gave me the time I needed, in my baby's absence, to allow myself to feel close to him and dedicated to our process. (Rebecca O., librarian)

Pumping at work is a beautiful break. Most of us do not take enough breaks at work. Pumping is a good excuse to just sit back and relax in the middle of your day. Some companies now are doing post-lunch power naps, some company yoga, and I did pumping. (Brenda H., pediatric resident)

Nursing—and Bonding—after Work

When planning your breastfeeding-at-work strategy, don't forget the reunion with your baby at the end of your workday. If you encourage your child-care provider not to feed the baby close to the end of the day, she will be hungry when she sees you, which will help maintain your milk supply—and support your breastfeeding relationship.

I would tell any mother returning to work to continue to breastfeed her baby for the obvious health reasons, but also because there is nothing like that bond and the feeling of connection between you and your baby. Especially if you are gone all day, coming home and relaxing with your nursing baby is one of the sweetest moments in life. (Rebecca S., program director)

THE PUMPING-AT-WORK SURVIVAL KIT

A complete pumping kit for work will include:

- A good electric pump or an easy-to-use manual pump that you can carry with you or leave at work
- All of the pump parts, including connections for pumping both sides at once if desired (If you don't have time to wash everything during the day, get an extra set for your second collection and bring it all home to wash later)
- Bottles to pump into, and lids
- A cooler with ice or cold packs to transport your milk home
- A photo, preworn little T-shirt, or used receiving blanket, to remind you of your baby (to help with letdown)
- A washcloth to pat yourself dry after pumping, and to clean up any spills
- Extra nursing pads (washable or disposable)
- A bottlebrush and dish soap, or specially designed pump-cleaning wipes, for cleaning the pump parts
- A clean blouse in case of leaks
- Extras: a pumping band or pump bra, to hold the double pump in place and free up your hands.

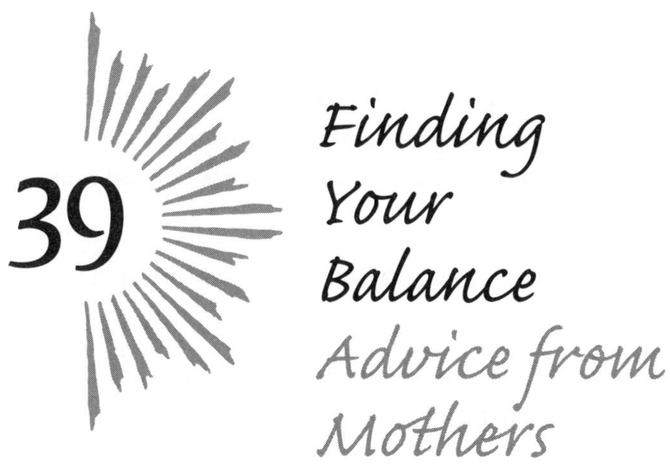

39 Finding Your Balance

Advice from Mothers

The topic of balancing work and motherhood could fill many books. Even though I can't begin to be that comprehensive here, several themes came up again and again during my interviews for this book: finding creative solutions to the inevitable challenges of caring for young children, attending to your personal needs, and most important, keeping perspective and a sense of humor through it all. In this chapter, I will share some of the different strategies that have worked for families dealing with the challenges of jobs and young children.

Be Proud of What You Are Accomplishing

Occasionally step back and look at all you have achieved. Although you may sometimes feel burdened by your busy schedule and by having to juggle so many responsibilities, this is a productive time of your life; by handling it all, you become a role model for your children and for the next generation.

> ***Even though you are not with your child every moment, you are setting a great example for your children. They will grow up to be proud of all their mother has accomplished and know the value of hard work. (Christi M., medical student)***

> ***Once they're older, the fact that their mother works, is independent, is bringing home an income, and has interests outside of the home is going to be important to them. (Linda S., creative director)***

There is a backlash of conservatism in this country that says women should stay home with their babies. But girls come up to me and they know that in our touring group women have babies, and they ask how we manage. (Annie F., classical violinist)

Remember, too, the aspects of working that are good for you and your children.

You are no less of a mom because you don't spend all day with them; in fact, you are doing quite a service by providing for them. (Brenda W., lawyer)

About ten years after having kids, I took an eight-week break from work. I realized that when I was home all the time, I became worked up over things like the kitchen floor. My family and I are all happier when I am working. (Jill H., gynecologist)

It's okay to enjoy your job. Enjoying your job and being happy with it does not make you a bad mother. In fact, I would argue that it makes you a better one. Kids with happy mothers (even those who work a lot) are likely to be happy kids. The reason is that they have a good role model. A mom who allows herself to be happy while working is doing her kids a favor, not harming them. (Heidi R., law professor)

I used to be away for a couple of nights at a time, so that was tough. But the kids have done great; they're very independent. They know when their parents leave that they are coming back. (Susan G., commercial airline pilot)

I try to remember that I had them so that they can grow up and leave . . . that if I do my job, they will move out, be independent, and never come back to live with me. And if that is the truth about what I have, I better make sure that I'm in pretty good shape, mentally, financially, emotionally, and physically, by myself. (Linda S., creative director)

Accept Your Emotions: You Will Sometimes Feel Guilty

Most working mothers experience feelings of guilt when they have to divide their time, attention, and loyalties between home and work. Even if you are clear about your priorities and know that you are doing your best, you will sometimes feel conflicted.

I feel conflict every time I walk out the door to go to work. (Rebecca S., program director)

If you're working, you feel guilty. If you're not working, you feel guilty. (Carolyn S., parenting educator)

There have been times I have had to choose between a work obligation and a child obligation. I still feel badly about the times I've chosen work over child, but the guilt about choosing child over work fades quickly. (Kendra F., civil litigator)

Everyone knows that they will love their baby, but what you don't know is that by the time you have to return to work, you will be IN *love with him. And when you're in love with somebody, it's hard to leave him there with a bunch of toddlers banging spoons on their heads. (Carolyn S., parenting educator)*

I put a picture on my desk at work. Whenever I feel guilty I call the daycare to check on them and then look at that picture of them smiling. They are okay and having fun. (Michele C., accountant)

Amazingly, my most comforting piece of advice was from my twenty-one-year-old nanny. She had recently graduated with a major in family studies. She was married, with a baby on the way. I was working sixty hours a week with two small children at home. When I lamented that I was no good as a full-time, stay-at-home mom, she reassured me. First, she said I was a good mom and my kids were wonderful. Then she said: "Studies have shown that kids do best (happy, well, adjusted) when mom is happy. So if mom is working and happy at work, or happy staying at home, kids do great." It was a relief and fit with what I saw. (Jill H., gynecologist)

What beliefs shape your image of how to be a mother? Fantasies about being the "perfect" mom often influence our expectations of ourselves. Remember to keep some perspective: try to make life easier, and don't create rules about doing things "right" that make your life more complicated and difficult. Manage your own expectations.

Relax standards about less important things even though you might not want to. (Andrea R., graphic artist)

Working mothers really, truly can't do it all. There are always choices to be made. Most often, we choose correctly. Sometimes we don't. Learn to forgive and then forget the mistakes. (Rebecca M., senior vice president, financial corporation)

At some point, I started letting myself have a break from the things that they don't find important, like a homemade lunch every morning. I mean, they really do care if I can make it to their games, but they don't care if I'm the room mom. And they do want me to come to their field trips, so I'll just make sure that I can get that day off. But I don't need to not work full-time for that. (Jill H., gynecologist)

When friends and family offer help, take it and don't feel guilty. I was very reluctant to take help when it was offered and ended up completely exhausted and unable to enjoy my daughter and tired at work. Once I realized that people wouldn't offer if they didn't want to help, my life got a million times easier. (Christi M., medical student)

It's great to have extended family. You lose some control and have to let people do things their way, but it really helps. Don't isolate yourself. It takes a village. Children are so adaptable they can do well with many different caregivers. (Annie F., classical violinist)

One thing for balancing home and work . . . lower your standards! My mom was a homemaker, and my dad had the demanding career, so those were my expectations. It's taken me ten or eleven years to realize that I can't be this Martha Stewart homemaker and have this full-on career. (Kristi V., professor)

Accepting the stereotype of the mother as the primary parent can conflict with the sharing of parental responsibilities that working mothers want and need.

If you really intend to share childcare equally (especially with a male partner), you need to give up being the "main," "primary," or "special" parent and really let him become the expert too. (Lori G., professor)

Think Creatively about Work Options

When possible, consider work hours that fit with your whole life. Are your job and financial situation amenable to part-time, flextime, or job-sharing? What about your spouse's job?

Working part-time in my own home-based consulting business gives me maximum freedom and flexibility to work (or not) around my children's schedules. I feel like I have been able to maintain a very healthy balance in my life between work and motherhood. (Lisa H., community planner)

My husband really wanted to have a major role in parenting. We chose not to have a baby until he could move into a less pressured job. (Maggie P., administrator)

I worked two hundred miles away from Monday through Thursday. Kate went to daycare three days a week, I had her on Fridays, and Joel took her on the train for his work in New York City on Wednesdays, where she spent the day with alternating grandmas. Joel organized a consulting career that was flexible, and other than "grandma Wednesdays" simply didn't take clients who required that he make out-of-town trips. (Lori G., professor)

For me the most important thing for going back to work was having some flexibility. Like I did some job-sharing, and when things were slow, I was able to say that I needed to go home. (Laurie M., budget manager)

For part-time, the most important advice I can give is that it is best to work full days though fewer of them. So work three full days a week instead of five half-days. It is crucial to find someone on site who can make decisions when you are not in the office. A job share situation works best. Otherwise, you will be distracted with phone calls while you are "off." Be prepared to work harder than the full-time people in the office on the days you work, as you will be catching up from the days you were not there. (Jenny K., internist)

The education field can be very accommodating to mothers. I was able to work on a very part-time basis (one to two days each week) when I was ready to return to work. (Edie U., school psychologist)

Often your needs change as your family enlarges, and as the children get older.

When they were babies, I didn't feel like I was missing anything, so I was able to work full-time. Then when they were three, four, and five years old, I thought they were just fascinating, so I cut back on work in order to spend more time with them. (Jill H., gynecologist)

I have a very flexible job as a professor, but during my pre-tenure years, our nanny pretty much worked full-time. By the time my youngest was in preschool five mornings a week, I would just arrange to teach my classes in the mornings. We haven't needed childcare since he was three years old because I've just done it. (Heidi R., law professor)

Negotiate for what you need. As I have said elsewhere, *Getting to Yes: Negotiating Agreement without Giving In* is a terrific resource on negotiating, available at your local bookstore or online.

Don't be afraid to ask them to rewrite the rules. If you want a four- or three-day week, ask for it, but make sure they see enough value in your work to be inclined to give it to you. (Jane J., advertising executive)

I'm really lucky because I work part-time from home, just twenty hours a week. I had worked at the company for several years before I got pregnant, so they trusted me and were willing to be flexible and work out these arrangements. I have several great babysitters who come over and watch Evelyn while I'm upstairs working. (Amanda O., meeting planner)

One benefit of being "advanced maternal age" is that I'm at a point in my career that I can make those decisions and have more control over my career. I have a group of people who work under me, so I can delegate when I need to. (Rebecca M., senior vice president, financial corporation)

Negotiate to work from home one day a week. Even if your child is in daycare or preschool for part of the day, and with a sitter for the rest, you

still get to see him more than usual and that time at home is great for catching up on random household things and phone calls. (Elizabeth S., online producer)

If you are in a hostile culture at work and can't change it, don't make yourself a target. Be professional and save your venting for friends and family.

As a woman, I don't think you want to be in the kind of job where there are mostly men who are in the type of relationship where he goes off to work and hunts and brings home the food, and the woman stays at home. (Cheryl P., radiologist)

I haven't felt a lot of validation that I am a serious professional since I have had children. There is always this underlying, unspoken feeling that prevails that since I am a mother of two small children, I must not be very committed to my job. (Rebecca S., program director)

I felt the pressure to work twice as hard when I came back to work, just to prove I was still in the game. And I did so at a huge personal cost. I took on several international assignments just to prove that I was at the same place in my career as I had been before, and as everyone else was. (Jane J., advertising executive)

Be prepared for male coworker comments like "My wife stays home with our kids; at least you get a break." When I hear comments or comparisons I say, "This is what works best for my family" and leave it at that. (Michele C., accountant)

Try not to complain at work that you are so tired because you were up three times last night feeding the baby and cried your entire drive into work, even though you are dead on your feet and feel like your heart is being ripped out because you miss your child. Your coworkers will tire of this very quickly and will soon proclaim you the office whiner. (Christi M., medical student)

When times are stressful, never complain; keep your mouth shut, head down, and focus. Never let them see you sweat. (Vivian V., oncologist)

But even as you cope with your current work situation, you can always consider trying to find a job that will make you feel supported and nurtured. Some companies are beginning to recognize that family-friendly environments are good for the bottom line. Check out *Working Mother* magazine's website, www.workingmother.com, for their annual report on the most family-friendly companies.

In terms of making it work, really look at your company. Look at your partners, especially look at the men, because what they have written down and what they actually believe about family time, etc., may really be different. (Cheryl P., radiologist)

I finally have a boss who is actually nursing her five-month-old, and does so during some of our meetings. (Hurray!) She is very flexible in terms of my mothering needs. Having this in place makes my work more rewarding and helps me to feel good about being at work. I don't feel as trapped and conflicted as I once did. (Rebecca S., program director)

Find Childcare That Works for Your Family

Learn about all your childcare options as early as possible, and pick the one that seems best for you and your family. When your childcare solution is working well, it will free you physically and emotionally to do your best on the job.

Find a daycare provider you trust. I could not do my job if I spent even one fraction of the day worrying about whether Natalie is safe. My daycare arrangement isn't perfect—the darn TV is on too much, my daycare provider knows all the secrets in the world to raising the perfect child as I am reminded regularly, and I receive a lecture every time I arrive late for pick-up at the end of the day (two-minute grace periods are provided—no more. I'm not kidding.)—but I absolutely, fundamentally know Natalie is safe and happy while I am at work. (Rebecca M., senior vice president, financial corporation)

Find a babysitter or nanny you trust and feel comfortable with. Have her come and spend time with you and the baby before you return to work. Introduce her to your friends in the neighborhood. This is a great way to create an instant community for her while alerting all of your friends and neighbors that you're going back to work and your child will be in this woman's care. (Elizabeth S., online producer)

If you can afford it, schedule slightly more childcare than you need for work, so you can take care of some of your personal needs. This way, while your child is safe and happy in a familiar setting, you can take a little time to refresh yourself.

> ***Try (if you can) to take a "regular business day" (or even half a day) off work once a month to catch up on all those little errands that take so much less time when you are solo and don't have to cart that little bundle of joy in and out of the car at every stop. I use this precious time to myself to get my hair cut, mail that belated birthday present, or shop for some clothes that actually fit me since I am unfortunately one of those women who is still trying to reach her pre-pregnancy weight. (Ann M., research scientist)***

> ***I saw that two of my male coworkers left early on Fridays to play squash, with no repercussions. So I started scheduling myself to come in late on Thursdays. I protected that time like it was already booked. I was able to get to know Dan's preschool teachers, and I had time for errands. I even took a pottery class. I still got all my work done, but the flexibility gave me breathing space. (Marge G., obstetrician)***

> ***Don't just pay a babysitter for the time you are at work—get out and exercise every day and have a date with your husband every week. (Peggy L., nurse-administrator)***

Appreciate your childcare providers as important employees. You know as a worker that feeling appreciated and respected by your boss makes you work that much harder. Consider paying her for vacations when you are away. At the holidays, a week's pay is a standard bonus for household staff. Thoughtfully chosen and timed personal gifts are nice, too. But the most important way you can ensure a healthy working relationship—and a continued nurturing environment for your baby—is to tirelessly show her that you value her work and never take her for granted.

> ***A happy nanny makes a happy baby; remember that she cares for your most precious asset; treat her with respect and kindness, even if you are running in the door frazzled from work . . . her job is just as hard. (Brenda W., lawyer)***

Have Backup Childcare Plans

Plan ahead for *when* (not if) a childcare crisis will develop. It helps to have family nearby; but if not, one parent may need to stay home if the child is ill or childcare arrangements fall through.

If possible, have a daycare backup ready for when you absolutely, positively cannot stay home from work. It's okay to ask for help from those you love and trust. (Rebecca M., senior vice president, financial corporation)

I'm not convinced that you can have a husband with a full-steam-ahead career and at the same time have a just as demanding career yourself. I am the backup plan because his work is less flexible than mine. Somebody has to be the backup parent, or you have to prearrange how you will handle crises. (Kristi V., professor)

Some communities' visiting nurse agencies provide "sniffle care" for a child too sick for school but not so sick that a parent needs to be home. Many moms suggested trading childcare with other families, especially in a pinch.

Build a network of friends who are parents and don't mind trading favors. (Susan G., commercial airline pilot)

Exchange support with other moms, especially stay-at-home moms. I often provide weekend/night babysitting for them and they sometimes pick up my kid from school during the week. (Andrea R., graphic artist)

One thing I haven't done that I wished I'd done more of is to form a network of other parents with kids that you can kind of trade off with, so that if you're in a bind, you always have a plan B. And you can help them out when they need it. (Kristi V., professor)

Work with your employer. Learn about the formal and informal rules at your workplace, so you can plan for different eventualities.

Be prepared to have a phone call from daycare on the worst days possible to come and pick up your child early. Because of this I made sure my boss knew the hours and rules that my daycare had. (Michele C., accountant)

Save your personal days for when you really need them—because you will. Your nanny will call in sick or your child will be too sick to go to daycare. (Elizabeth S., online producer)

I've made it clear at work, to the extent that I can, that my family is the priority. I get the kids out the door in the morning for school. So if there is an 8 AM meeting, that means I would have to leave the house at 7. I'll just say I can't do that; there are enough of us with young children where I work that it's made it okay. So we have our meetings at 10:30, which works out fine. (Kristi V., professor)

Make sure you don't use all your sick time during your maternity leave. You may need to take a day off if the baby is not feeling well. (Mary Ellen M., pediatric nurse)

Chances are the daycare/preschool will have vacations, so you'll need to plan yours accordingly. (Elizabeth S., online producer)

Your spouse has parental rights at work too. Talk to your partner ahead of time to define who is the emergency backup parent for any given day.

Choose a partner who will work hard to share fully in every aspect of child raising, not only in doing childcare itself, but in making it clear at work that he/she is equally a primary parent. (Lori G., professor)

Domestic Responsibilities: Don't Go It Alone

Many of the tips from moms in this chapter reflect the expectation (which we often put on ourselves) that the mother is the primary parent, ultimately responsible for childcare or childcare arranging. But this assumption limits your options, and can lead to unnecessary stress when you run up against the reality that you can't do it all. Single moms, who by necessity shoulder most of the burden, especially benefit from prearranging help and support.

Don't think of it—or call it—a "motherhood" challenge. If one has a spouse or partner, expect and insist that that person be an equal partner in caring for the home and children. That includes BOTH parents doing the day-to-day

stuff, taking the time off from work when necessary, making career sacrifices, communicating with teachers, etc. To be honest, I think that our society's continued insistence on thinking of this as a women's issue, rather than a family issue, contributes to the pressure on mothers. (Janet G., attorney)

My friends that seemed to be able to make it work had the luxury of full-time help in the house (nanny and/or housekeeper) plus very supportive spouses who could pick up the domestic slack. (Lisa H., community planner)

Make sure your spouse is willing to do at least 50 percent of the work. That includes housework of all sorts. This will be ongoing forever—the whole partnership thing! (Andrea S., nurse)

Many women commented on the importance of having their partners participate fully as parents. The corollary is that you need to allow the baby's father to become competent. If you see yourself as the better parent and try to control how he takes care of the kids, he will never become the confident, capable parent that you need him to be.

Having a supportive partner (or another adult who you can rely on) is the key to keeping the kids healthy and happy and the career on track. I am saying this since I just submitted my first major research grant and Jeff essentially took care of the kids and household for five weeks so I could focus on writing it. (Ann M., research scientist)

Because I had a two-hundred-mile commute to work, and would be away from home for four days a week, Joel had to share infant care in a way that not many men did. It was often harder on him than me, but he wanted to have children at least as much as I did, and we were both committed to raising them together, so we thought it was fair. (Lori G., professor)

Trust that dad will get used to childcare, crying babies, and housework. Don't give in to him when he calls you your first day back at work and you hear the baby crying, and he begs you to come home and make the baby stop crying! (Andrea S., nurse)

When my first child was born, being a working mom was a little less common. I had a husband who was well ahead of his time, had work flexibility

as I did, and who equally shared all the responsibility of parenting and home making. (Loree R., school psychologist)

Leave the baby alone with him and don't look back. (Lori G., professor)

Another theme for the domestic work front that emerged from the interviews was paying for services. If funds are tight, you may not have options, but many families don't think about how to use money to make their lives easier. Dry cleaners, drugstores, and groceries deliver. The teenager next door might love to get paid to mow your lawn. Shopping online saves time. Full-time employment and being a mom can be seen as two whole jobs: figure out which tasks are making your life hard, and delegate.

Hire as much help as you can possibly afford. You have to hire a wife. (Cheryl P., radiologist)

Don't be so strong that you can't ask for help—maids, personal shoppers, drive-throughs—it's okay! (Susan G., commercial airline pilot)

It's important to delegate. I know not everyone can pay someone to clean her house, but at least pick and choose. I mean, if you absolutely have to make the homemade birthday cake, order take-out for dinner. (Kristi V., professor)

During her job interview, our future nanny said: I think the essence of this job is to do whatever it takes to make your lives easier. Hired! She would go to the supermarket, do laundry, clean up after breakfast, even chop up the ingredients for dinner—AND Dan loved her. Between Ida and the fact that my husband did all the cooking, I actually felt my life was balanced most of the time. (Marge G., obstetrician)

I have a nanny, a housekeeper, and a part-time cook. My nanny has a college degree in education. I get home at six and there's dinner on the table and the homework is done, so I have three uninterrupted hours with my kids before they go to bed. (Vivian V., oncologist)

Be Efficient and Allow Yourself to Be "Good Enough"

Do a good job at work: the more indispensable you are, the more likely they are to try to accommodate your needs. Spending the last few minutes of the workday preparing for the next morning will increase your productivity. Efficiency can compensate for fewer hours worked.

There is always the suspicion that you're not going to be back once you have a baby, and that you're now going to be a mom and not be as good at your job, when actually it's the opposite—having a baby makes the use of your time more efficient. (Peggy L., nurse-administrator)

I've noticed that those of us with younger children at home want to be efficient in our use of the workday. We will often work through lunch or grab a quick sandwich and bring it back to the office so we can continue working, while our colleagues with fewer family responsibilities will take an hour out to have a full lunch in the dining room. (Kristi V., professor)

Minimize calls home during the day. Chances are your child and your caregiver are getting on just fine. Let them call you if something comes up, otherwise you'll always be thinking about what you're missing at home and not fully engaging in the workday. (Elizabeth S., online producer)

I come in to work each day knowing exactly what I want to accomplish. Usually I make a list the night before, so that I can really focus on what's important that day. (Kristi V., professor)

Stay organized at home, too.

Keep only ONE calendar and coordinate with your spouse at the beginning of each week—having work responsibilities listed on one calendar and children's doctors' appointments, etc. on another is a recipe for disaster, not to mention the scheduling your spouse adds for late/early meetings, work-travel, etc. Sleep deprivation is a good excuse for forgetting meetings or appointments, but you can only use that one for so long. (Ann M., research scientist)

We keep an online calendar that my husband can add to, my daughter can add to, I can add to. (Cheryl P., radiologist)

A schedule is key; if the baby and nanny set one during the week, do the nanny a favor and follow it on the weekend to make her job on Monday easier; it also eases stress for the working mom by making things more predictable. (Brenda W., lawyer)

Think about how you can manage your life to make it easier. Putting out clothes for the next day and making lunches ahead speeds you up in the morning. Straighten the house and pick up toys just once a day.

No matter how tired you are, get everything ready the night before. It will save a ton of time. (Michele C., accountant)

Pack bags the night before—your work bag, your child's day bag . . . (Elizabeth S., online producer)

Take Time to Meet Your Personal Needs

The topic of how to get personal needs met generated by far the most interest among the moms I interviewed. I think these lessons are often hard-learned. When life gets really busy, you need to schedule time for yourself, or you won't get it.

The important thing is that you take some time for yourself. Even if it's just a bubble bath and a glass of wine with the door closed. Carve out some time for you because no one else will, and if you never get any, you'll be left tired and resentful. (Susan G., commercial airline pilot)

Take five to ten minutes a day to practice whatever it is that makes you feel connected to the earth and the universe just by yourself. It's that connection that must be preserved and nurtured, even while you are breastfeeding a baby and trying to get tenure/make partner/advance to the next level. (Deb L., writer)

Always make time for yourself, even if it's giving yourself a five-minute time out—with such a busy schedule you tend to worry about everyone but you. (Dana W., network technician)

Don't forget about yourself in the process. Do something just for you a couple times a week. Commiserate with other mothers; watch a "chick flick" when your child's asleep; paint your toenails! (Tracy G., police officer)

I didn't live somewhere where I could go to a gym and get back in shape with other moms. That would have been the best, but the best thing I ever did was get the jogging stroller. At first I would just walk. Then I started jogging and really started to feel good about myself. (Susan G., commercial airline pilot)

Condense the hour-and-a-half yoga routine from before motherhood into a series of stretches while the coffee brews. (Deb L., writer)

Take time for yourself during the workday. Take a walk at lunch and listen to music or just think. It's amazing what a little time alone does to waken the senses and the brain. (Elizabeth S., online producer)

If you are in a relationship, nurture it.

A happy marriage makes a happy baby; continue to invest in your relationship with your spouse; remember, your child will eventually move on and it will be just the two of you. (Brenda W., lawyer)

My parents used to go out of town for the weekend once or twice a year and leave us kids with relatives or friends. Since our children's grandparents live out of town, we trade babysitting with close friends. This way one set of parents can go out on a date without the added expense of a babysitter, and the kids get a play date. (Ann M., research scientist)

Many moms described how their lives ran much more smoothly once they had developed some boundaries and set aside some grown-up time. Try to get everyone on a schedule so you and the baby know what to expect. Bedtime rituals also help ease the transition to sleep—for babies and for parents.

Try to set a real schedule for bedtime for baby and mom. Even if it is too early for mom to go to sleep, she can still have some quiet-time for herself/ spouse. (Andrea S., nurse)

If you are tired, go to bed when the baby goes to bed. There may be laundry to fold, dishes to wash, or toys to pick up, but that can wait. Rest is important. (Mary Ellen M., pediatric nurse)

This one I learned from my parents who were married for over thirty-five years. Make time to be with your spouse. I know everyone says this, but I believe parenting is one of the most difficult things I have ever done and making time to be with your spouse and TALK without interruptions from work or the kids is very important to maintaining a strong relationship. (Ann M., research scientist)

It helped us as a couple once we could set a schedule to get the kids to bed so we had time for us together. (Jennifer A., secretary)

Be Realistic

Periodically reassess how your arrangements are working for yourself and your family as a whole. If you are miserable, make changes.

Your job is not forever; your child is. If your life is too busy, slow it down—put on the brakes. You're no good to anyone if you can't remember your own name! Don't risk your health and well-being to get those cupcakes made or meet that deadline ahead of your coworkers. There's a time to excel and a time to just get by. (Tracy G., police officer)

For someone like me who waited this long to get married and have children, candidly, priorities are very clear to me, and it's easy to put my family first. Granted, it's not always easy to bolt out of the office to meet the daycare provider, but I make it work. (Rebecca M., senior vice president, financial corporation)

I don't think it is possible to "do it all," at least not all at the same time. I've watched enough of my smart, highly educated, professional girlfriends have complete meltdowns while trying to balance demanding careers, young children, long commutes, and husbands to convince me of this truth. (Lisa H., community planner)

It's easy to let your organization dictate what you want, instead of thinking about what's really important to you. I have a demanding career, but I'm not willing to miss my kids' childhoods to build up my CV. (Kristi V., professor)

Say "no" to people (family/friends/coworkers) who want you to do more than you are comfortable handling. (Andrea S., nurse)

Learn how to say no to requests not in line with your goals. One trick I learned is to have a plan ahead of time for how to decline. First, "Thanks for thinking of me." Second, a generic reason why it is not possible right now. (Don't be too specific if you don't want to have the requestor trying to solve your "problem.") Third, either open the door—"Please call me if something like this comes up next year when I may have time"—or close the door: "Good luck!" If you find yourself leaning toward saying yes, ask for time to think about it. (Marge G., obstetrician)

Finding that balance continues to be a struggle. I'm better at it today than I was six months ago, and I was better at it six months ago than I was six months before that. I just work on keeping a very clear focus on what my priorities are, and the top priority is my family. (Rebecca M., senior vice president, financial corporation)

Remember to Enjoy Your Life

It is easy to get so scheduled, frazzled, and distracted that you forget to pay attention and enjoy time together as a family.

Whenever I feel that I have to justify the limits I've set on my work schedule, I tell myself that I deserve to enjoy my life. My family is better off if I'm happy, and so are the residents and students I work with, who look at me and see their futures. (Marge G., obstetrician)

Schedule periodic vacations—whether they be long or short, do it. You need them and your spouse needs them and your kid needs them. (Susan G., commercial airline pilot)

Take pleasure in your children—they grow up quickly.

Be fully engaged when you are at home. At the end of the day, change clothes to signal to yourself that you are "off duty." Try to spend some time with your kids right after work, even if that means having take-out. Make this a special time without interruptions. (Maggie P., administrator)

Coming home I would always take my baby and the first thing we would do is nurse. It would be our time to reconnect. (Brenda H., pediatric resident)

If you can afford it, hire someone to clean your house so you can spend time away from work playing with your kids—that is until they get old enough to help clean the house and think it's fun. I recently bought one of those Swiffers and Garret and Alaina fight over who gets to clean the hardwood floors. Best fifteen dollars I ever spent! (Ann M., research scientist)

Enjoy the good, bad, and ugly, because they grow up too fast. (Anne C., radiologist)

Don't see your kid as a chore; see her or him as a human being and friend you can't wait to get to know better. (Susan G., commercial airline pilot)

All day I would look forward to my after-work time with my son. I felt like a high school girl with a new little boyfriend. (Maggie P., administrator)

My mom told me to "Enjoy your son while he's a baby. The time will move fast." She was right, and sometimes I can't help but remember those words when I'm looking UP at him. (Val P., administrative coordinator)

Most Important: Keep Your Sense of Humor

Remember that what people say to you reflects on them, not on you.

The biggest advice: learn to be flexible and laugh off the small stuff. Without this a working mom will drive herself crazy. (Michele C., accountant)

When Emily was two months old, I was optimistic that I could drive the babysitter home and get back before she woke for her midnight nursing. I was always pretty good at speeding. The very young Wisconsin police officer came to the side of my car. "Oh officer, I am so sorry. I had been going exactly the speed limit until I felt my milk coming in (now pointing to my breasts). You see, I have the milk and my husband is home with the baby." And before I could finish adding any other touches he said, with a ruby red face, "Just go home . . . sorry to stop you." (Kathy C., family therapist)

Sometimes you just have to say F—k. (Vivian V., oncologist)

Never lose your sense of humor. Late one evening, before I was slated for an 8 AM presentation to a large group, my daycare provider called saying she'd forgotten to tell me that Natalie had used her last diaper. Two options, given that my husband was out of town: I could wake Natalie up and head to the store, or hit the grocery early the next morning. Clearly the only choice was the morning pickup. We walked into the grocery at 6:50 AM, found the diapers, paid in cash, and headed back to our car in four minutes flat. As I buckled Natalie in, congratulating myself on my well-executed plan, I realized she had just made good use of her diaper [and it] didn't quite hold up. Plow ahead for the thirteen-minute drive to daycare and deliver a dirty baby, or return home—five minutes away—to clean her up? I arrived at the office at 8:15. My opening line to the group: "Sometimes shit happens." (Rebecca M., senior vice president, financial corporation)

Just as there isn't a perfect time to have a baby, there isn't a perfect, one-size-fits-all solution to the challenges of juggling career and family demands. I hope these stories and bits of advice will help you as you negotiate your next decade or two, and that you will find approaches that work for you and your family. Live well and love deeply—these are amazing years!

Appendix A
Pre-Pregnancy Resources

Preparing to conceive a baby is an emotional decision with practical implications. You may be amazed at how much there is to learn beforehand about pre-pregnancy health and genetic testing. But there is no need to feel overwhelmed—just turn to this section when you need more detailed information. The lists and other resources here will help you understand the process of conception and will provide information to help you work with your doctor, midwife, or genetic counselor. Here I have provided:

- A table to calculate your body mass index (a measure of your body weight in relation to the optimal range)
- A list of health conditions that may affect pregnancy
- Genetic tests that may be recommended based on your geographic heritage and ethnicity
- Tests that may be included in the fertility workup
- Common fertility treatments

Health Conditions That May Affect Pregnancy

Some medical conditions that affect the gynecological system, or the body as a whole, can have a profound effect on pregnancy. Learning your personal risk factors will help you to anticipate—and hopefully head off—any problems.

GYNECOLOGICAL ISSUES

- Prior cervical cone biopsy or LEEP treatment for abnormal Pap test or cervical dysplasia

  Concerns: Risk of weakened cervix

  What you should know: Most cancer-free women with prior cervical biopsies have full-term uncomplicated pregnancies. Generally you will be followed more closely during pregnancy, and there is a greater chance that you will need bed rest or treatment to try to prevent preterm delivery.

Body Mass Index Calculator

Pounds	Height 5'0"	5'1"	5'2"	5'3"	5'4"	5'5"	5'6"	5'7"	5'8"	5'9"	5'10"	5'11"	6'0"
100	20	19	18	18	17	17	16	16	15	15	14	14	14
105	21	20	19	19	18	18	17	16	16	16	15	15	14
110	22	21	20	20	19	18	18	17	17	16	16	15	15
115	23	22	21	20	20	19	19	18	18	17	17	16	16
120	23	23	22	21	21	20	19	19	18	18	17	17	16
125	24	24	23	22	22	21	20	20	19	18	18	17	17
130	25	25	24	23	22	22	21	20	20	19	19	18	18
135	26	26	25	24	23	23	22	21	21	20	19	19	18
140	27	27	26	25	24	23	23	22	21	21	20	20	19
145	28	27	27	26	25	24	23	23	22	21	21	20	20
150	29	28	27	27	26	25	24	24	23	22	22	21	20
155	30	29	28	28	27	26	25	24	24	23	22	22	21
160	31	30	29	28	28	27	26	25	24	24	23	22	22
165	32	31	30	29	28	28	27	26	25	24	24	23	22
170	33	32	31	30	29	28	27	27	26	25	24	24	23
175	34	33	32	31	30	29	28	27	27	26	25	24	24
180	35	34	33	32	31	30	29	28	27	27	26	25	24
185	36	35	34	33	32	31	30	29	28	27	27	26	25
190	37	36	35	34	33	32	31	30	29	28	27	27	26
195	38	37	36	35	34	33	32	31	30	29	28	27	27
200	39	38	37	36	34	33	32	31	30	30	29	28	27
205	40	39	38	36	35	34	33	32	31	30	29	29	28
210	41	40	38	37	36	35	34	33	32	31	30	29	29
215	42	41	39	38	37	36	35	34	33	32	31	30	29
220	43	42	40	39	38	37	36	35	34	33	32	31	30
225	44	43	41	40	39	38	36	35	34	33	32	31	31
230	45	44	42	41	40	38	37	36	35	34	33	32	31
235	46	44	43	42	40	39	38	37	36	35	34	33	32
240	47	45	44	43	41	40	39	38	37	36	35	34	33
245	48	46	45	43	42	41	40	38	37	36	35	34	33
250	49	47	46	44	43	42	40	39	38	37	36	35	34

Underweight < 18.5
Healthy 18.5–26
Overweight > 26
Obese 30–39
Very Obese > 39

INFECTIONS

- History of gonorrhea, chlamydia, or pelvic inflammatory disease (PID)
  Concerns: Increased chance of ectopic (tubal) pregnancy
  What you should know: No special treatment is needed prior to pregnancy, but you should *call your doctor or midwife as soon as you know you are pregnant.* An ultrasound around four weeks after conception (what we call six weeks pregnant) can help assure that the embryo is where it should be. If bleeding or pain develops in early pregnancy, see a doctor right away.
- Genital herpes
  Concerns: An active infection can be transmitted to the baby during a vaginal birth (the greatest risk occurs if the mother catches genital herpes for the first time during pregnancy; see Chapter 21 for more information).
  What you should know: No special treatment is needed prior to pregnancy. If a herpes sore is present during labor, a cesarean section will be recommended to protect the baby from catching herpes during birth. Women with herpes can take antiviral medication during their last month of pregnancy to help prevent outbreaks.
- HIV
  Concerns: Women who are HIV positive can transmit this infection to their babies, particularly at the time of vaginal birth.
  What you should know: *Talk to your HIV doctor before becoming pregnant.* Antiviral medications can help prevent transmission of HIV to the baby.

NEUROLOGICAL CONDITIONS

- Headaches
  Concerns: Headaches often get worse in pregnancy, and some migraine medications aren't safe to take while pregnant.
  What you should know: Talk to your practitioner about which medications are safe to use.
- Epilepsy
  Concerns: Both epilepsy and the medications used to treat it may increase the chance of birth defects. The risk is greatest for women who

have uncontrolled seizures, are taking high doses of medications, or take multiple drugs for seizure control. Even so, 90 percent of babies born to women with epilepsy are healthy and free from major birth defects.

What you should know: *Consult your neurologist and obstetrician before you get pregnant.* Do not take yourself off of your medicines without a doctor's supervision. Having seizures during pregnancy is often riskier than being on medications. Taking a vitamin supplement with 1 mg of folic acid *before* and through early pregnancy can prevent the birth defects caused by some of the drugs; vitamin K during the last month of pregnancy may help prevent medication-related blood-clotting problems in the newborn. The North American AED Pregnancy Registry (1–888–233–2334) is collecting information on pregnancy outcomes of women with epilepsy.

CARDIOVASCULAR ISSUES

- Hypertension (high blood pressure)

  Concerns: Poor fetal growth, preterm birth, placental abruption, and worsening of blood pressure at the time of delivery (called superimposed pre-eclampsia) are all more likely in mothers with hypertension. Borderline blood pressure elevations don't pose much risk, but severe hypertension and high blood pressure complicated by kidney disease often lead to problems.

  What you should know: *Consult your obstetrician before getting pregnant.* Some blood pressure medications are unsafe for the fetus, but many safe medicines are available. Pregnant mothers with high blood pressure may need to take time off from work for bed rest or hospitalization.
- Congenital heart disease (valve or other structural problems)

  Concerns: The pregnancy risk *to the mother* of congenital heart disease varies from minimal to life-threatening. In general, maternal congenital heart conditions with normal oxygen flow don't cause severe pregnancy complications, but cyanotic heart disease can lead to poor fetal growth and preterm birth. Mitral valve prolapse, the most common valve condition, typically doesn't increase risk.

  What you should know: *Consult a cardiologist and obstetrician before becoming pregnant.* Some heart defects are so dangerous that women who have them should never become pregnant. Men and women with congenital heart disease are at increased risk for having children with heart abnormalities, but the structural changes may be different from the parent. A special type of ultrasound called a fetal echocardiogram can be done in the second trimester to look at the fetal heart.

- Prior or current blood clots in the leg or lung (deep venous thrombosis or pulmonary embolism)

  Concerns: Pregnancy increases the chance of blood clots in the legs or lungs. The blood thinner Coumadin (Warfarin) causes birth defects and shouldn't be taken in early pregnancy.

  What you should know: *Discuss plans for pregnancy with your practitioner before conceiving.* If you become pregnant, expect to be on daily self-injected blood thinners for nine months.

RESPIRATORY PROBLEMS

- Allergies

  Concerns: Many mothers-to-be find they are more congested during pregnancy.

  What you should know: Avoid known allergy triggers. Check with your practitioner for which medications are safe to use.

- Asthma

  Concerns: Around 4 to 8 percent of pregnant women have asthma. In about one in three cases, asthma will worsen during pregnancy; any low oxygen levels that result will be unsafe for the baby.

  What you should know: *Be sure your asthma doctor knows you are planning to conceive, and get in your best possible health before getting pregnant.* Most asthma medications are probably safe in pregnancy, but more is known about the older drugs than about some of the newer ones. Plan ahead with your doctor so you know what to do if you develop symptoms during pregnancy.

GASTROINTESTINAL ISSUES

- Inflammatory bowel disease (IBD)

  Concerns: Inflammatory bowel disease, if quiescent at the outset of pregnancy, generally doesn't cause problems for the baby. The risk of preterm delivery and miscarriage are higher in women who have active Crohn's disease.

What you should know: *Talk to your gastroenterologist and obstetrician before getting pregnant.* Waiting until remission before trying to conceive is best. Although most drugs used for IBD are safe in pregnancy, some can be dangerous to a developing fetus.

BLOOD CONDITIONS

- Sickle-cell disease (including sickle-thal and sickle-c)

  Concerns: Miscarriage, poor fetal growth, preterm birth, and fetal demise are not uncommon with sickle-cell disease, and pain episodes may be more frequent during pregnancy.

  What you should know: *Talk to your doctor before you get pregnant.* Because of the genetic risks, a woman with sickle-cell anemia should have her partner's blood tested (including a complete blood count and hemoglobin electrophoresis) before attempting pregnancy. If possible, obtain your prenatal care from a doctor experienced with sickle-cell disease.
- Sickle-cell trait

  Concerns: One in ten women of African ancestry carries the recessive gene for sickle-cell disease. If the father also carries an abnormal hemoglobin gene, the baby could develop sickle-cell disease.

  What you should know: *Talk to your doctor or midwife before you get pregnant.* Just as with sickle-cell disease, women known to be carriers of sickle trait should have their partners' blood tested (complete blood count and hemoglobin electrophoresis) before attempting pregnancy. Kidney infections are more common in pregnant women with sickle trait.
- Von Willebrand disease (vWD)

  Concerns: Von Willebrand disease does not affect fetal growth or development. Pregnancy boosts clotting factors and makes vWD temporarily less severe, but excess bleeding may be a problem after delivery.

What you should know: Your hematologist can help the obstetric team make a plan to manage any excess bleeding after childbirth.

ENDOCRINE (HORMONAL) PROBLEMS

- Thyroid disease

  Concerns: Too much or too little thyroid hormone can lead to miscarriage, poor fetal growth, and preterm birth. Low thyroid may put the baby at risk of impaired intellectual development. New guidelines advise supplementing thyroid hormone to keep the TSH under 2 or 2.5, to best protect the baby. Untreated hyperthyroidism increases birth defects, and may lead to life-threatening complications in the mother.

  What you should know: *Talk to your thyroid doctor and your obstetrician before becoming pregnant.* If you have hypothyroidism, blood tests should show that you are perfectly controlled before becoming pregnant; you should expect to adjust medications in early pregnancy and follow thyroid tests every trimester. If you suffer from hyperthyroidism, consider definitive treatment with radioactive iodine or surgery before conception.
- Preexisting diabetes

  Concerns: Birth defects are much more common in infants of diabetic mothers; *the higher the blood sugars in early pregnancy, the more likely the baby is to have a severe birth defect.* Although infants of diabetic mothers can be very large, causing difficulties at delivery, mothers-to-be with longstanding insulin-dependent diabetes and vascular disease are actually at risk of poor fetal growth and premature birth. (For information on gestational diabetes, which develops only during pregnancy, see Chapter 21.)

  What you should know: *All diabetic women should plan their pregnancies with their diabetes doctors and obstetricians.* Perfect glucose control is essential before and during pregnancy. Taking a vitamin with 1 mg of folic acid before conception may help prevent birth defects. Expect to work hard at glucose control during pregnancy, and don't be surprised if you need to be admitted to the hospital at times. Many insulin-dependent diabetics find it hard to hold a job while pregnant—taking care of the diabetes may be a job in itself.

EMOTIONAL AND BEHAVIORAL ISSUES

- Depression and anxiety

  Concerns: Both depression and anxiety are common among women in their childbearing years. Pregnancy and parenting a newborn can be stressful, and may exacerbate depression and anxiety. New mothers with a history of depression, for example, are more likely to experience postpartum depression.

  What you should know: *Before you try to get pregnant, talk to your doctor or midwife;* you'll want to be sure you are emotionally ready for pregnancy before discontinuing your birth control method. Counseling is often as effective as drugs for treating mild to moderate depression or anxiety. If you do need medication, the prenatal risks of antidepressants aren't clear, but medications may be safer for the mother and baby than untreated depression.
- Substance use, abuse, or addiction

  Concerns: Cigarettes, alcohol, and drugs are unsafe for developing fetuses and can cause infertility, miscarriage, birth defects, poor fetal growth, premature birth, and other serious complications. Cocaine can cause fetal demise with just one use.

  What you should know: *Get help before you get pregnant.* Your doctor or midwife can help you to quit smoking or refer you to a drug or alcohol treatment program. If you use alcohol sporadically, limit drinking as soon as you are off of birth control and watch carefully for signs of pregnancy so you know when to stop altogether: the embryo's organs start developing before most women even know they are pregnant.
- Eating disorders

  Concerns: To ensure good fetal growth and nutrition, you will need to gain weight. Although vomiting is common in early pregnancy, self-induced vomiting is not healthy and can lead to electrolyte disturbances, poor nutrition, and dental problems.

  What you should know: *Women with eating disorders should be in remission before getting pregnant.* Even after treatment for an eating disorder, many women struggle with the full, bloated feeling that often accompanies the growth of the uterus, and with allowing themselves to gain the weight that is necessary for a healthy pregnancy. Have a therapist lined up in case symptoms recur in pregnancy, and tell your doctor or midwife of your history so they can be sure that the baby is growing well.

AUTOIMMUNE DISORDERS

- Lupus and other autoimmune collagen-vascular diseases

  Concerns: With the exception of rheumatoid arthritis, autoimmune diseases increase the risk for poor pregnancy outcomes, including miscarriage, poor fetal growth, preterm birth, and fetal demise.

  What you should know: *Talk to your doctors before getting pregnant.* At least six months of remission is recommended before conception, to ensure the best pregnancy outcome. Your doctor can test for anticardiolipin antibodies and other factors in the blood that increase the chance of pregnancy complications. Low-dose aspirin and/or daily injections of blood thinners may offset the risk. Mothers-to-be with lupus should expect to be monitored more closely during pregnancy, with frequent office visits and fetal testing.

URINARY TRACT PROBLEMS

- Kidney stones

  Concerns: Kidney stones don't pose risk to the baby, but episodes of pain can require strong medications and sometimes hospital admission.

  What you should know: Calcium supplementation doesn't increase the risk of kidney stones, but becoming dehydrated does. Women with a history of kidney stones need to be careful to stay well hydrated during pregnancy.

ADVANCED MATERNAL AGE

- Maternal age over thirty-five

  Concerns: Fertility decreases and miscarriage risk increases with age. Down syndrome and other chromosomal variations are more common, but the chance isn't as high as many people believe (see Chapter 17).

  What you should know: Women over age thirty-five should seek medical care if they are not pregnant after six months of trying. Women over age forty should do the same after three months. Once pregnant, think ahead about how much prenatal genetic testing you want to do for chromosomal problems, and what you would do if an abnormal result were found. For more information, see Chapters 12 and 17.

PRIOR PREGNANCY COMPLICATIONS

- Miscarriage

  Concerns: Of those women who have had a first trimester miscarriage, 90 to 95 percent will have no problem in the next pregnancy. Generally no special evaluation is warranted. Even after three miscarriages, the chance of the next pregnancy going full term is around 70 percent.

  What you should know: Women who have had two first trimester miscarriages in a row or any second-trimester loss should talk to the doctor before trying to conceive again. Some causes of miscarriage can be identified only when a woman isn't pregnant, and a treatment plan can be made that may help the next pregnancy succeed.
- Prior preterm birth (fewer than thirty-seven completed weeks)

  Concerns: Women with a prior preemie are at risk for delivering early again. Sometimes the history or testing reveals a treatable cause of prematurity.

  What you should know: *Before pregnancy, talk to your doctor;* some tests for prematurity risk factors can only be done when the woman isn't pregnant. If no specific cause is identified, expect to be monitored closely in the next pregnancy. You might have to take time off from work to rest. Recent studies have demonstrated benefit of 17-alpha-hydroxyprogesterone injections during the second and third trimesters.

Genetic Testing

Your ancestry can influence the chance of having certain genetic conditions occur in your offspring. Recommendations may expand as new tests become available. Remember that for all these recessive conditions, *both parents* must be carriers for children to possibly be affected. Carriers typically have no symptoms or signs of the condition and don't know that they carry the genetic trait. It is

Recommended Genetic Tests by Ancestry

Ancestry	*May carry a gene for:*	*Incidence of gene in people without symptoms or signs*	*Description of condition (if both parents carry the gene)*
African	Sickle-cell anemia	1 in 10	Blood disorder of the oxygen-carrying protein hemoglobin; causes anemia (decreased red blood cells), pain episodes, and trouble fighting infection
	Alpha thalassemia	1 in 30	Blood disorder of the oxygen-carrying protein hemoglobin
	Beta thalassemia	1 in 100	Blood disorder of the oxygen-carrying protein hemoglobin; can lead to severe anemia (decreased red blood cells) and shortened life expectancy
Caucasian (Northern European)	Cystic fibrosis	1 in 29	Affects the tissues that produce mucus. Usually lung disease is severe, requiring long-term antibiotics, daily physical therapy, and multiple hospitalizations

Recommended Genetic Tests by Ancestry (Continued)

Ancestry	*May carry a gene for:*	*Incidence of gene in people without symptoms or signs*	*Description of condition (if both parents carry the gene)*
Mediterranean	Beta thalassemia	1 in 30	Blood disorder of the oxygen-carrying protein hemoglobin; can lead to severe anemia (decreased red blood cells) and shortened life expectancy
	Alpha thalassemia	1 in 25	Blood disorder of the oxygen-carrying protein hemoglobin; most severe form can be lethal to fetus or young infant
Southeast Asian/ Southern Chinese	Alpha thalassemia	1 in 20	Blood disorder of the oxygen-carrying protein hemoglobin; most severe form can be lethal to fetus or young infant
Hispanic	Sickle-cell anemia	1 in 12	Blood disorder of the oxygen-carrying protein hemoglobin, causes anemia (decreased red blood cells), pain episodes, and trouble fighting infection

Recommended Genetic Tests by Ancestry (Continued)

Ancestry	*May carry a gene for:*	*Incidence of gene in people without symptoms or signs*	*Description of condition (if both parents carry the gene)*
French Canadian or Cajun	Tay-Sachs disease	1 in 30	An enzyme deficiency leads to severe, progressive neurological disease; most children don't live past age four
Eastern European Jewish	Tay-Sachs disease	1 in 30	An enzyme deficiency leads to severe, progressive neurological disease; most children don't live past age four
	Panel of Jewish genetic diseases: Canavan disease and familial dysautonomia are usually included; sometimes Niemann-Pick disease, Gaucher disease, Fanconi anemia, and Bloom syndrome	1 in 10 to 1 in 100	Many of these conditions are caused by enzyme deficiencies with consequent accumulation of toxic byproducts. Some cause neurological degeneration similar to Tay-Sachs disease
	Cystic fibrosis	1 in 29	Affects the tissues that produce mucus; usually lung disease is severe, requiring long-term antibiotics and multiple hospitalizations

best to test for these genes before pregnancy; if both parents are found to carry the gene, several options are available to prevent having a baby with a severe disease. Talk to your doctor or genetic counselor for more information.

The Fertility Workup

The fertility evaluation can be intimidating; many women worry about what will be done and what might be found. Not all tests are employed in all situations. Use this list to look up tests that are recommended to you, so you will know what to expect.

- Physical examination. A pelvic examination will allow your practitioner to assess the size and shape of your uterus, and to check for signs of endometriosis or other problems with your reproductive organs.
- Basal body temperature charting. Graphing your daily morning temperature can establish if and when you are ovulating. A day or so after ovulation, your temperature will rise by about one degree. This result doesn't help with getting pregnant that month, since the temperature rises after the egg is released, but it can help predict ovulation for the next month, and can help with the timing of other fertility tests.
- Ovulation detection. A urine test can check for luteinizing hormone (LH), which rises sharply the day before ovulation. Although this test may have false positives (detecting ovulation when it hasn't happened) and false negatives (missing ovulation), it can be useful for monitoring fertility treatment and for timing intercourse. If you don't get a clear-cut result, your doctor can use blood tests, endometrial biopsy, or ultrasounds to identify ovulation. For more information on ovulation testing, see Chapter 4.
- Blood tests for thyroid hormone and prolactin. Abnormal levels of these two hormones can interfere with ovulation.
- Day 3 blood test for follicle stimulating hormone (FSH). FSH starts to rise during the years preceding menopause. Elevations in FSH levels on cycle day 3 indicate a decreased likelihood of getting pregnant with your own eggs, and may influence decisions about fertility treatment. But home

testing for FSH can be misleading; for an accurate reading, you will need to have a physician supervise the testing and interpret the result.

- Progesterone level. After ovulation, the ovary makes the hormone progesterone, which is needed to sustain the lining of the uterus until the pregnancy starts to make its own hormones. A progesterone level drawn the week before the period is due is the easiest way to document that ovulation has occurred.
- Endometrial biopsy. The purpose of this test is to see whether the uterine lining has been hormonally prepared for implantation of a pregnancy. Endometrial biopsy has become controversial, since it is often difficult to interpret and because the findings may not help to target treatments.
- Semen analysis. For a semen analysis, a sample is collected by masturbation, then viewed under a microscope to check sperm number, shape (called morphology), and motility (swimming ability). Men who have religious or personal difficulties with collection should talk to the doctor—an SCD (semen collecting device) is a special nontoxic condom that may also be used to obtain sperm. Semen analysis explains 30 to 40 percent of all fertility issues. It is a valuable part of the fertility workup and should not be omitted, even if it is embarrassing or difficult. Often if one sample is subpar, a second sample is obtained, since even fertile men can occasionally have an abnormal result.
- Post-coital test (PCT). For this test, the couple has sex two to twenty-four hours before the examination. Then, using a speculum just like for a Pap test, fluid is collected from the woman's cervix and looked at under the microscope to check the quality of the cervical mucus and how the sperm are faring. The value of this test is controversial, but it may help identify couples who would benefit from hormone supplementation or intrauterine insemination. PCT can also give an indirect estimate of semen quality if the partner can't or won't get a semen analysis.
- Transvaginal ultrasound. During this test, an ultrasound probe is placed into the vagina to allow a close view of the ovaries, so that the follicle, which houses the egg, can be measured. Ultrasound can be also used to check on the size and shape of the uterus and to evaluate the uterine lining.

- Saline sonogram. A saline sonogram creates a clearer image of the inside of the uterus than is possible with transvaginal ultrasound alone. The doctor uses a speculum to see inside the vagina and inserts a small tube into the cervix. Saline fluid is injected into the uterus to make the inside easier to see with transvaginal ultrasound. Cramping may be felt during this part of the exam. Saline sonograms can detect polyps (outpouchings of tissue), fibroids (benign tumors), scarring, or an unusual uterine shape that may affect fertility.
- Hysterosalpingogram (HSG). A hysterosalpingogram creates an image of the inside of the uterus and checks that the tubes are open. The doctor uses a speculum to see into the vagina, then instills X-ray dye through the cervix and up into the uterus. X-rays are taken to see the shape of the uterine cavity and the flow of dye out of the fallopian tubes. Because of the X-ray exposure, it is important not to be pregnant when this test is done, so schedule it for right after a period. Some women experience bad cramping during HSG. A normal test is good evidence that the uterus and the tubes are open. If a tubal blockage is seen, further testing with laparoscopy can help determine if there really is an obstruction. Some experts believe that even having the HSG test improves fertility for a month or two. The thought is that the dye may temporarily open up slightly obstructed tubes.
- Hysteroscopy. During hysteroscopy, a telescope is placed into the vagina and through the cervix, to look inside the uterus. The test can be performed either in the office or under anesthesia in the operating room. Hysteroscopy can see the inner contour of the uterine cavity, allowing the doctor to check for polyps, fibroids, or a septum (dividing wall).
- Laparoscopy. Laparoscopy is usually performed in the operating room under general anesthesia. A small incision is made near the belly button, and the laparoscope (a surgical telescope) is inserted, giving the doctor a view of the reproductive organs. Laparoscopy can check for endometriosis, a condition in which the tissue that lines the uterus grows in abnormal locations, and can assess the condition of the uterus, ovaries, and tubes. If the HSG was abnormal, laparoscopy can be used to document with greater certainty whether the tubes are open or closed,

because sometimes a tubal spasm during HSG can make the tube appear blocked when it isn't.

Fertility Treatments

If your doctor has encouraged you and your partner to pursue treatment to enhance your fertility, don't panic. Many treatments are available to increase your chances of having a baby. Your fertility team's specific recommendations will depend on your specific fertility problems and financial resources.

LIFESTYLE MODIFICATIONS

- Timed intercourse
  One of the simplest fertility "treatments" is to make sure you are having sex at your most fertile time. Ovulation detection using an over-the-counter urine testing kit will help you know when you are about to release an egg, and having sex one to three days before ovulation will give you your greatest chances of becoming pregnant.
- Quitting smoking
  Becoming a nonsmoker (for the man and especially for the woman) improves the effectiveness of any fertility treatment. Talk to your doctor if you need help quitting. Many excellent Internet smoking cessation sites can be found by searching under "smoking cessation," or try the American Lung Association at www.lungusa.org.
- Weight loss
  Women who have problems with ovulation because of excess body weight (defined as a body mass index greater than 27) are more likely to get pregnant if they lose weight. Dropping just twenty to thirty pounds may get the ovaries cycling again and help fertility treatment succeed.
- Weight gain
  Women who have problems with ovulation due to low body weight (defined as a body mass index less than 18.5) are more likely to get pregnant if they gain weight. Many women find that they have a threshold weight over which they cycle normally.

- Limiting exercise

  Exercising for more than an hour a day can disturb ovulation; switching to a lower-intensity program can help achieve pregnancy.

FERTILITY DRUGS

- Ovulation induction with clomiphene citrate (Clomid)

  Clomiphene citrate is a medication designed to improve ovulation; it is taken orally for five days early in the cycle. Clomiphene conveys a 5 to 10 percent chance of twins and a very small chance of triplets. Usually the cycle is followed closely, with monthly exams or ultrasounds, to see what dose is necessary to promote ovulation and to be sure that large ovarian cysts don't develop. If this treatment does not succeed within a few months, most fertility specialists will recommend adding intrauterine insemination or switching to a different treatment.
- Ovulation induction with gonadotropins

  Gonadotropins are medications used to induce multiple eggs to develop at once, usually in conjunction with intrauterine insemination (IUI) or in vitro fertilization (IVF). These drugs, which cost hundreds or even thousands of dollars a month (and have some medical risks), are also those famous for causing high-order multiple pregnancies—more than twins. Only reproductive endocrinologists or specially trained ob-gyns treat patients with gonadotropins, which require daily injections and must be closely supervised, with frequent blood hormone levels and transvaginal ultrasounds of the developing follicles. Your doctor will talk to you about the risks, including the possibility of having twins or more, before you start these potent drugs.
- Metformin (Glucophage)

  This medication is for women who are insulin resistant, a prediabetic state that is often part of the hormonal condition polycystic ovarian syndrome (PCOS). Some studies have shown that women with PCOS ovulate better when taking metformin, either by itself or in addition to other fertility medications.
- Bromocriptine

  The daily oral medication bromocriptine, or any of several similar drugs, diminishes the level of prolactin in women who overproduce it. Prolactin interferes with ovulation and can cause a milky discharge from the breasts.

- Progesterone supplementation

  The ovarian hormone progesterone usually maintains the uterine lining until the pregnancy starts making its own hormones. In some cases, supplemental progesterone is taken to sustain the early pregnancy. Except when used as part of IVF treatment, the benefits of progesterone supplementation are controversial. But there is consensus that there is no risk.

- Supplemental hCG

  HCG is similar in structure to LH, the hormone that causes ovulation. HCG may be used midcycle to stimulate ovulation, or during the second half of the cycle, to help the ovary continue to make progesterone until a pregnancy is established.

ASSISTED REPRODUCTIVE TECHNIQUES (ART)

- Intrauterine insemination

  In intrauterine insemination, or IUI, sperm are collected by masturbation, prepared ("washed"), and then instilled into the uterus through the cervix. For the woman, this feels much like a Pap test. IUI can use sperm from the male partner or from a sperm donor. Compared to other methods of fertility treatment, IUI is relatively inexpensive: it costs a few hundred dollars a month.

- In vitro fertilization (IVF)

  For in vitro fertilization, ovulation is stimulated with gonadotropins; when the eggs are ready they are removed, usually by inserting a needle through the back of the vagina while watching with ultrasound. The eggs are then mixed with sperm in the lab, and a few days later the tiny embryos are transferred back to the woman's uterus. In vitro was invented to bypass obstruction in the fallopian tubes, but it is also effective for many other causes of infertility. IVF is expensive, averaging $10,000 per cycle, with an 8 to 60 percent chance of success each time, depending on the mother's age and other factors.

- ICSI

  Intracytoplasmic sperm injection, or ICSI, is a variation of in vitro fertilization that is particularly useful when only a few sperm are available, such as when the father has a low sperm count. Using IVF techniques, eggs are removed from the mother, and then, while watching under a microscope, one sperm is injected into the egg. The embryos are incubated and then transferred back to the woman's uterus a few days later.
- Donor sperm

  If the male partner has no sperm at all or chooses not to do ICSI, donor sperm can be used to achieve pregnancy through intrauterine insemination or in vitro fertilization. Donor insemination is also an option for lesbian couples and single mothers. Sperm banks supply samples from donors who have been tested for sexually transmitted infections and screened for genetic diseases.
- Donor eggs

  Using IVF techniques, eggs can be retrieved from a donor and fertilized with the father's sperm, then implanted into the mother. Egg-donor IVF allows women who are postmenopausal (have no eggs left), or are otherwise unable to ovulate, to have a baby. Most of the older celebrities having babies on the news have become pregnant with donated eggs.
- Gestational carrier

  In situations where the mother can't carry a pregnancy, in vitro techniques can be used to create embryos that are carried for her by another woman, sometimes known as a "surrogate mother." The embryos can be created with the mother's eggs, or if that isn't possible, with those from an egg donor.

SURGERY

- Hysteroscopic removal of fibroids, polyps, or a uterine septum

  If the uterus is deformed by uterine fibroids (benign muscular tumors), polyps (outpouchings of the uterine lining), or a septum (a fibrous wall within the uterine cavity), surgical removal may improve the chances for pregnancy. This surgery is usually done vaginally, using a transcervical telescope called a hysteroscope, in the operating room under general anesthesia.

- Surgical treatment of endometriosis

  Most doctors will treat endometriosis, in which uterine lining tissue grows on the ovaries and other abnormal sites, if they find it at the time of laparoscopy, but surgical treatment is only clearly beneficial if the endometriosis is obstructing the tubes. Ovulation induction combined with IUI is often effective for women with mild or moderate endometriosis.

- Varicocele repair

  Varicoceles are enlarged veins in the scrotum that may interfere with sperm development. In a man with a varicocele and an abnormal semen analysis, surgery to repair the varicocele may help, although its effectiveness is controversial. If other fertility factors indicate a need for IVF, the sperm problem can usually be overcome by the IVF procedure, and surgery on the man won't further improve the chance of success.

- Tubal surgery

  If tubal obstruction is the only problem, surgical reconstruction is an alternative to in vitro fertilization, with less risk of multiple pregnancy (and perhaps better health insurance coverage). Sometimes after you weigh the cost, risks, and benefits, however, IVF turns out to be a better choice, especially if the tubes are very damaged. If a tube is swollen and full of fluid, called a hydrosalpinx, removal of the tube before IVF may increase fertility rates.

- Reversal of sterilization

  "Infertility" caused by a prior male or female sterilization procedure can sometimes be reversed with a surgical operation. The chances for success depend on the age of the mother, the type of sterilization procedure, and several other factors. After you weigh the cost, risks, and benefits of reversing sterilization, IVF or ICSI may turn out to be a better choice.

Appendix B
Additional Information for Pregnant Moms

I know that reading about every pregnancy symptom, test, or potential negative outcome can be distressing. Much of what is listed here won't be relevant for most mothers because complications are rare. But it also can be reassuring to have information at your fingertips if you are concerned about test results or a developing problem. Here, then, you will find information about:

- Common early pregnancy symptoms and suggestions for how to ease them
- The Food and Drug Administration's risk categories for medication use in pregnancy
- Miscarriage and ectopic (tubal) pregnancy and their treatments
- Environmental and infectious exposures in the workplace and how you can assess your risk
- Abnormal findings on first trimester ultrasound, including markers for genetic conditions
- Diagnosis and treatment of vaginal and urinary tract infections during pregnancy
- Common late pregnancy symptoms and what you can do to feel better
- Special tests that may be necessary in the third trimester
- Diagnosis and treatment of complications during late pregnancy
- Fetal positions at term, and external cephalic version, the procedure used to turn a breech baby

Common Early Pregnancy Symptoms

Although you may have spent months longing for a baby and are thrilled to be pregnant, it can be tough when pregnancy starts off with a bang. Many women experience at least some of the following symptoms during the earliest weeks:

- Breast soreness. Your breasts may start to be sore even before the first missed period, due to the hormone progesterone. The achiness usually resolves in a few weeks. If you need to ease the pain, wear a supportive bra during the day and consider a soft bra at night.
- Absent periods. For many moms-to-be, the first sign of pregnancy is a missed period. Although a little spotting is normal during the early stages, you shouldn't have a full-fledged period during pregnancy. That's because the pregnancy hormone hCG keeps progesterone levels high throughout a healthy pregnancy, preventing the uterine lining from shedding. If you do experience mild spotting during early pregnancy, always use a pad, not a tampon. You should also call your doctor right away if you bleed as much as a period in the first trimester or have any bleeding at all between sixteen and thirty-five weeks. Light, painless bleeding in the first trimester should be reported to your doctor or midwife but you can usually wait until regular office hours to call in. Missed periods with a negative pregnancy test are not caused by pregnancy.
- Mild cramps. No one knows why some women experience mild cramping during early pregnancy, but thankfully, they usually resolve in a few weeks. It is best not to take medications, so hang in there for mild cramps, and call your doctor if you experience severe or one-sided pain.
- Fatigue. Many moms feel wiped out during their first few weeks. The best treatment is to rest when possible, even adjusting your work schedule if necessary (see Chapter 8 for suggestions). And you can look forward to feeling more energetic during the second trimester—fatigue usually resolves on its own by then.
- Frequent urination. It is common during the first trimester to have to visit the bathroom more frequently, because of pregnancy hormones. But don't be tempted to limit your fluid intake to relieve this symptom—instead listen to your body and drink as much as you need. If you feel pain when urinating, be sure to tell your doctor: you may have a bladder infection.
- Sensitivity to odors. Another common first sign of pregnancy is having a strong response to smells, such as when cooking. The cause is not

known, but you can help yourself get through it: you might try controlling your environment as much as possible, or even carrying something with you that has a pleasant odor so you'll have something else to sniff if you're feeling overwhelmed by a strong smell.

- Nausea or vomiting. We all know women who have struggled with nausea or vomiting during pregnancy: about 70 percent of pregnant women suffer from these symptoms. Although no one knows why these side effects occur, it is clear that the early weeks are usually the most troublesome, and that they are more common in situations like twins, where the mom has high levels of the pregnancy hormone hCG. If you're suffering, try to avoid triggers; eat several smaller meals over the course of the day rather than fewer large meals (and never let your stomach get empty); drink fluids separately from trying to eat; stick with easy to tolerate foods like toast, dry cereal, potatoes, and pasta (or whatever goes down easily for you); and keep a supply of plain crackers, like saltines, with you to nibble on if they help to make you feel better. (See Chapter 8 for more ideas.)
- Change in appetite. During your pregnancy, for unknown reasons, your appetite may increase or decrease. My best advice is to try to eat healthful foods in normal quantities.
- Constipation. It can be frustrating to have your digestive system slow down due to the hormone progesterone. To prevent constipation, which can occur at any point during pregnancy, drink lots of fluids, exercise, and eat fiber-rich foods. If you are stopped up, take a mild laxative like Milk of Magnesia until things are working, then start a fiber supplement like Metamucil or Citrucel every day. If you start at a low daily dose and slowly increase each week, you won't get as gassy as you will if you jump right to the full dose. If this strategy doesn't resolve the problem, talk to your doctor or midwife—we have many more tricks to improve constipation in pregnancy.
- Lightheadedness. If you're feeling lightheaded, it may be due to low blood sugar (a common side effect of pregnancy) or, more commonly, a drop in blood pressure when getting up or standing a while (because during pregnancy your leg veins hold more blood than normal and

prevent its circulation). If you think you may be lightheaded from low blood sugar, have a snack, especially one with a significant amount of protein: high-protein foods tend to keep your blood sugar more stable than sugary foods do. Move from foot to foot if you are standing in one place, and get up slowly when you have been sitting or lying for a while. If you feel like you might faint, find a place to sit or lie down immediately—don't be polite and risk a fall.

- Mood swings and overemotionalism. Hormonal changes, relationship issues, the significance of being pregnant—or all three—can supercharge your emotions during early pregnancy. It may be disconcerting to feel this way when you want to feel professional and on top of things, but the experience is normal. You might try counting to ten before reacting; taking a step back from the situation to see if you are being rational; and working hard to control your responses in critical situations. See Chapter 13 for more ideas.
- Difficulty concentrating. Some women have a hard time settling in to do tasks that require their full concentration, which can be unnerving in a professional setting. No one knows for sure why this happens, but the cause may be hormonal or the distraction of knowing that your life is about to change. If you're struggling to concentrate, you might try to figure out when in the day you are at your best and plan important activities for during that time.
- Feeling totally normal. Some women have no significant pregnancy symptoms and feel just like they always do. Usually this is just due to good luck. Occasionally, though, it is an indication that hCG levels are low and the pregnancy is destined to miscarry. Your doctor or midwife can investigate if you have concerns.

The Food and Drug Administration's Risk Categories for Medication Use in Pregnancy

The Food and Drug Administration (FDA) uses categories A through D, and X, to describe the risks of taking particular medications during pregnancy.

Category A: Studies on pregnant women did not demonstrate a risk to the fetus in the first trimester (and there is no evidence of risk in later trimesters); the possibility of fetal harm seems remote. Folic acid is an example of a category A drug.

Category B: Either pregnant animal studies have not shown risk (and there are no human studies) or animal studies have shown a problem that hasn't occurred during human studies. Acetaminophen (Tylenol) is an example of a category B drug.

Category C: Either animal studies have shown a problem and there are no studies in pregnant women, or tests haven't been done on pregnant animals or people. Category C drugs should be given only "if the potential benefits outweigh the potential risks." Most medications fall into category C, because good studies to prove safety often don't exist. The asthma medicine metaproterenol (Alupent) is an example of a category C drug.

Category D: Risk to humans has been shown, but benefits may outweigh risks under certain circumstances. Some drugs for epilepsy fall into this category.

Category X: The risk in pregnant women clearly outweighs any potential benefit, so the drug should not be used in pregnancy. Isotretinoin (Accutane), a drug for acne, is category X.

(Note that as of this printing, the FDA was still using these five categories, but experts are working toward a rating system that will be clearer about risks from animal studies and human data. Then doctors will be able to make better judgments about potential risks and benefits. For an excellent web resource, go to www.motherisk.org.)

Miscarriage

When a miscarriage completes on its own, the woman usually has heavy bleeding and cramps for six hours or so, passes somewhat solid-appearing tissue, and then feels better. The bleeding will gradually stop a few days to a couple of weeks later. If you think you have miscarried, you should let your doctor or midwife know the next day so they can check to be sure that it is complete, and that you don't need any further treatment. In addition, if your blood type is Rh-negative you should receive an injection of the medication Rhogam within a day or two to prevent you from developing antibodies that could harm future pregnancies.

Miscarriage may be diagnosed before the pregnancy is expelled—and in this case is sometimes called a missed or incomplete abortion. (Although in common use the word abortion refers to voluntary termination of pregnancy, in medical terms abortion refers to any pregnancy loss. Don't be offended if your miscarriage is referred to as a spontaneous abortion in your doctor's records.)

The traditional treatment for miscarriage is dilation and curettage, or D&C. This surgical procedure uses a suction tube to remove the embryo and placenta from inside the uterus, usually with the mother under sedation or asleep. This gets it over with quickly and avoids worries about when the bleeding and cramping will occur, but does involve the risks of surgery and anesthesia, and may be more expensive than the other options.

Medicines that cause uterine contractions also can hasten the expulsion of a miscarriage. One medication, misoprostol or Cytotec, is taken either orally or vaginally, in one to four doses, depending on the protocol; the pregnancy usually passes within a few days. Some women like this option because it is more private than coming into the hospital, and seems more natural. Others don't like the idea that they won't know exactly when the pregnancy will pass. Note that with medications, sometimes the miscarriage still won't complete or bleeding will become prolonged and heavy; if this happens, a D&C will be necessary.

Many miscarriages will complete on their own, if given enough time. This is certainly the most natural approach, but it may involve a greater risk of infection and excess blood loss, if the uterus doesn't empty in short order.

If you experience a miscarriage, you should know that early pregnancy loss is very common—about one in eight pregnancies (and even more in older moms) ends in miscarriage. Most first trimester miscarriages occur because the pregnancy isn't developing properly, due to abnormal chromosomes or some other factor outside of anyone's control. Usually first trimester miscarriage isn't due to any failure on the part of the parents, and the likely outcome of the next pregnancy is a healthy baby. If you have a miscarriage, be sure to talk to your practitioner about why it occurred. Parents often harbor concerns about things they did that they believe led to the loss, but most miscarriages are not preventable. Obtaining accurate information can be a step toward healing and being ready to try again.

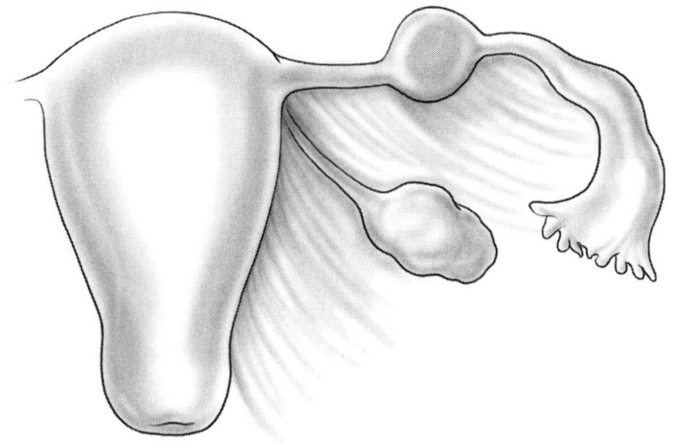

Tubal ectopic pregnancy

Ectopic Pregnancy

About 1 percent of pregnancies implant and grow outside of the uterus. These "ectopic" or out-of-place pregnancies are usually located in the fallopian tubes and so may be referred to as tubal pregnancies. Tubal pregnancies cannot survive, and their continued growth can burst the tube, leading to internal bleeding. First trimester bleeding or pelvic pain may be the first sign of an ectopic pregnancy.

Ultrasound and/or measurements of the "pregnancy hormone," hCG, can sometimes identify an ectopic pregnancy even before symptoms develop. If an ultrasound scan can't detect the pregnancy anywhere in the pelvis, blood pregnancy tests that measure hCG may differentiate an ectopic from a really early pregnancy that is too small to see with ultrasound. If the situation still isn't clear, hCG measurements taken a few days apart may be needed. Usually the diagnosis can be made for certain within a few days.

A pregnancy growing outside the uterus must be removed or destroyed to avoid rupture of the tube and internal bleeding. Tubal pregnancies can be treated with surgery or with a medication called methotrexate, which kills the dividing cells. Your doctor will discuss the pros and cons of the options before treatment. If the ectopic ruptures, surgical removal of the tube is usually necessary.

The chance of ectopic pregnancy is greater for women who have had gonorrhea or chlamydia, pelvic inflammatory disease (PID), pelvic surgery, prior ectopic pregnancy, or infertility, and for those rare women who get pregnant with an IUD in place. Women with significant risk factors should have an ultrasound between five and seven weeks to locate the pregnancy. In most cases, once an ultrasound shows that the pregnancy is within the uterus, or as soon as a fetal heartbeat is heard, ectopic pregnancy can be ruled out.

Environmental and Occupational Exposures

Workplaces can expose pregnant women to solvents, smoke, and other environmental toxins. If you have concerns about potentially dangerous exposures at your job, talk to your doctor or midwife, preferably before you become pregnant.

Occupational exposures to infectious agents also worry many healthcare workers and others who may be at risk.

Herbal medications may be unsafe in pregnancy. If you think about it, anything that can have a biological effect can in theory have a negative effect. Herbals aren't typically researched with the same rigor that is required of medications, and even with medications we sometimes find out about risks late in the game. Exposures have the greatest potential for damage in the first trimester when fetal organs are forming. Known unsafe herbal supplements include:

- Arbor vitae (Thuja occidentalis)
- Beth root (Trillium erectum)
- Black cohosh (Cimicifuga racemosa)
- Blue cohosh (Caulophyllum thalictroides)
- Cascara (Rhamnus purshianus)
- Chinese angelica, dong quai (Angelica sinensis)
- Cinchona (Cinchona sp.)
- Cotton root bark (Gossypium herbaceum)
- Feverfew (Tanacetum parthenium)
- Ginseng (Panax ginseng)
- Golden seal (Hydrastis canadensis)
- Juniper (Juniperus communis)
- Kava kava (Piper methysticum)
- Licorice (Glycyrrhiza glabra)
- Meadow saffron (Crocus sativus)
- Pennyroyal (Mentha pulegium)

- Poke root (Phytolacca americana)
- Rue (Ruta graveolens)
- Sage (Salvia officinalis; may be used to suppress lactation)
- Senna (Cassia senna)
- Tansy (Tanacetum vulgare)
- White peony (Paeonia lactiflora)
- Wormwood (Artemisia absinthium)
- Yarrow (Achillea millefolium)
- Yellow dock (Rumex crispus)

Some sources recommend blue cohosh and black cohosh for labor stimulation or pain; research hasn't established if their use is safe for mother or child. I don't recommend experimenting on yourself and your baby.

Environmental Exposures in the Workplace

Type of chemical	*Types of jobs*	*Details*	*Protective measures*
Lead	Remodeling older houses, jobs with exposure to lead, living near a smelter, or residing in a developing country are all risk factors for high lead levels	Lead exposure has been associated with high blood pressure, miscarriage, premature delivery, and learning disabilities. Pregnancy blood lead levels <10 mcg/dl are considered safe, although previous lead exposure (that doesn't show up in blood testing) can still pose a risk, since lead can be stored in the mother's bone and released to the baby during pregnancy	Blood lead levels measure current exposure. Oral calcium supplements taken during the second half of pregnancy may prevent lead in the mother's bones from being released to the baby
Pesticides	Agricultural workers, crop dusters	May make infertility, miscarriage, poor fetal growth, and some birth defects more	Wearing proper protective clothing, including a respirator, and good hand wash-

Environmental Exposures in the Workplace (Continued)

Type of chemical	*Types of jobs*	*Details*	*Protective measures*
Pesticides (continued)		likely, but the studies are conflicting	ing before eating and before going home may help prevent exposure
Chemotherapy agents	Nurses and other hospital personnel	Exposure may lead to higher rates of pregnancy loss	Established guidelines for handling these toxic agents provide protection
Inhaled anesthetic agents	Operating room personnel, particularly in pediatric or open-mask cases	Increases the chance of miscarriage	Pregnant personnel and those trying to conceive should avoid open-mask cases and be sure that proper room ventilation procedures are being followed
Organic solvents	Medical equipment sterilization; painting; some hobbies; printing; dry cleaning; scientific research; and manufacturing of textiles, paint, rubber, semiconductors, and many other products	Children of workers who use these chemicals in pregnancy are more likely to have birth defects, growth restriction, and learning disabilities. These complications are much more common in situations in which the mother has headaches, dizziness, or other symptoms of solvent exposure	Proper ventilation and protective gear prevent solvents from entering your system. You can get data pages on each chemical, called MSDS sheets, from your employer, your union representative, or the Internet at www.ilpi.com/msds
Secondhand smoke	Workers in bars and restaurants	Secondhand tobacco smoke affects the fetus just like smoking does. Children of women who work in smoke-filled environments are at risk for poor fetal growth and asthma	Although U.S. laws limit secondhand smoke exposure in the workplace, women who live with smokers or who work where smoking is allowed should stay away from smoke as much as possible

Occupational Exposures to Infectious Agents

Type of infection	*Types of work*	*Risks*	*Prevention*
Chicken pox	Teachers, healthcare workers, mothers. Unimmunized women who don't remember having chicken pox in childhood should be tested to see if they are immune, because many people who never had clear-cut chicken pox nevertheless have protective antibodies	Chicken pox poses two major risks—women can become particularly sick if they acquire chicken pox during pregnancy, and occasionally a fetus will catch it from the mother	If you are exposed to a person with chicken pox or touch the skin of a person with shingles, talk to your practitioner about getting tested to be sure you are immune. If you had chicken pox in childhood or were immunized, you and your baby are not at risk
Cytomegalovirus (CMV)	Childcare workers who change diapers, mothers of children in daycare, healthcare workers. Many adults have had CMV in the past. Some cases of CMV transmission to the fetus are from mothers who were infected long ago	CMV can infect the fetus through the placenta, causing birth defects, deafness, mental retardation, and stillbirth. Recent infection poses a greater risk than infection in the past	Good hand washing works well at preventing acquisition of CMV. Healthcare workers are less likely than daycare workers to get CMV, probably because of better hand washing practices. No treatments have been shown to protect the baby once the mother is infected

Occupational Exposures to Infectious Agents (Continued)

Type of infection	*Types of work*	*Risks*	*Prevention*
Hepatitis B, hepatitis C, and HIV	Jobs that involve direct contact with body secretions, especially blood: healthcare workers, police, firefighters, tattoo artists, body piercers	Maternal illness can be severe. Hepatitis B, HIV, and possibly hepatitis C can be transmitted to the baby before or during birth	All healthcare workers and others at risk should be immunized against hepatitis B. The vaccine is safe in pregnancy. Universal precautions (prevention of contact with blood and body secretions) help protect against viral transmission. If you are inadvertently exposed during pregnancy, talk to your doctor or infection-control nurse about your options
Influenza	Anyone who has a lot of contact with people, particularly sick people	Pregnant women may become more ill from the flu than other adults do	All pregnant women should be immunized during flu season
Parvovirus B19 (slap face or fifth disease)	Teachers, daycare workers, mothers	This virus can pass through the placenta, occasionally leading to fetal anemia, heart failure, and stillbirth. It is important to remember, though, that most fetuses exposed to this virus have no problems	By the time a child has the rash, they have been infectious for a few days, and others may have already been exposed. Your titers of antibody against parvovirus can be checked if you get exposed; it may be clear that you already had this infection and are immune. Inform your practitioner if you think you have been exposed to parvovirus

Occupational Exposures to Infectious Agents (Continued)

Type of infection	*Types of work*	*Risks*	*Prevention*
Toxoplasmosis	Animal workers, cat owners, agricultural workers. Interestingly, research has shown that veterinarians are no more likely to have been infected with toxoplasmosis than are members of the general public. When cats and their litter are handled properly, the chance of infection is low. Fruit or vegetables can be contaminated from soil containing animal feces	Toxoplasmosis can infect the fetus through the placenta, leading to miscarriage, birth defects, or stillbirth	It takes one to five days for the eggs to form spores after excretion by the cat; the feces are not infectious before then. Women who work in veterinary settings may be safer than those at home, since the litter in a clinic is changed frequently. Those who work with cats should wear gloves for changing the litter, and anyone who might come in contact with toxoplasmosis spores should practice good hand washing

Abnormal Findings on a First Trimester Ultrasound

Most pregnant women have an ultrasound scan at some point during pregnancy. It isn't unusual to find something on the ultrasound that is out of the ordinary. If concerns come up, use the table on pages 520–521 to better understand your situation.

Another possible ultrasound finding is the two-vessel umbilical cord. Usually the cord has two arteries and a slightly larger vein. But in about one in two hundred newborns (and more frequently in twins), there are only two vessels. For most babies, the finding of a two-vessel cord is inconsequential. But sometimes it indicates other structural variations, perhaps in the urinary tract or heart. If problems are seen in the structure of other organ systems, further evaluation for chromosomal disorders may be necessary. And all babies who are known to have only two vessels in the cord should be followed closely during pregnancy to assure that they are growing well.

Abnormal Ultrasound Findings

First trimester ultrasound finding	*Description*	*What does it mean?*
Possible miscarriage	Sometimes the ultrasound sees the pregnancy but can't tell if it is okay or going to miscarry. Usually this uncertainty occurs when the pregnancy is so small that a heartbeat can't be seen. Sequential blood levels of the pregnancy hormone hCG, taken a few days apart, or another ultrasound a week later, can help clarify the situation	It may just be an early and viable pregnancy, but if it was expected to be bigger by now, miscarriage is likely
Retroplacental clot (may also be termed subchorionic bleed or subchorionic hemorrhage)	Sometimes the ultrasound shows a collection of blood behind the placenta. This finding is commonly associated with vaginal bleeding	The clot may resolve, or the pregnancy may go on to miscarry. This finding also indicates a slightly higher risk of preterm birth later on
Miscarriage	Sometimes the ultrasound shows a pregnancy that is big enough so that a heartbeat would normally be seen but none is present. Alternatively, the sac can look irregular, like it is collapsing. Such findings may definitively indicate miscarriage	Most first trimester miscarriages are random events that aren't caused by anything the mother did, and are not likely to recur

Abnormal Ultrasound Findings (Continued)

First trimester ultrasound finding	*Description*	*What does it mean?*
Possible ectopic pregnancy	The pregnancy may be seen outside of the uterus, or no pregnancy may be found, despite a positive pregnancy test. If no pregnancy is found but the suspicion for ectopic pregnancy is low, sequential blood levels of the pregnancy hormone hCG taken a few days apart and/or another ultrasound several days later can help distinguish between possibilities	If the pregnancy is outside of the uterus, it is an ectopic pregnancy. Ectopics, which cannot survive, usually are located in the fallopian tube. Untreated ectopic pregnancies can rupture, leading to internal hemorrhage in the mother
Ovarian cyst	A cyst is a fluid-filled sac that is often seen on the ovary early in pregnancy	The great majority of ovarian cysts resolve within a few months. If pain develops or the cyst remains, surgery may become necessary
Other anatomical findings	Sometimes early ultrasound finds evidence of other anatomical variations	Depends on what is seen

First trimester ultrasound can give indications of genetic disorders as well. If an abnormality is identified at your ultrasound, use this table to help you to understand the implications.

Vaginal and Urinary Tract Infections during Pregnancy

Vaginal and urinary symptoms are common in pregnancy, and their prevention and treatment depend in part on the cause. If you're experiencing trouble, consult the table on pages 523–524 for answers to some typical questions.

Genetic Markers Detected on First Trimester Ultrasound

Finding	*Description*	*What does it mean?*
Nuchal translucency	An increased echo-free area seen at the back of the fetal neck between ten and fourteen weeks' gestation. These measurements are difficult to determine, and a few millimeters can be the difference between calling the result normal or abnormal. Inexperienced ultrasonographers can underestimate or overestimate the measurement	Indicates an elevated chance for Down syndrome or other chromosomal variations, and is associated with structural alterations in the heart. Some older women use the results of this test to decide whether to test for Down syndrome with chorionic villus sampling (CVS), which can be done at eleven weeks, rather than waiting for amniocentesis, which can't be performed until about sixteen weeks. Combining nuchal translucency with blood testing for PAPP-A and hCG, called "first screen," improves the accuracy of risk assessment
Absent/small nasal bone	The fetal nasal bone is visualized by ultrasound with the face in profile. These measurements are difficult, and small variations can be the difference between calling the result normal or abnormal. Inexperienced ultrasonographers can underestimate or overestimate the result	Most but not all fetuses with Down syndrome have a small or absent nasal bone. About 5 percent of white babies with normal chromosomes, and a greater percent of babies of African heritage, have this finding as well, which also does not mean that the baby's nose will be abnormal

Vaginal and Urinary Tract Infections

Diagnosis	Symptoms	Tests	Treatment	Notes
Vaginitis				
Yeast	Itching or discharge	Secretions can be tested in the office or lab	Over-the-counter or prescription creams or suppositories	Yeast is not dangerous to the baby or the pregnancy
Trichomonas	Irritation or discharge (may have no symptoms)	Secretions can be tested in the office or lab	Oral antibiotics	Trich, as it is called, is sexually transmitted. The mother's partner(s) should be treated and condoms should be used for the remainder of pregnancy
Bacterial vaginosis	Fishy odor	Secretions can be tested in the office or lab	Oral or vaginal antibiotics	BV is not an infection, but rather an imbalance of the normal bacteria of the vagina. For unclear reasons, women with BV are at a slightly increased risk of preterm birth

Vaginal and Urinary Tract Infections (Continued)

Diagnosis	*Symptoms*	*Tests*	*Treatment*	*Notes*
Urinary tract infection				
Bladder infection (also called UTI or cystitis)	Frequent urination and urgency are common, but these symptoms occur in normal pregnancy too. Some bladder infections occur without any symptoms	Urine culture or urine analysis in the office or lab	Oral antibiotics	Recurrent urinary tract infection requires suppression with a small dose of antibiotic every night at bedtime for the remainder of the pregnancy
Kidney infection (pyelonephritis)	Back or side pain, fever, and nausea or vomiting	Urine culture	Usually requires hospital admission for intravenous antibiotics	Kidney infections can lead to serious illness and also preterm birth. Once treated, you will be prescribed a small dose of antibiotic to take every night at bedtime to prevent recurrence

Common Late Pregnancy Symptoms

As you're coming into the home stretch, sometimes new discomforts crop up. If you're feeling some new and unwelcome sensations, you might check below to get a better understanding of what they mean and what you can do about them.

SKIN DISCOMFORTS

- Dry, itchy skin on the abdomen. The stretching of your abdominal skin across your growing baby can make it feel dry and itchy. Lotions or oils can be soothing.
- Stretch marks. More than half of all moms develop pregnancy stretch marks or "striae gravidarum"; they occur most commonly in women who developed striae on their thighs or breasts during puberty and whose family members have stretch marks. The cause is primarily genetic. Stretch marks may look bright pink during and right after pregnancy, but they usually fade and become more silvery over time. Unfortunately, despite advertisements to the contrary, I can't find any scientific studies that show that any cream or treatment truly helps prevent stretch marks. Some studies indicate that starting off pregnancy overweight or gaining excess weight makes stretch marks more likely; other studies, though, have shown that striae aren't any more likely in heavy women.
- Rashes. About one in two hundred women gets an itchy rash that starts on the abdomen, called PUPPP—for Pruritic (itchy) Urticarial (hive-like) Papules and Plaques (bumpy rash) of Pregnancy—or "polymorphic eruption of pregnancy." The cause is unknown, but we do know that they are most common in a first pregnancy. They can be treated with anti-itch medicine, topical steroids, and time—the rash always resolves after the baby is born.

SYMPTOMS CAUSED BY WATER RETENTION

- Swollen legs. It is common to retain water in your legs during pregnancy, but it also can be a sign of pre-eclampsia, a condition characterized by high blood pressure and protein in the urine. Call your practitioner if you experience a sudden increase in water retention, particularly if your face and hands become swollen. If you have puffy legs, avoid very salty foods, keep your legs elevated, and swim for exercise. Why swimming? It seems that the water pressure on your body pushes excess tissue fluid back into the blood vessels, where it is then carried to your kidneys and exits through your urine.

- Carpal tunnel syndrome. Carpal tunnel syndrome, a numb achy feeling along the thumb side of the hands, is caused by a buildup of fluid in the wrist. This fluid compresses the nerve as it travels through its small space. Angling the hand back, like when you are typing or on the phone, can make symptoms worse. Carpal tunnel symptoms also can flare at night, when the fluid that has settled to your feet redistributes throughout the body. Your best bets for prevention and treatment: position yourself carefully when at the keyboard—with a good upright posture and gel pads for the wrist if needed. Using a speakerphone or headset instead of holding the phone may also help. The best position for your wrist is with your hand straight out. A splint can be fitted by a physical therapist or medical supply shop to keep your hand in that neutral position.

CIRCULATION ISSUES

- Varicose veins. Between hormonal changes and the weight of the baby, your circulation may get sluggish as pregnancy moves along. Varicose veins occur when the valves that help push blood along stop functioning, and blood pools in the veins, making them swollen and achy. You can get varicosities in the legs, vulva, and rectal area (hemorrhoids are varicose veins of the rectum). Allowing blood to pool makes varicose veins worse. Standing is bad. Constipation makes hemorrhoids worse because you have to strain, increasing the blood flow into that area. Compression, by contrast, often gives great relief, and may prevent worsening of the varicosities. Support hose are the mainstays of compression for leg veins. You can try regular maternity support pantyhose, but many women need heavy-duty compression—the kind you can get from prescription compression hose. Garments that put pressure against the vulva can be helpful for vulvar varicosities. Talk to your doctor or midwife about your options. Usually insurance will help to pay for prescription compression hose.

- Blood clots. Deep venous thrombosis (DVT, or blood clots in the deep veins of the legs), which may be caused by the extra clotting factors and sluggish blood flow of pregnancy, is a dangerous condition. If one leg becomes swollen and painful, tell your practitioner right away. Sudden shortness of breath can be a sign of a blood clot in the lung, also called pulmonary embolism, or PE. Again, call your practitioner right away or go to the emergency room if you think you might have a blood clot in your legs or your lungs. The doctor will most likely treat a DVT or PE with blood thinners, which allow the clot to dissolve. Women who get a DVT or PE generally have to take blood thinners until six weeks after delivery and again during every subsequent pregnancy. They also should not use estrogen-containing birth control.

PROBLEMS WITH THE DIGESTIVE TRACT

- Bleeding gums. Bleeding while brushing or flossing is usually caused by gingivitis, or inflammation of the gums, a common problem during pregnancy. Good dental care, including flossing regularly (even if it causes bleeding) and seeing your dental hygienist should improve the swelling and irritation that leads to bleeding.
- Heartburn. Pregnancy hormones, especially when combined with the pressure of the baby pushing on the stomach, can lead to reflux of acid up the food pipe, or esophagus. This can cause heartburn (a burning sensation or pain in the chest), a sore throat, or a cough. Caffeine, alcohol, spicy and fatty foods, and lying down right after eating make heartburn worse. If you're dealing with heartburn, try to avoid foods that make symptoms worse, don't eat before you go to bed, and sleep with your head raised, but antacids will probably be necessary. Tums and other chewable calcium-based antacids only work for about an hour, so liquid antacids like Mylanta or Maalox are better. The dose isn't critical—you can take a sip or two right out of the bottle at night if necessary (you don't have to get up to measure out teaspoons). If you are still suffering, talk to your doctor or midwife about other effective treatments.

BLADDER CONTROL ISSUES

It is not rare to leak urine, particularly in second and subsequent pregnancies. Usually just a little trickle comes out with a cough or sneeze. Sometimes women who leak a little bit of urine wonder if their water has broken. But amniotic fluid smells more like Comet cleanser, and urine smells like . . . urine. If you are leaking, you need to strengthen your pelvic floor. To do the famous "Kegel exercises" that work on this area, you will first need to identify the Kegel muscles. This you can do while urinating—Kegels are the muscles that can stop the flow. But it isn't good for your body to practice during urination, so once you learn where these muscles are, start doing your Kegels at other times in sets of five or ten, frequently throughout the day. Contrary to popular belief, Kegel exercises will not help with labor or birth, but they can keep you dry if you practice enough.

Special Tests That May Be Necessary in the Third Trimester

If a test has been recommended for you during your third trimester, this list will give you some general information about it, but be sure to ask your doctor about the test's risks and why it is right for you and your baby. You'll see, too, that some tests are only done under special circumstances, like if you are showing signs of preterm labor, or if the size of your uterus seems bigger or smaller than expected.

- Glucose tolerance test. The glucose tolerance test is performed to find out whether women with an abnormal one-hour screening test have gestational diabetes.

  How it is done: The glucose tolerance test is more time-consuming and annoying than the one-hour test because you have to get your blood tested at four points in time: after fasting overnight, and at one, two, and three hours after drinking glucola, a glucose solution.

  What it tests: If two or more of the four measurements are high, you have gestational diabetes; one high value would be considered borderline. If the results are normal and your original screening test wasn't too high, you're off the hook.

Risk: Glucola makes some people queasy.

- Fetal fibronectin. Fibronectin is a protein released from the uterus, and fetal fibronectin (fFN) testing can be useful in a mother-to-be who is showing some signs of preterm labor (like frequent contractions) in order to know whether treatment, like medications or bed rest, is necessary.

  How it is done: Using a speculum to see into the vagina, secretions from near the cervix are collected on a cotton swab.

  What it tests: When fetal fibronectin is absent (a negative test), preterm delivery is very unlikely within the next two weeks. A positive fetal fibronectin test, though, means preterm delivery is more likely. While there are few false negatives, there are many false positives—in other words, if you have a negative result you can be pretty confident that you will not deliver soon, but if you have a positive result you still may not deliver early.

  Risks: No direct risks. The test is expensive, although usually covered by insurance. False positive test results can lead to worry and unnecessary treatment.

- Ultrasound for cervical length. Like the fetal fibronectin test, cervical length can be used to screen for mothers who are likely to deliver early.

  How it is done: The ultrasound wand is placed into the vagina to get a close-up view of the cervix.

  What it tests: A short cervix may be a sign that the baby is going to come early. A cervix longer than thirty millimeters (a little over an inch) is normal.

  Risks: Ultrasound itself has little if any risk. A borderline cervical measurement, however, can be confusing and lead to overtreatment.

- Third trimester amniocentesis: The amniotic fluid can be tested to assess fetal lung maturity before thirty-nine weeks, to help decide if the baby is ready to be born. This technique may be useful before a scheduled cesarean, or if considering induction of labor for medical reasons.

  How it is done: A needle is placed through the mother's abdomen under ultrasound guidance, to draw fluid out from the amniotic sac. (See Chapter 17 for more information on amniocentesis.)

  What it tests: Substances in the amniotic fluid correlate with the chance of respiratory distress syndrome and other complications of premature birth.

Risks: Although amniocentesis always has some risk, the risk to the baby from amnio during the third trimester is less than when amnio is done earlier in the pregnancy because if a complication (such as rupture of membranes) occurs, the baby can usually be delivered safely.

Tests of Fetal Well-Being

If you have risk factors such as diabetes or hypertension, if your baby isn't growing well, or if you are progressing past your due date, your doctor may recommend a test of fetal well-being. The choice of test is a judgment call that your doctor or midwife will make. If you want to watch your baby more closely, fetal movement tracking is a safe and effective measure of fetal well-being, and can be done at home.

- Non-stress testing (NST). In non-stress testing, the fetal monitor is used to measure the baby's heartbeat and any contractions. Non-stress testing provides information about the frequency of contractions and how the baby is doing.

  How it is done: Two fetal monitoring belts are placed around the mother's abdomen; one feels for contractions and the other listens to the baby's heartbeat.

  What it tests: Characteristics of the fetal heartbeat will tell the medical team about your baby's well-being. When the baby moves inside of you, the heartbeat normally speeds up. Results can be reassuring or "non-reassuring." If results are worrisome, further testing is warranted. Regular contractions before thirty-six weeks can be a sign of preterm labor.
- Biophysical profile. The biophysical profile, or BPP, assesses fetal well-being with a score of two, four, six, eight, or ten.

  How it is done: A transabdominal ultrasound is used to watch fetal activity. The test may take up to one hour and is sometimes combined with non-stress testing.

What it tests: Points are assigned based on four ultrasound characteristics: fetal tone, fetal movement, fetal breathing activity, and whether enough amniotic fluid is present. Two more points are given if the nonstress test is reassuring.

- Fetal movement counts. It is easy to assess fetal well-being at home using fetal movement counts.

  How it is done: Depending on your medical team's protocol, you will be asked to count fetal movements either three times a day for a half hour, or once a day.

  What it tests: Fetal movement is a sign of fetal well-being. A baby who isn't moving may just be asleep, but a baby who doesn't move for more than two hours may be in trouble. If the baby doesn't move within the time allotted, the mother will be told to go to the office or hospital for further fetal assessment.

- Third trimester ultrasound of fetus and placenta. Ultrasound may be recommended when the uterine size is bigger or smaller than expected, when there have been unexplained contractions or bleeding, or when the doctor wants to follow up on ongoing questions about the baby or placenta.

  How it is done: The ultrasound probe is used transabdominally or transvaginally to look at the baby and placenta.

  What it tests: A third trimester ultrasound can check on the size and position of the fetus, the amount of amniotic fluid, the location of the placenta, and some fetal and placental problems.

- Ultrasound Doppler flow. You may undergo an ultrasound Doppler flow test if your medical team wants to assess if and why a baby isn't growing well.

  How it is done: A special ultrasound machine is used to measure the flow of blood in the uterine blood vessels.

  What it tests: The amount of blood flowing through the uterine arteries determines in part how much oxygen and nutrients are delivered to the baby. Knowing how much blood is flowing will help the doctor understand whether your fetus is receiving enough oxygen and nutrients to stay healthy.

Late Pregnancy Complications

The list that follows is designed to help mothers-to-be who have been diagnosed with problems; these concerns will not apply to most women. To avoid unnecessary worry, I suggest using the index to look up anything relevant for your care, then reading only the applicable section. If you have an obstetrical complication, you should of course also ask your doctor for individualized information and recommendations.

GESTATIONAL DIABETES

Pregnancy can interfere with a woman's sugar levels, making her temporarily diabetic. Gestational diabetes is pretty common; it occurs in 2–14 percent of women.

What is the risk?

Untreated gestational diabetes can lead to excessively big babies who may be difficult to deliver, and rarely, stillbirth.

What are the signs?

Most women with gestational diabetes have no symptoms; routine testing helps to identify moms with gestational diabetes.

How is it treated?

If you are diagnosed with gestational diabetes, you will need to check your blood glucose and carefully control your diet for the remainder of your pregnancy. Pregnant women should strive for completely normal blood sugars: typically under 100 before eating and under 120 after meals. When diet alone isn't enough to maintain normal blood sugar levels, insulin treatment can help prevent complications for mother and baby. It may sound overwhelming to think of watching your diet all the time, or sticking your finger to check your sugar, or giving yourself injections of insulin—but remember it is for a good cause, and temporary. Gestational diabetes usually resolves as soon as the baby is born, although many women with gestational diabetes will become diabetic again later in life.

LARGE-FOR-DATES BABY

Babies who are going to be over the ninety-fifth percentile in size may be identified by ultrasound or by the practitioner's estimated weight during a prenatal visit. Overweight moms, those who have gained excess weight during pregnancy, mothers who gave birth to large babies in the past, and diabetic women whose sugars have been high are most likely to have larger babies.

What is the risk?

A larger baby may have trouble getting through the birth canal, leading to a difficult birth. If the head delivers but the shoulders don't fit easily, shoulder dystocia may result. Cesarean is also more likely.

What are the signs?

Measurements of the mom's abdomen at a prenatal appointment may be greater than expected, leading to an ultrasound to check the baby's size. Unfortunately, ultrasound isn't as accurate as we would like, and the estimated weight can be off by as much as 15 percent, which means a baby who weighs nine pounds could be estimated as anywhere from seven-and-a-half to over ten pounds. But ultrasound combined with the clinical assessment is often the best we have to go on.

How is it treated?

Babies thought to be really big are often watched more closely during labor; if the size seems bigger than eleven pounds (or ten pounds if the mom is diabetic, since infants of diabetic mothers have bigger shoulders), some doctors will recommend doing a cesarean without trying for a vaginal birth, to prevent a traumatic delivery. You might think that early induction of labor would decrease the chance of needing a cesarean, but because induction itself increases the chance of cesarean, the benefits are cancelled out.

THREATENED PRETERM BIRTH

Regular contractions or changes in the cervix can make preterm birth seem likely, although the correlation is far from perfect: about one in five women shows some signs of preterm labor, but most of these won't deliver until term. Women with a prior preemie, twins or more, second or third trimester vaginal bleeding, a known abnormality of the uterine shape, or who have a cerclage suture holding the cervix closed are more likely to deliver early.

What is the risk?

Of all babies born, 11 percent come early. Most are born after thirty-two weeks, and do very well, although they may need to be admitted to a newborn intensive care unit at first. Extremely premature babies often have prolonged hospitalizations, and may suffer long-term problems with their breathing and/or with neurological and intellectual development. Despite tremendous research on preventing and treating prematurity, treatments don't always work; many babies still come early.

What are the signs?

All women should be aware of the signs of preterm labor (see Chapter 19). Cervical changes (on exam or ultrasound) or a positive fetal fibronectin test would suggest an increased risk.

How is it treated?

New research has indicated that premature birth can sometimes be prevented if progesterone is administered to mothers at risk before preterm labor begins. Once preterm labor has been diagnosed, medications can be given to quiet contractions, and bed rest is often used to try to keep the baby in.

SMALL-FOR-DATES BABY

Babies below the fifth percentile for size are said to be "small for dates." Although some babies (like some parents) are just little, this finding can indicate that the baby is not getting the nutrients it needs (perhaps because of insufficient maternal weight gain or inadequate blood flow to the placenta).

What is the risk?

Babies who aren't getting enough nutrients are at risk for oxygen deprivation, poor brain development, fetal distress, and stillbirth.

What are the signs?

If the mom's abdomen is smaller than expected, an ultrasound scan is usually done to check on the baby's size. Although ultrasound alone isn't exceedingly accurate at estimating weight, a combination of the estimated weight, the volume of amniotic fluid, and Doppler studies of uterine blood flow can help assess the situation.

How is it treated?
Bed rest can sometimes improve blood flow to the baby, although if the baby is near full term, delivery may be the best choice. If the situation is dire, even a very early preterm baby may need to be delivered, to be cared for outside the womb.

PRE-ECLAMPSIA AND GESTATIONAL HYPERTENSION

Pre-eclampsia, which used to be called toxemia of pregnancy, occurs in about 5 percent of first-time moms. This condition is characterized by high blood pressure, swelling, and protein in the urine. Gestational hypertension is diagnosed if your blood pressure is up without the protein in the urine or other signs of pre-eclampsia.

What is the risk?
If severe, the high blood pressure that accompanies pre-eclampsia can cause problems in the mother's other systems, including the blood's clotting system, the liver, the kidneys, and the brain; it also can stress the baby. Rarely, the mother may have a seizure, or "eclampsia."

What are the signs?
Increased blood pressure; swelling in the hands, face, or feet; and protein in the urine are the classic signs of pre-eclampsia. Blood tests and a twenty-four-hour urine collection for protein can sometimes aid in differentiating pre-eclampsia from gestational hypertension.

How is it treated?
If your blood pressure starts to go up, you will be followed more closely, and may be asked to rest at home or in the hospital. The cure for pre-eclampsia is delivery, so typically labor will be induced if the mother is near term, or if the pre-eclampsia becomes severe. During labor and for about a day afterward, magnesium is given intravenously to the mother to prevent seizures.

TOO LITTLE AMNIOTIC FLUID

Amniotic fluid is mostly composed of fetal urine. Too little fluid, or "oligohydramnios," may indicate that the baby isn't urinating as much as expected, possibly because the baby is dehydrated, which may be caused by inadequate blood flow to the placenta. Decreased amniotic fluid can also result from ruptured membranes, or from an obstruction in the baby's urinary tract.

What is the risk?

The risks vary according to the cause of the decreased fluid. A baby who isn't getting enough blood flow from the placenta may also be low on nutrients and oxygen. Lung development can be compromised if fluid levels are very low during the late second and early third trimesters because lung development depends on the fetus breathing amniotic fluid in and out of the lungs.

What are the signs?

Decreased fluid is usually identified by ultrasound.

How is it treated?

The treatment depends on the cause. If the baby is full term, labor induction will often be the best choice.

TOO MUCH AMNIOTIC FLUID

The amount of amniotic fluid around the baby is determined by how much the fetus adds to the fluid with urination and takes away through swallowing. If the baby is urinating more than expected, as sometimes happens with gestational diabetes, or (more rarely) is not swallowing well, too much amniotic fluid (also known as "polyhydramnios" or "hydramnios") can result—sometimes, though, the reason for the polyhydramnios is undetermined.

What is the risk?

Mild increases in fluid don't pose much risk. In severe polyhydramnios, however, the mother can become extremely uncomfortable, and the overdistended uterus can initiate preterm labor. Babies with swallowing difficulties need evaluation from a specialist after birth, and may require surgery.

What are the signs?

Increased fluid may be identified by a larger-than-expected uterus, or by ultrasound.

How is it treated?

If the distension becomes a problem, removing some fluid with a needle (therapeutic amniocentesis) can help.

PLACENTA PREVIA

Placenta previa occurs when the placenta grows across the inside opening of the cervix. Placenta previa can be marginal, in which the placenta is just at the edge of the cervix; partial, where the placenta covers some of the cervix; or complete. Placenta previa is more common when the placenta is big, like in a twin pregnancy, or (for unknown reasons) in mothers who have had prior cesareans.

What is the risk?

Marginal or partial placenta previas diagnosed early in pregnancy often resolve as the uterus grows and the placental edge moves away from the cervical opening. Placenta previa can bleed as the cervix starts to open during labor, if the woman has sex, or after a vaginal examination. Although the first episode of bleeding usually isn't heavy, hemorrhage can be severe and sudden. Complete placenta previa requires cesarean delivery.

What are the signs?

Placenta previa is often found incidentally at the time of routine ultrasound; partial and marginal previas often resolve by the seventh month or so. Third-trimester bleeding is the most serious sign of placenta previa.

How is it treated?

If there is no bleeding and the baby isn't full term, no treatment is necessary. Bed rest and "pelvic rest" (no sex) are often recommended if activity or direct contact is likely to cause bleeding. Heavy bleeding usually requires cesarean delivery.

PLACENTAL ABRUPTION

Placental abruption occurs when the placenta partially separates from the inside wall of the uterus.

What is the risk?

Since the baby is getting oxygen and nutrients through the placenta, abruption can lead to fetal distress and even stillbirth. Small separations can lead to poor fetal growth.

What are the signs?

Vaginal bleeding and preterm labor are the most common signs of placental

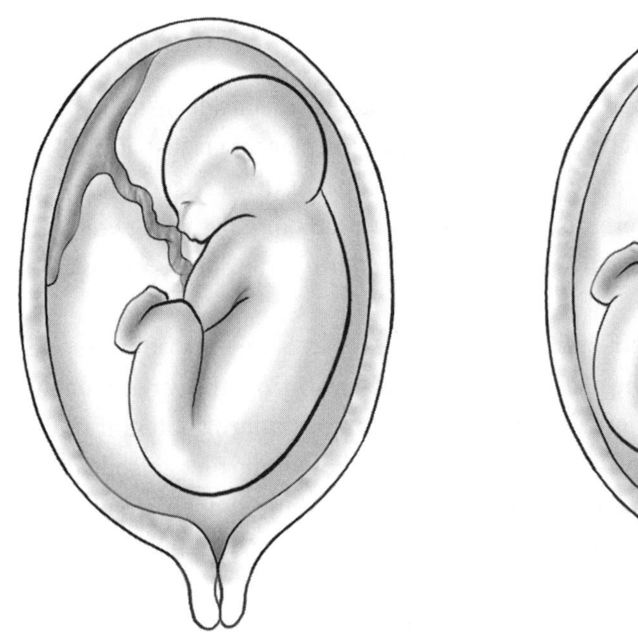

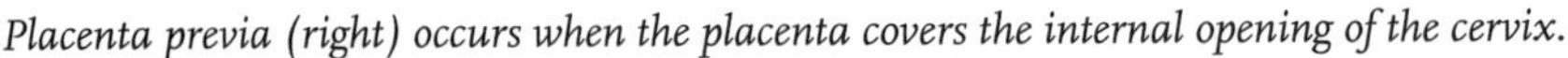

Placenta previa (right) occurs when the placenta covers the internal opening of the cervix.

abruption. Other causes of third trimester bleeding include placenta previa, cervical dilation, and irritation of the cervix.

How is it treated?

In mild abruptions before full term, the baby usually is watched closely with fetal monitoring, serial ultrasounds, or other techniques. At full term, or if the baby starts showing problems, delivery is the best treatment. Often, abruption causes labor, and the baby delivers fairly quickly.

BREECH AND OTHER "MALPRESENTATIONS"

Most babies are born headfirst through the birth canal. Breech means that the baby is bottom first, and transverse lie, which is quite unusual, means the baby is lying sideways in the uterus.

What is the risk?

Transverse babies cannot be delivered vaginally. They would have to fold in half in order to get out, and wouldn't fit. Breech vaginal birth is more controversial. Recent research indicates a slight safety advantage for delivering all breech

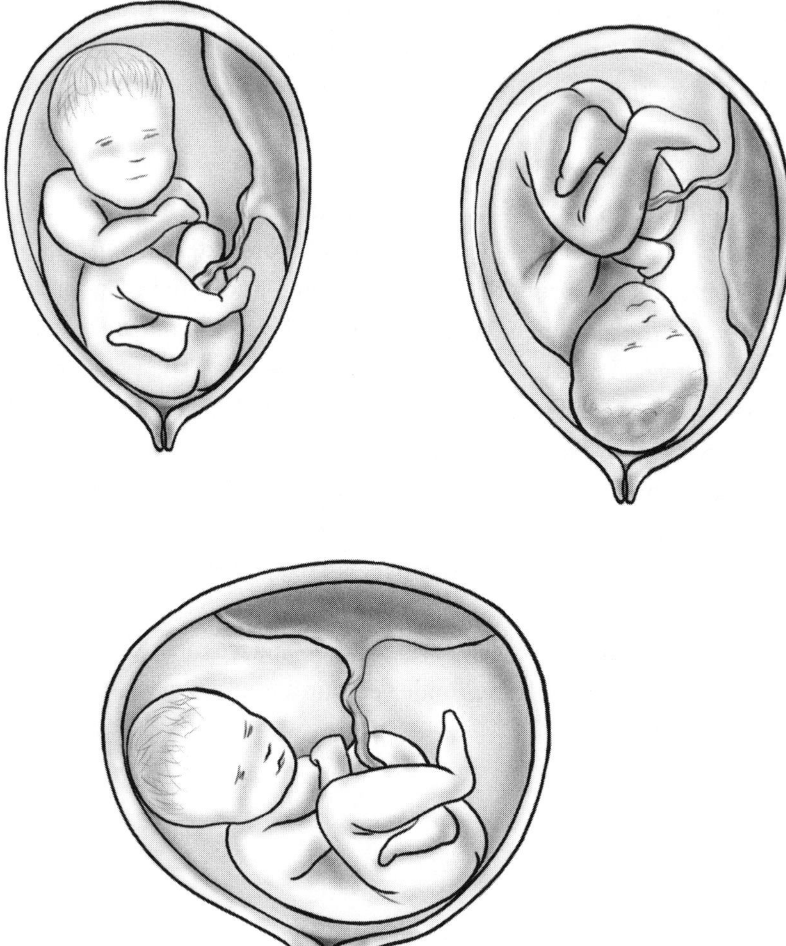

Fetal positions (clockwise from top left): breech, cephalic, and transverse lie

babies by cesarean because rarely a serious complication of breech vaginal birth, such as cord prolapse or head entrapment, will occur.

What are the signs?

You may notice that you feel kicks down low, or feel the hard ball of the head up under your ribs, or your doctor or midwife may be able to assess the baby's position. Ultrasound also can show that a baby is breech.

How is it treated?

Options to help the baby turn to a headfirst position include exercises you can do at home, moxibustion (a Chinese herbal treatment that requires an experienced practitioner), or a procedure called external cephalic version.

In external version, the doctor pushes on your abdomen to move the baby either in a forward roll or a back flip, trying to rotate your little one to head first. The experience is fairly uncomfortable for the mother, but remember you can always ask to stop if necessary, and it is usually better than having a cesarean. Some doctors give medications to quiet the uterus before external version, so you don't have contractions during the brief procedure, and some even give an epidural to help relax the abdomen. When it goes well, version may take just a minute, although repeated attempts are sometimes necessary. The risk is minimal, but we usually do versions on the labor unit so medical help is nearby if a problem develops. Note that a temporary slowing of the baby's heartbeat is not unusual or dangerous. Sometimes, too, the fetus can't be budged. Versions are most successful in non-obese mothers who have given birth before, whose abdomens are relaxed and soft, and whose babies are not yet engaged into the pelvis.

If the baby is still breech at term or when labor starts, most doctors will recommend cesarean, although some, under certain circumstances, will offer breech vaginal delivery.

Recommended Reading

ON GETTING PREGNANT

American Society for Reproductive Medicine. "State Infertility Insurance Laws." www.asrm.org/patients/insur.html. This site lists the laws about insurance coverage for infertility for many states and provides information on how to get involved in legislative efforts to improve insurance coverage for fertility care.

Centers for Disease Control. "Assisted Reproductive Technology." www.cdc.gov/reproductivehealth/art/index.htm. Objective information on fertility treatments is provided here, including in vitro statistics and links to other fertility resources.

Consumer Reports. "The Fertility Window." February 2003. Here you'll find reviews of the various brands of ovulation tests.

Consumer Reports. "When the Test Really Counts: Earliest Pregnancy Detection." February 2003. This site reviews pregnancy tests by brand, and provides home pregnancy test and ovulation predictor test information and images.

Resolve: The National Infertility Association. www.resolve.org. Resolve is the largest national fertility support group; its website provides a lot of information and a link to your local Resolve chapter.

Swire-Falker, Elizabeth. *Infertility Survival Handbook.* New York: Riverhead Trade, 2004. This book addresses the emotional and physical aspects of trying to conceive. It may be a bit scary because the author really went through a lot, but the information is good and acknowledging the emotional difficulties can be validating.

www.peeonastick.com. This website really cracked me up. The site's author is an expert on all aspects of pregnancy testing, and a great storyteller as well.

GOOD BOOKS AND CDS ON PREGNANCY AND BIRTH

Clapp, James F. *Exercising through Your Pregnancy.* Omaha: Addicus Books, 2002. Written by a world expert on exercise during pregnancy, this book makes a good case for getting moving.

Douglas, Ann. *The Mother of All Pregnancy Books.* New York: Wiley, 2002. This is my favorite of the standard comprehensive pregnancy books. Ann Douglas covers it all, accurately and with common sense.

Greenberg, Sindy, Elyse Kroll, and Hillary Grill. *Dreaming for Two.* New York: Penguin Putnam, 2002. This book explores, through the dreams of different mothers-to-be, the psychic stresses and changes brought by pregnancy.

Greenfield, Marjorie. *Dr. Spock's Pregnancy Guide.* New York: Pocket Books, 2003. This small book covers all of the basics from conception through birth. It's nice to carry along for quick reference.

King, Janie McCoy. *Back Labor No More!! What Every Woman Should Know before Labor.* Terrell, Tex.: Plenary Systems Publishing, 1994. A must for any woman who has significant back pain in labor, this book explains the causes of back labor and what you can do about it.

Koren, Gideon. *Everyday Risks in Pregnancy and Breastfeeding.* Toronto: Robert Rose, 2004. A good reference, this book gives you accurate information about everything that might concern you (although if you tend to worry a lot, you might want to stay away from a book like this). In any case, use it for reference, don't read it cover to cover.

Naparstek, Belleruth. *Health Journeys* series. Audio CDs. New York: Time Warner AudioBooks. (Varied years). These soothing CDs on topics such as infertility, stress, sleep, and wellness will help you use your own mind to control anxiety and fear.

Tracy, Amy E. *The Pregnancy Bed Rest Book: A Survival Guide for Expectant Mothers and Their Families.* New York: Berkley Publishing Group, 2001. This reassuring book offers specific "how to's" for mothers-to-be who are prescribed bed rest.

PREGNANCY INFORMATION ON THE WEB

http://embryo.soad.umich.edu/index.html. Amazing detailed photos, including 3D renderings of every stage of embryo development, can be found at this site. For additional incredible time-lapse images of the growing embryo, see www.pbs.org/wgbh/nova/odyssey/clips.

www.babycenter.com. Good basic information. If you supply your due date, you can sign up for an email newsletter tailored to how far along you are in the pregnancy.

www.drspock.com. I wrote most of their pregnancy articles, which are aimed at providing accurate information without being too scary. This site also features wonderful articles on child health and parenting.

www.duematernity.com is a fun website about maternity fashion, with a large assortment of clothing for sale as well as links to magazine images of famous preggies and what they are wearing this week.

www.marchofdimes.com. This is a terrific source of accurate information about health promotion before and during pregnancy, and about pregnancy complications.

www.motherisk.org. This site offers great science-based information about the safety of specific medications during pregnancy and breastfeeding.

www.nationalcordbloodprogram.org. This website, by the New York Blood Center, provides the basics on what umbilical cord blood can do, and is a good starting point for considering cord blood donation or banking.

www.nlm.nih.gov/medlineplus/pregnancy.html. A wonderful collection of trustworthy sources is offered here.

www.phac-aspc.gc.ca/hp-gs. Take a look at the Canadian government's website on healthy pregnancy.

www.pregnancy.about.com. See this site for loads of good basic information.

www.sidelines.org. At this site, the National High Risk Pregnancy Support Network provides resources for women with high-risk pregnancies. The information on how to cope with bed rest is very helpful, but I don't agree with some of their medical information. I would recommend relying on your doctor or midwife for accurate information regarding preterm labor or other pregnancy problems.

CHILDBIRTH PREPARATION RESOURCES ON THE WEB

Birth Works classes: www.birthworks.org.

Birthing from Within: www.birthingfromwithin.com.

Bradley method: www.bradleybirth.com.

Childbirth teachers: www.icea.org.

Doulas: www.dona.org.

Hypnobirthing: www.hypnobirthing.com.

Lamaze classes: www.lamaze.org.

PREGNANCY INFORMATION WITH WORKING MOMS IN MIND

Boyd, Hilary. *Working Woman's Pregnancy*. London: Mitchell Beazley, 2001. This small, visually attractive book published in Great Britain addresses work issues in detail.

Hall, Nancy. *Balancing Pregnancy and Work: How to Make the Most of the Next Nine Months on the Job*. New York: Stonesong Press, 2004. This book offers helpful and detailed advice on everything from clothing during pregnancy to maternity leave laws.

Interactive Learning Paradigms, Inc. "Where to Find Material Safety Data Sheets on the Internet." www.ilpi.com/msds. Although your employer is responsible for providing official MSDS sheets regarding your work exposures, this site can help you locate resources about different chemicals. It includes a program called the "demystifier" that links terms on the MSDS sheets with a glossary.

National Partnership for Women and Families. "Guide to the Family and Medical Leave Act." www.nationalpartnership.org. You can find specifics on the FMLA and other laws under the "legislation" tab.

Sara, Lauren. *Expecting Style*. New York: Bulfinch Press, 2003. A beautifully photographed book of sexy, stylish looks for expectant moms.

Working Mother. "100 Best Companies." Every October, *Working Mother* magazine rates the best companies for working parents, based on criteria that include parental leave policies, breastfeeding support, and flexible scheduling. The information may be useful for job hunting, or for showing your employer what forward-thinking companies are doing to recruit and retain the best employees.

www.lizlange.com has great options for professional maternity attire.

FOR FATHERS AND OTHER PARTNERS

Brott, Armin, and Jennifer Ash. *The Expectant Father.* 2d ed. New York: Abbeville Press, 2001. While sometimes a bit patronizing, this book does have helpful information about pregnancy and birth from the father's point of view.

Simkin, Penny. *The Birth Partner: Everything You Need to Know to Help a Woman through Childbirth.* 2d ed. Boston: Harvard Common Press, 2001. I love this book! Aimed at the natural childbirth audience, it is dead-on accurate about the birth experience and what the support person can do to be truly helpful.

GENERAL HEALTH AND NUTRITION INFORMATION

Body Mass Index calculator: www.cdc.gov/nccdphp/dnpa/bmi/calc-bmi.htm. Enter your height and weight to find out your BMI.

Family medical history chart: www.hhs.gov/familyhistory. This fun website allows you to create a printable family tree of your (or your partner's) medical history.

Family violence resources: www.ncadv.org or 1–800–799-SAFE. For help keeping yourself safe, click the "protect yourself" or "resources" tab. In a family violence emergency, dial 911.

Food safety: www.foodsafety.gov or call 1–888–SAFEFOOD. This site has resources like videos that cover all areas of how to store and prepare food safely; it includes some information specifically for pregnant women. The Canadian government's health site www.hc-sc.gc.ca is also useful, and provides a different perspective than that offered on the U.S. government site.

Nutrition: www.mypyramid.gov. The food pyramid isn't specifically for pregnancy, but it is a good starting point for thinking about which foods are the most healthful.

Quitting smoking: www.smokefree.gov. This website provides practical tips and resources for people thinking about stopping smoking.

Weight control: www.amihungry.com. This is a proprietary program that has the right idea about how to help people have a healthier relationship with food. Take the quiz and learn about yourself. If you are interested, you can get the book or seek out a program in your area.

TIPS FOR RELATIONSHIPS AT HOME AND AT WORK

Cockrell, Stacie, Cathy O'Neill, and Julia Stone. *Babyproofing Your Marriage.* New York: Harper Collins, 2007. This book offers funny examples and terrific advice for helping your relationship thrive through the joys and jobs of raising a family. The subtitle is "how to laugh more, argue less, and communicate better as your family grows."

Fisher, Roger, William L. Ury, and Bruce Patton. *Getting to Yes.* 2d ed. Boston: Houghton Mifflin, 1992. This is my favorite book about negotiating for what you need—it offers useful tips for dealing with employers, coworkers, and even your spouse and kids. This book comes on tape and CD, if you want to listen in the car. It is well worth it.

Gray, John. *Men Are from Mars, Women Are from Venus.* New York: Harper Paperbacks, 2004. This book explains, often humorously, how we sometimes seem to speak a different language than those of the other sex.

HELPFUL PARENTING BOOKS

Jana, Laura, and Jennifer Shu. *Heading Home with Your Newborn: From Birth to Reality.* Chicago: American Academy of Pediatrics, 2005. This practical guide to those first few months is written with humor and insight.

Karp, Harvey. *The Happiest Baby on the Block: The New Way to Calm Crying and Help Your Newborn Baby Sleep Longer.* New York: Bantam, 2005. Karp has patented his system for calming newborn babies. You may also be able to find "happiest baby" classes in your area.

Spock, Benjamin, and Robert Needlman. *Dr. Spock's Baby and Child Care.* 8th ed. New York: Pocket Books, 2004. This classic on raising healthy children, updated and expanded by a specialist in child behavior, covers health and parenting issues from birth through early adolescence. It even may help with adult ailments: my mother diagnosed my father's appendicitis from an older edition of this book (it was the only medical book she had in the house!).

GOOD PARENTING RESOURCES ON THE WEB

Baby names: www.babynamewizard.com/namevoyager. This fun website allows you to see timelines of names' popularities, as well as browse a large number of names.

Postpartum depression: www.postpartum.net. Information on postpartum depression, including links to local resources, can be found here.

Postpartum doulas: Check out the Doulas of North America website, www.dona.org, or the Childbirth and Postpartum Professional Association at www.cappa.net, for help locating a postpartum doula.

BREASTFEEDING ADVICE

Mohrbacher, Nancy, and Kathleen Kendall-Tackett. *Breastfeeding Made Simple: Seven Natural Laws for Nursing Mothers.* Oakland: New Harbinger, 2005. Instead of a lot of instructions, this book lays out principles to help you understand how to make breastfeeding work for you and your baby.

www.breastfeeding.com. This site has it all—from tips, to humor, to listings of lactation consultants by region.

www.kellymom.com. Here you will find reliable information about breastfeeding, sleep, and parenting.

www.lalecheleague.org: La Leche is the original breastfeeding support network, and its website offers updated help on breastfeeding and the return to work.

www.motherwear.com. If you're a breastfeeding mom, you'll want to see Motherwear's collection of nursing bras, tops, nightwear, swimwear, and dresses, all designed with your special needs in mind.

RESOURCES ADDRESSING MATERNITY LEAVE AND RETURNING TO WORK

Connell, Linda H. *The Childcare Answer Book.* Naperville, Ill.: Sphinx, 2005. This very practical and user-friendly book includes a cost-benefit analysis of both parents working versus one staying home, information on all types of childcare arrangements, and some tips on how to deal with problems that arise.

Holcomb, Betty. *The Best Friend's Guide to Maternity Leave.* Cambridge: Perseus, 2001. The well-written practical advice in this book focuses on making the most of time "off" after the baby.

www.childcareaware.org. Childcare Aware is a nonprofit organization with information and connections to daycare.

www.naccrra.org. The National Association of Childcare Resource and Referral Agencies provides lists of accredited daycare centers by location.

www.workandpump.com. Comprehensive information about working and breastfeeding is available at this helpful website.

www.workingmother.com. The website of *Working Mother* magazine features many ideas and resources for working families.

Acknowledgments

This book has been a labor of love, but it has been a long labor. I gestated longer than an elephant, whose journey from conception to birth takes twenty-two months. And like childbirth, it has taken help, support, and teamwork. First off, I would never have attempted to write, if not for the support and instruction from the team at The Dr. Spock Company, including Dr. Laura Jana, Dr. Robert Needlman, and editor extraordinaire Mona Behan. This book could not have been born without my writing doulas: my agent, Regina Brooks, and my editor, Jean Thomson Black. Thanks for your confidence in me, and for your patient guidance.

My views on pregnancy and birth have been shaped by my training and experiences, extensive reading, and innumerable conversations with physicians, midwives, nurses, doulas, and parents. I am particularly indebted to Patsy Harman, CNM; Karen Kapela, CD; and John Kennell, MD. Many professionals reviewed sections of the book for accuracy and clarity: thanks to Christina Smillie, MD, and her team from Breastfeeding Resources, Tina Schulin, RN, IBCLC; Leslie Kushner, RN; Sandy Piderit, PhD; Libby Svoboda, RN, IBCLC; Noreen Roman, CD; Francisco Arredondo, MD; Sandy Stewart, RN; Leslie Cohen, MS; and Elizabeth Brandewie, MD. Particular thanks to Susan Sprigg, CPM, for providing evidence and clarity on the subject of direct-entry midwifery and home birth. I also appreciate the wonderful ultrasound images supplied by Carmela Entsminger, RDS; Noam Lazebnik, MD; and Molly Gallogly.

Special thanks to Kathy Cole-Kelly, MS, MSW, for help with relationships (and help writing about them too), and to my terrific Case Western Reserve University medical students for substantial contributions through their research over a two-year time span: Dr. Sarah Hutchinson, class of 2005; Drs. Abigail Tucker, Lindsey Hower, Julia Keith, and Kira Mattison, class of 2006; and Drs. Shani Muhammad and Jill Minger, class of 2007.

To a stellar ob-gyn resident, Rebecca Flyckt, MD, I can only say that I lucked out telling you about this project at that applicant dinner. Who knew you were a skilled (and gentle) editor?

To my mom, thanks for believing in me, and Dan, thanks for teaching me to be a mom. And to my friends Drs. Elisa Ross and Kristi Victoroff, your patience, support, and practical help as I perseverated over this project deserve a permanent state of thankfulness and at least a dozen more Tony-dinners.

Finally, to the parents who have let me into their lives, shared their stories, and given me their trust: gratitude always.

Index

Page numbers in *italics* refer to illustrations. **Bolded** page numbers indicate the most complete information on that topic.